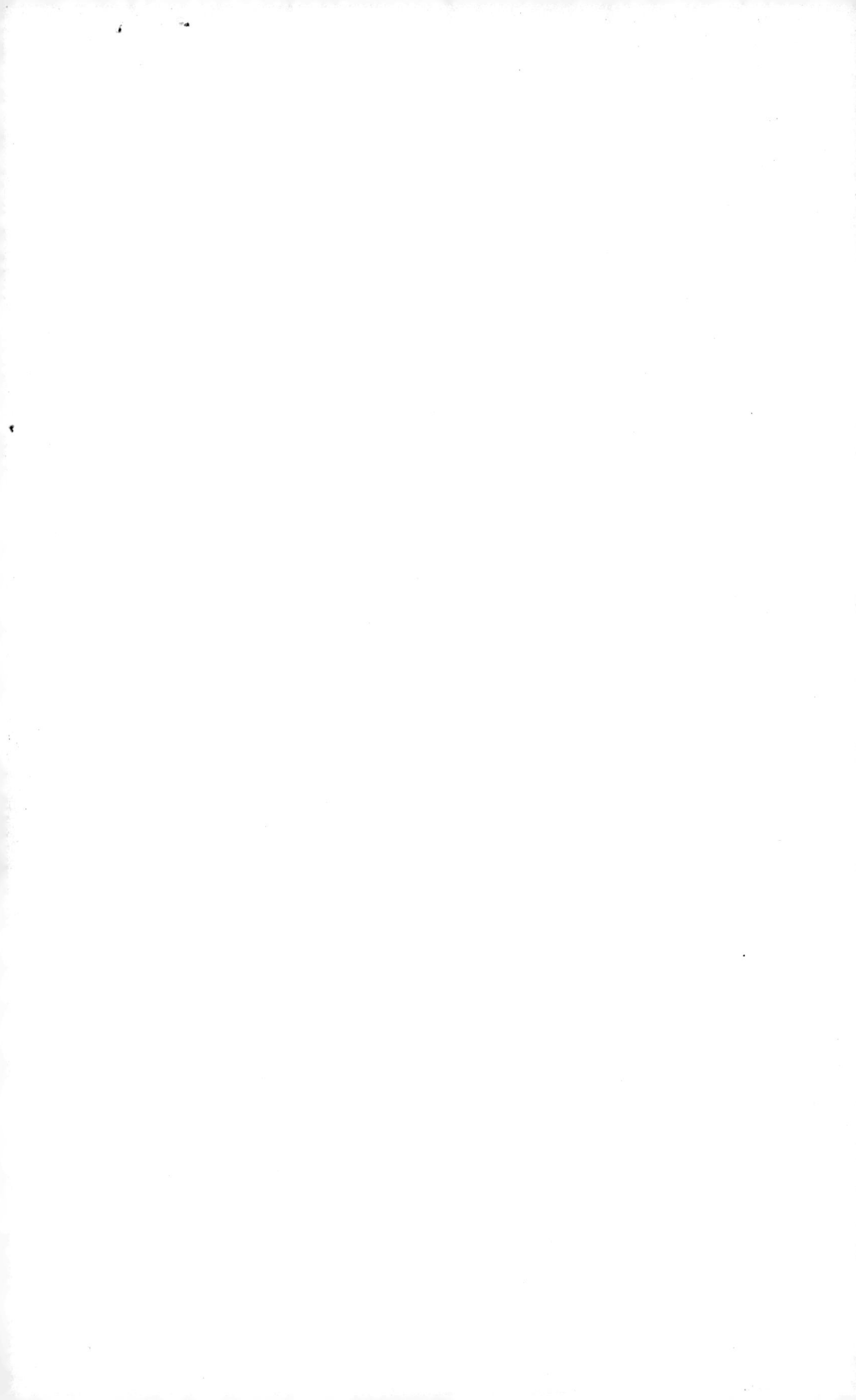

Current Topics in Microbiology 230 and Immunology

Editors

Springer
Berlin
Heidelberg
New York
Barcelona
Budapest
Hong Kong
London
Milan
Paris
Santa Clara
Singapore
Tokyo

Specificity, Function, and Development of NK Cells

NK Cells: The Effector Arm of Innate Immunity

Edited by K. Kärre and M. Colonna

With 22 Figures and 17 Tables

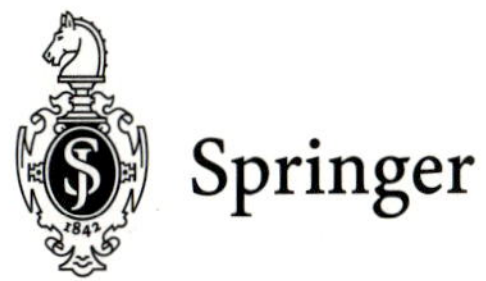

Dr. Klas Kärre
Microbiology and Tumor Biology Center
Karolinska Institute
S-17177 Stockholm
Sweden

Marco Colonna, M.D.
Basel Institute for Immunology
Grenzacherstraße 487
CH-4005 Basel
Switzerland

Cover Illustration: NK cells (in red) attack EBV-transformed B cells that lack MHC class I molecules (in green).

Special thanks to Marina Cella and Mark Dessing for confocal microscopy pictures of NK cells.

Cover Design: Design & Production GmbH, Heidelberg

ISBN 0070-217X
ISBN 3-540-63941-1 Springer-Verlag Berlin Heidelberg New York

Library of Congress Catalog Card Number 15-12910
Printed in Germany

SPIN: 10558209 27/3136 – 5 4 3 2 1 0 – Printed on acid-free paper

Preface

Our understanding of the molecular basis of natural killer cell function has greatly advanced in the past few years. The discovery of multiple natural killer cell inhibitory receptors specific for MHC class I molecules has explained how NK cells perceive expression of "self" on neighboring cells and, hence, discriminate between normal class I-bearing cells and transformed or virus-infected cells that lack expression of class I molecules. Upon engagement with class I molecules, inhibitory receptors recruit protein tyrosine phosphatases via cytoplasmic immunoreceptor tyrosine-based inhibitory motifs (ITIMs) and deliver a negative signal that blocks cytotoxicity. Stimulatory counterparts of inhibitory MHC class I receptors have been also found. These receptors lack intrinsic signaling ability and require associated proteins to trigger cell activation as, for example, CD16 requires CD3ζ or FcεRI-γ for signal transduction. Although the physiological role of activating MHC class I receptors is still puzzling, it is now clear that NK cell activation is controlled by a balance between opposing signals transduced by distinct MHC class I receptors. When this equilibrium is altered, the NK cell activation threshold is overcome and NK cell-mediated lysis is switched on. A similar mechanism modulates activation threshold, signaling and function of a small subset of T cells expressing MHC class I NK cell receptors (T-NK cells).

Along with the discovery of MHC class I receptors, cumulative evidence suggests that NK cell functions are also regulated by a variety of other receptors. Fc receptors mediate antibody-dependent cell-mediated cytotoxicity (ADCC), which allows NK cells to kill antibody-coated target cells. Adhesion molecules, abundantly expressed on NK cells, can sense an abnormal distribution of their ligands caused by tranformation or infections of target cells. C-type lectin receptors, such as NKR-P1, may recognize carbohydrate ligands. Finally, costimulatory molecules like 2B4 potentiate NK cell recognition and Fas-Fas-ligand interactions may mediate lysis of several target cells *in vivo*.

The great number of receptors on NK cells raises the question of how and when NK cells acquire the optimal balance between stimulatory and inhibitory receptors required to mediate normal effector functions yet avoid autoreactivity. There is evidence that

NK cells begin to express MHC class I receptors during development and are educated to become self-tolerant. NK cells originate from a bone marrow-derived progenitor under the influence of both stromal cells and soluble factors (including IL-2, IL-12, and IL-15) and develop their repertoire in a thymic-independent manner. Two mechanisms of education have been proposed. According to one hypothesis, cells expressing an optimal combination of inhibitory and stimulatory receptors are positively selected from a pool of cells expressing a pre-formed, randomly generated repertoire. Alternatively, NK cell progenitors may sequentially express NK cell receptors; only when an optimal balance is reached, do progenitor cells mature and proliferate.

While the mechanisms underlying NK cell recognition, effector function and development are being elucidated, the role of NK cells in anti-viral and anti-tumor host defense is also under active investigation. Inhibitory MHC class I receptors probably play a role in host defense against viruses and tumor cells that down-regulate MHC class I molecules to evade host T cell immunity. Accordingly, genes for resistance to cytomegalovirus (CMV) infection in the mouse map within the NK receptor complex. In addition, CMV and other viruses encode MHC class I-like proteins in an attempt to suppress NK cell-mediated lysis of virus-infected cells. NK cells also mediate host resistance to viruses, intracellular bacteria and parasites, as they may be the first source of interferon-γ in peripheral tissues, and, thereby, stimulate microbicidal activity in macrophages and drive a Th1 immune response. Whether NK cells can be effectively used in tumor therapy is still under evaluation. However, the dramatic rate of research in the NK field, in particular our recent understanding of how activating and inhibitory signals control NK cell recognition, should soon allow us to exploit the therapeutic potential of NK cells in diseases.

Stockholm, Basel

KLAS KÄRRE
MARCO COLONNA

Contents

A. NK Receptors and Coreceptors

B. Activation of NK Cells and Effector Functions

List of Contributors

(Their addresses can be found at the beginning of their respective chapters.)

Bejarano, M.T. 53
Bellón, T. 41
Bennett, M. 161
Binstadt, B.A 103
Brumbaugh, K.M. 103
Carretero, M. 41
Chambers, B.J. 53
D'Andrea, A. 25
Helander, T.S. 89
Hengartner, H. 123
Herberman, R.B. 221
Kägi, D. 123
Kumar, V. 161
Lanier, L.L. 25
Leibson, P.J. 103
Ljunggren, H.G. 53
Llano, M. 41
López-Botet, M. 41
Markovic, K. 53
Mingari, M.C. 15
Moretta, A. 15
Moretta, L. 15
Navarro, F. 41
Pérez-Villar, J.J. 41
Perussia, B. 63
Ponte, M. 15
Puzanov, I. 161
Raulet, D.H. 135
Salcedo, M. 53
Sivakumar, P.V. 161
Sivori, S. 15
Szomolantyi-Tsuda, E. 193
Tay, C.H. 193
Timonen, T. 89
Van den Broek, M.F. 123
Vance, R.E. 135
Vujanovic, N.L. 221
Wang, L.L. 3
Welsh, R.M. 193
Whiteside, T.L. 221
Williams, N.S. 161
Wilson, J.L. 53
Yokoyama, W.M. 3

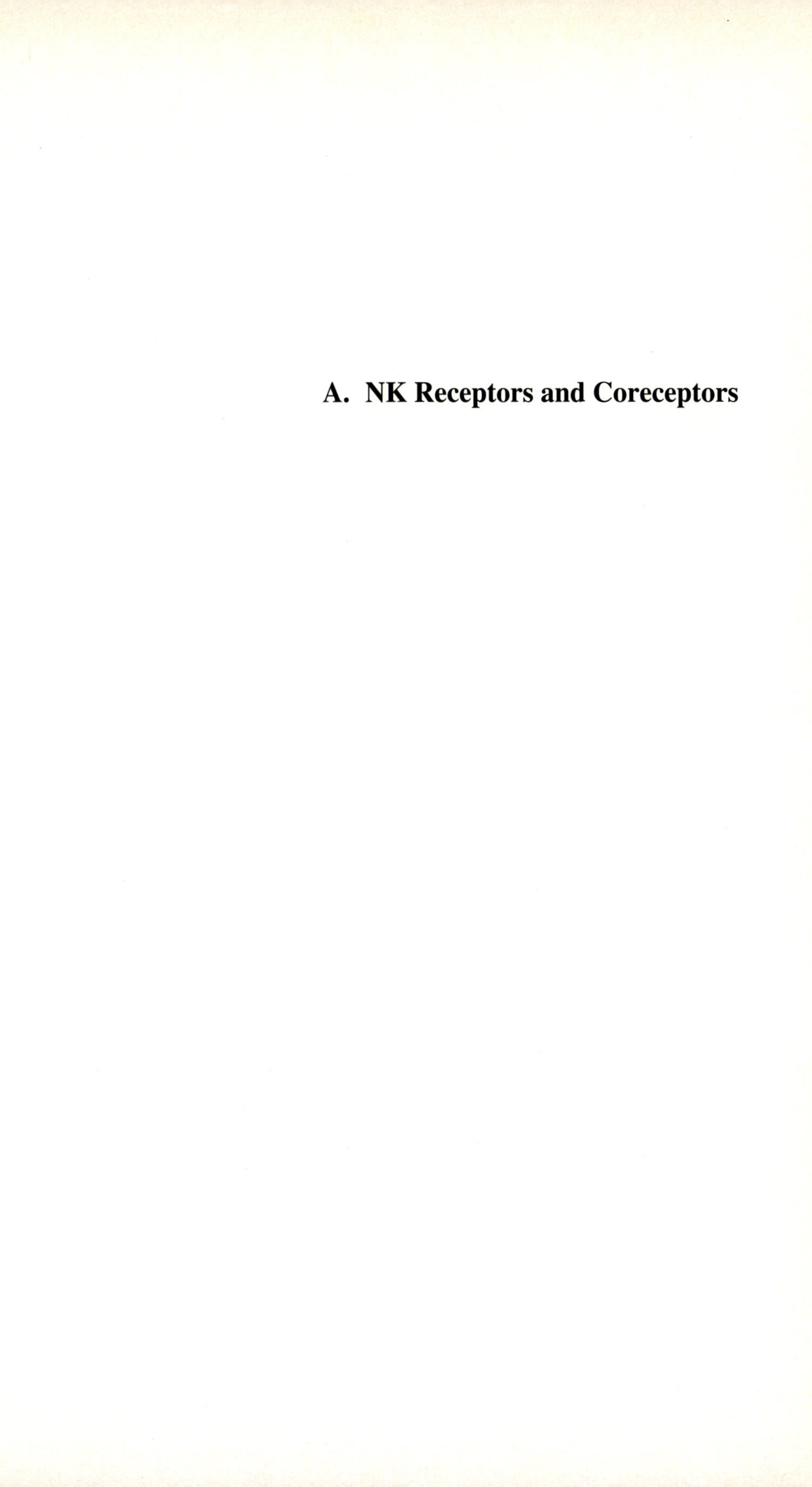

A. NK Receptors and Coreceptors

Regulation of Mouse NK Cells by Structurally Divergent Inhibitory Receptors

L. L. WANG and W. M. YOKOYAMA

1 Introduction

Natural killer (NK) cells contribute to the natural host defense mechanism by lysing certain virally infected and tumor cells and by releasing cytokines that promote an inflammatory immune response. NK cell specificity and the activation events resulting in NK cell stimulation remain poorly understood. However, from parallel studies in rodents and humans it is becoming increasingly evident that a major mode of NK cell specificity is through regulation of NK cell activation by a series of inhibitory receptors specific for MHC class I molecules.

While the presence of such inhibitory receptors on mouse and human NK cells is well established, it is still unknown how these receptors evolved in the two species. Our laboratory has been involved in the characterization of inhibitory receptors on mouse NK cells, specifically the Ly-49 family of receptors. Members of the Ly-49 receptor family are type II integral membrane proteins with homology to C-type lectins (YOKOYAMA and SEAMAN 1993). In contrast, human NK receptors belonging to the killer inhibitory receptor (KIR) family are structurally distinct from the Ly-49 receptors (COLONNA and SAMARIDIS 1995; WAGTMANN et al. 1995a,b). KIRs are type I integral membrane proteins belonging to the immunoglobulin (Ig) superfamily. Since homologues of Ly-49 and KIR had not yet been discovered in the reciprocal species, speculation arose that mouse and human NK cells evolved structurally distinct receptor systems to subserve the same function (GUMPERZ and PARHAM 1995).

Rheumatology Division, Department of Medicine and Pathology, School of Medicine, Washington University, 660 South Euclid Avenue, St. Louis, MO 63110, USA

However, recent reports support the view that both structural types of receptors are expressed on human and mouse NK cells. This contribution reviews our most recent work demonstrating that mouse NK cells express a putative inhibitory receptor known as gp49B1 which, like receptors in the KIR family, belongs to the Ig superfamily. Therefore current models of NK cell regulation invoking structurally distinct receptors require consideration of receptor systems utilizing both structural types of receptors on a single NK cell.

2 Recognition of MHC Class I by NK Inhibitory Receptors

NK cells share with T cells the ability to recognize specific MHC class I molecules through surface bound receptors. MHC class I specific NK receptors differ from T cell receptors in three major ways. First, NK receptors appear to deliver signals which suppress NK cell activation (KARLHOFER et al. 1992). Hence, NK cells may be activated by target cells which have lost MHC class I expression, as first proposed by LJUNGGREN and KÄRRE (1985). This feature of NK cell cytotoxicity is consistent with the known ability of NK cells to lyse certain virally infected and tumor cells which often exhibit aberrant MHC class I expression. Second, NK cells do not express physically rearranged receptors. In mice with mutations in the genes encoding components of the recombinase machinery – including the enzymes DNA-PK (*scid*), RAG-1, or RAG-2 – involved in physical rearrangement of antigen receptor genes, NK cell receptors appear to be normal (DORSHKIND et al. 1985; MOMBAERTS et al. 1992; SHINKAI et al. 1992). However, many NK receptors are highly polymorphic and thus may have unique specificities toward MHC class I alleles. Lastly, while conventional T cell receptors recognize a specific peptide in the context of an MHC molecule, some NK receptors appear to recognize MHC independently of peptide (CORREA and RAULET 1995; ORIHUELA et al. 1996). This inability of MHC class I specific NK receptors to discriminate between self and foreign peptides is consistent with the role of these receptors as general monitors of "absence of self" as defined by the missing-self hypothesis (LJUNGGREN and KÄRRE 1990).

3 Murine NK Inhibitory Receptors

The best characterized murine NK inhibitory receptor is the Ly-49A molecule, which has homology to C-type lectins and is expressed on the cell surface as a disulfide-linked homodimer (YOKOYAMA et al. 1989). Transfection of otherwise susceptible target cells with H-2D^d or H-2D^k can protect such targets from killing by Ly-49A$^+$ C57BL/6 interleukin (IL)-2 activated NK (LAK) cells; cytotoxicity can be restored by addition of antibodies specific for MHC class I or Ly-49A (KARLHOFER et al. 1992). A physical interaction between Ly-49A and H-2D^d has been demonstrated

(DANIELS et al. 1994a,b; KANE 1994), and H-2D^d specifically downregulates Ly-49A expression in vivo (KARLHOFER et al. 1994). Taken together, these data clearly substantiate that Ly-49A is an NK cell receptor for H-2D^d (and H-2D^k).

The finding that Ly-49A is expressed on only a subset of NK cells implied the existence of other NK receptors. We now know that Ly-49A is a member of a growing family of receptors currently consisting of Ly-49A through Ly-49I (SMITH et al. 1994; WONG et al. 1991; BRENNAN et al. 1996a,b). Although the ligands for many of the Ly-49 family members remain to be elucidated, it is likely that they engage MHC class I. Consistent with this, the C57BL/6 form of Ly-49C appears to recognize H-2K^b (STONEMAN et al. 1995; YU et al. 1996), whereas Ly-49G2 apparently recognizes H-2D^d or H-2L^d (MASON et al. 1995). Further complicating these studies is the high degree of polymorphism of Ly-49 genes (YOKOYAMA et al. 1990). The aforementioned studies each examined only one allele of a given Ly-49 gene. However, it is possible that other alleles have different specificities toward MHC class I. In support of this, recent reports suggest that the BALB/c allele of Ly-49C has a broader MHC specificity than the C57BL/6 allele (YU et al. 1996; BRENNAN et al. 1996a,b). Another potential mechanism for increasing the class I repertoire of Ly-49 molecules is through heterodimerization of different family members. BRENNAN et al. (1996a,b) failed to see pairing between Ly-49A and Ly-49C monomers when these cDNAs were transfected into COS cells. On the other hand, we have seen evidence of heterodimers when anti-Ly-49A immunoprecipitates from LAK cells were run on 2-D gels (SMITH et al. 1995). However, it is possible that these represent differentially glycosylated forms of Ly-49A. Thus the Ly-49 family of molecules appears to represent a diverse repertoire of NK cell receptors for MHC class I.

Consistent with the ability of Ly-49 receptors to discriminate between MHC alleles, Ly-49A is known to interact with the polymorphic α_1/α_2 domains of MHC class I (KARLHOFER et al. 1992). However, unlike the TCR, Ly-49 receptors do not bind peptide directly but instead interact with a peptide-induced conformational determinant of MHC class I (CORREA and RAULET 1995; ORIHUELA et al. 1996). Another unique feature of the Ly-49/MHC interaction is the requirement for MHC class I glycosylation. This carbohydrate recognition may not contribute to specificity toward MHC alleles by Ly-49 receptors but may instead strengthen the Ly-49/MHC interaction (DANIELS et al. 1994a,b; BRENNAN et al. 1995, 1996a,b). According to this model, Ly-49 has two binding sites, one involved in contacting oligosaccharide and the other recognizing a polypeptide determinant, but this has not yet been established.

4 Human NK Receptors Specific for MHC Class I

Human NK cells express inhibitory receptors belonging to the KIR family which may be grouped into 3 subtypes based on HLA specificity. The most extensively studied KIRs are those which are HLA-C responsive. Cloning of these receptors revealed that they are members of the Ig superfamily and contain two Ig domains (COLONNA and SAMARIDIS 1995; WAGTMANN et al. 1995a,b). KIRs specific for HLA-B also belong to the Ig superfamily but contain three Ig domains (DANDREA et al. 1995; WAGTMANN et al. 1995a,b). PENDE et al. (1996) have recently identified and cloned an HLA-A specific KIR which, like the HLA-B specific forms, has three Ig domains. It appears to be unique among the KIRs by its expression as a disulfide-linked dimer. With this finding of an HLA-A specific KIR, we now know of KIRs with specificities toward all of the classical HLA class I groups.

KIRs differ from Ly-49 molecules not only in structure but also in other important characteristics (YOKOYAMA 1995). In contrast to Ly-49 receptors, KIRs display little polymorphism although multiple family members do exist. Additionally, the two families of receptors appear to recognize different regions of the MHC class I molecule. The ability of p58 KIR to discriminate between HLA-C alleles is governed by amino acid residues 77 and 80 in the α_1 domain of MHC class I (COLONNA et al. 1993). As mentioned above, Ly-49A appears to recognize a region of the α_1/α_2 domains of MHC class I. There is also evidence that KIRs have some specificity toward peptide (MALNATI et al. 1995), though recent data challenge this (MANDELBOIM et al. 1996). Finally, whereas Ly-49 genes map to the mouse natural killer gene complex (NKC), genes encoding KIR map to chromosome 19 instead of the human NKC located on chromosome 12. Therefore, although KIR and Ly-49 receptors seem to be functionally homologous, there are important differences between the two classes of molecules, implying that they do not subserve the identical function.

Although less well characterized, receptors homologous to C-type lectins, including CD94 and members of the NKG2 family, have been identified on human NK cells but appear not to represent Ly-49 homologues. Their specificity in NK cell recognition remains controversial (PÉREZ-VILLAR et al. 1995; PHILLIPS et al. 1996). However, the recent finding that CD94 forms dimers with NKG2 members may alleviate much of this confusion (LAZETIC et al. 1996).

Despite the obvious structural differences between KIRs and CD94/NKG2 they likely signal through a similar mechanism. Both families contain receptors which have immunoreceptor-based tyrosine inhibition motifs (ITIM) in their cytoplasmic tails, a motif which was originally identified in the B cell FcγRIIB1 receptor as a negative regulatory region which can bind to the cytoplasmic tyrosine phosphatase SHP-1 (MUTA et al. 1994; DAMBROSIO et al. 1995). Several groups have subsequently shown that the KIR ITIMs can bind SHP-1 and thereby mediate inhibition (BURSHTYN et al. 1996; CAMPBELL et al. 1996; OLCESE et al. 1996). Furthermore, a dominant negative form of SHP-1 can block the inhibitory signal delivered by KIRs (BURSHTYN et al. 1996). Although Ly-49 receptors also contain ITIMs, and representative Ly-49A phosphopeptides can bind SHP-1 (OLCESE et al. 1996; Wang and Yokoyama, unpublished data), a physiological interaction between Ly-49 and SHP-1 has not yet been demonstrated. Nevertheless, the structurally distinct NK cell inhibitory receptors appear to utilize the same signaling mechanism to regulate NK cell function – ITIM recruitment of SHP-1 to dephosphorylate molecules involved in activation pathways.

5 Identification of a Murine Ig Superfamily NK Inhibitory Receptor

We were interested in determining whether a KIR homologue exists in mice. To this end we used degenerate primers against conserved regions of p58 KIR to clone by reverse transcriptase (RT) polymerase chain reaction (PCR) a murine structural homologue of p58 KIR (Fig. 1). Sequence analysis of the primary PCR product revealed a cDNA with 100% homology to gp49B1, a previously identified mast cell specific transmembrane protein with unknown function (ARM et al. 1991; CASTELLS et al. 1994). We further evaluated gp49 expression in mouse NK cells by northern blot analysis and found specific message in LAK cells from all strains of mice tested as well as in NK cell clones (WANG et al. 1997). FACS analysis using the anti-gp49B1 monoclonal antibody (mAb) B23.1 (LEBLANC et al. 1982; KATZ et al. 1996) confirmed surface expression of gp49B1 on LAK cells and NK cell clones. Furthermore, FACS analysis demonstrated that gp49B1, unlike members of the KIR and Ly-49 families, is expressed on all LAK cells. Thus mouse NK cells express gp49B1.

As mentioned above, Ly-49 members are polymorphic while KIRs are relatively nonpolymorphic, although DÖHRING et al. (1996) have recently cloned KIR alleles. Previous studies suggested that gp49 is nonpolymorphic (ARM et al. 1991). Our results confirm this, as we detected no restriction fragment length polymorphisms on Southern blot analysis of genomic DNA from four inbred strains of mice (Fig. 2). Furthermore, our gp49B1 full-length sequence, derived from a C57BL/6 LAK cDNA library, was identical to sequence from the C3H mouse strain (CASTELLS et al. 1994). These results further demonstrate the lack of polymorphism of the gp49B1 gene.

While its function was not known, its similarity in structure to p58 KIR, including the presence of two Ig domains and two ITIMs, strongly suggested that gp49B1 is also an inhibitory receptor. The sequences of and the spacing between the gp49B1 ITIMs differ slightly from that of p58 (Fig. 3, Table 1). The p58 sequence is $YxxL(x)_{26}YxxL$ while that of gp49B1 is $YxxV(x)_{18}YxxL$. However, the difference in spacing between the ITIMs is not critical for binding. FRY et al. (1996) have deleted

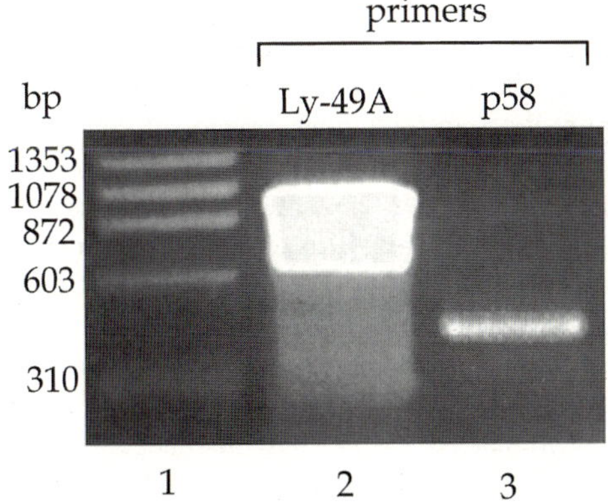

Fig. 1. RT-PCR results from degenerative priming for KIR (p58). cDNA from C57BL/6 LAK cells were amplified with primers specific for: *lane 2*, Ly-49A with an expected product of 1 kb; *lane 3*, degenerative primers for residues 601938 of cl-6/NKAT2 representing a human KIR (p58) (COLONNA and SAMARIDIS 1995; WAGTMANN et al. 1995). The 400-bp product is identical to nucleotides 595996 of gp49B1 (CASTELLS et al. 1994). PCR conditions were as previously described (WANG et al. 1997)

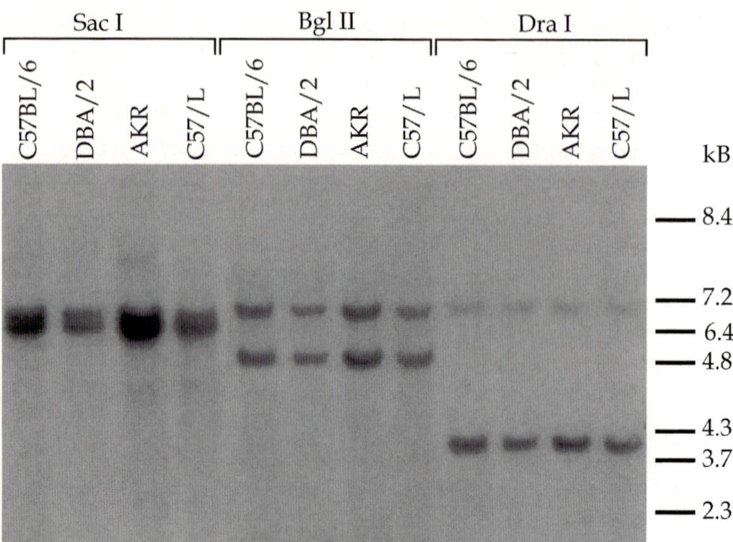

Fig. 2. Southern blot analysis of mouse genomic DNA with cDNA for gp49B1. The results reveal lack of restriction fragment length polymorphisms between several inbred mouse strains providing evidence that gp49B1 is not polymorphic

large portions of the intervening sequence between the KIR ITIMs and have not been able to abrogate binding to SHP-1. Addressing the replacement of the first conserved leucine with valine in the first gp49B1 ITIM, we have preliminary evidence that a phosphopeptide representing this polypeptide sequence can bind to SHP-1, albeit to a lesser degree than the YxxL sequence of gp49B1 (Wang and Yokoyama, unpublished data). Interestingly, the Ly-49A ITIM also contains a YxxV sequence (Fig. 3) which is known to interact with SHP-1 (Olcese et al. 1996; Wang and Yokoyama, unpublished data).

The ITIMs strongly suggest that gp49B1 functions as an inhibitory receptor on NK cells. Although we have not yet demonstrated this, recent published reports have addressed the function of gp49B1. Katz et al. (1996) show that mAb mediated co-cross-linking of FcεRI and gp49 on mast cells results in diminished granule exocytosis, as defined by β-hexosaminidase and leukotriene C4 release, compared to stimulation through FcεRI alone. Furthermore, Rojo et al. (1997) have used a vaccinia expression system to demonstrate that a fusion protein containing the cytoplasmic tail of gp49B1 is able to mediate inhibition in mouse LAK cells. Without knowledge of the ligand for gp49B1, however, it is currently difficult to address the function of gp49B1 in a physiological setting. Nevertheless, these two studies, along with our recent finding that the gp49B1 ITIMs can associate with SHP-1, suggest that gp49B1 is a new member of a growing list of murine NK cell inhibitory receptors, and the first belonging to the Ig superfamily.

Alternatively, gp49 may also act as an activation receptor. The gp49A isoform, which has an extracellular region almost identical to that of gp49B1, lacks an ITIM

S I H pY S E L V Q F mCD22 (Y5)
T V S pY A I L R F P mCD22 (Y2)
E D V D pY V T L K H mCD22 (Y6)
Ac- P H L K pY L Y L V V S D K mEpoR
G S L E pY L C L P A G D K hIL-3βR
E A E N T I T pY S L L K H FcγRIIB1
D E Q D P Q E V T pY A Q L N H p58 (N term)
S E Q E V T pY S M V R F Ly-49A
V x pY x x L x H Consensus
G I V Y A Q V K P gp49B1 (N term)
D V T Y A Q L C I gp49B1 (C term)

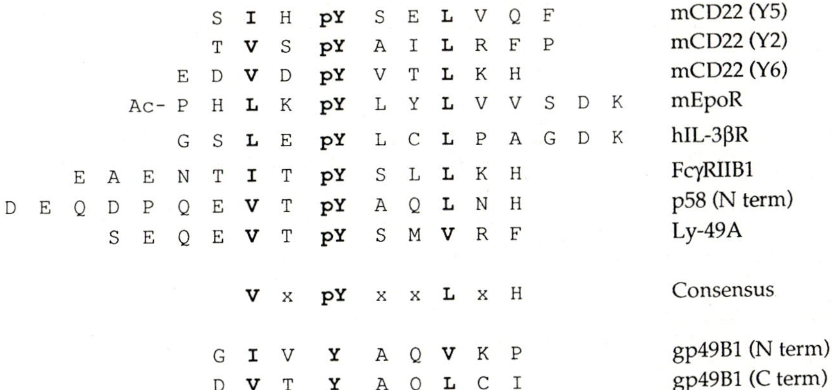

Fig. 3. Comparison of ITIM sequences. Alignment of phosphopeptides known to bind and activate SHP-1 (DOODY et al. 1995; PEI et al. 1994; DAMBROSIO et al. 1995; OLCESE et al. 1996) with the gp49B1 ITIMs (CASTELLS et al. 1994).

Table 1. Comparison of human KIR with mouse gp49B1

	Human KIR *(cl-6/NKAT2)*	*Mouse gp49B1*
Ig domains	2	2
Size (sequence)	320 amino acids	312 amino acids
Size (SDS/PAGE)	58 kDa	49 kDa
Cytoplasmic tail	76 amino acids	74 amino acids
ITIMs (with spacing)	$VxYxxL(x)_{24}IxYxxL$	$IxYxxV(x)_{16}VxYxxL$
Homologues without ITIM	+ (p50)	+ (gp49A)
Mast cell expression	?	+
NK cell expression	+ (subset)	+ (all)
Chromosomal location	19	?
Polygenism/polymorphism		
Family members	>10	2
Allelism	Minimal	Minimal
Ligand(s)	HLA-C	?
Binds SHP-1	+	+ (phosphopeptides)
Inhibits NK cells	+	+ (fusion protein)

(ARM et al. 1991) and therefore may serve as an activation receptor, much as the p50 form of KIR (MORETTA et al. 1995). While we were not able to detect a full-length gp49A cDNA from an NK cDNA library, ROJO et al. have identified sequences corresponding to gp49A by RT-PCR analysis of mouse NK mRNA. However, surface expression of gp49A has not yet been confirmed because mAb B23.1 is specific only for gp49B1 (Katz et al. 1996). Ly-49 family receptors may also be involved in activation. Mason et al. (1996) report that Ly-49D, which lacks the ITIM contained by the other Ly-49 members, activates NK cells. It is not known why NK cells appear to express stimulatory and inhibitory forms of gp49 and Ly-49 simultaneously. The two forms may have different ligand specificities, or alternatively, expression of each isoform may be differentially regulated.

While gp49B1 bears many similarities to KIR (Table 1), it may not represent the mouse homologue of KIR, based on several lines of reasoning. Rojo et al. (1997) have identified a novel human cDNA which is 50% homologous to gp49B1 (compared to KIR which is 35% identical to gp49B1) and is therefore a stronger candidate for the human homologue of gp49B1. Additionally, the expression patterns of KIR and gp49B1 are different. Most notably, although they are both expressed on NK cells, gp49B1 is also expressed on mast cells while KIRs are found on T cell subsets. Finally, gp49B1 is expressed on all LAK cells whereas KIRs are expressed on overlapping subsets of NK clones.

Our description of a mouse NK inhibitory receptor belonging to the Ig superfamily further complicates the murine NK cell receptor field. Instead of considering only Ly-49 receptors, we must now entertain another putative inhibitory receptor, gp49B1, on mouse NK cells. The simplest scenario is that gp49B1 resembles Ly-49 functionally and acts as an MHC class I specific inhibitory receptor. As with human NK cells, mouse NK cells would utilize structurally distinct receptors for the same function. Alternatively, gp49B1 may have a completely different ligand which remains to be identified. It is also possible that gp49B1 may act as a coreceptor with Ly-49. This hypothesis is especially appealing if we consider that Ly-49 is polymorphic while gp49B1 is monomorphic. Specificity toward MHC class I may be conferred by Ly-49 which, with one ITIM, can deliver only a weak inhibitory signal. If Ly-49 is complexed with gp49B1, which possibly binds to a conserved region of MHC class I, the inhibitory signal delivered by this complex, including the two gp49B1 ITIMs, could then fully paralyze NK cell killing. This coreceptor hypothesis is analogous to the relationship between the highly variable T cell receptor and the monomorphic CD8 coreceptor. A resolution to this issue will come with the identification of a ligand for gp49B1.

6 Similar Regulatory Mechanisms Shared by Mouse Mast Cells and NK Cells

It is becoming apparent that inhibition as a means of regulating immune cell function is a primary mechanism by which immune responses are controlled. Our study, in addition to those by others, suggests that mast cells and NK cells, by their expression of gp49B1, utilize similar regulatory mechanisms. Furthermore, mast cells express MAFA, a type II integral membrane protein with structural homology to Ly-49 receptors, which also acts as an inhibitory receptor (Guthmann et al. 1995). A better understanding of gp49 function and especially identification of its ligand will provide insight as to how NK cell killing and mast cell activation may be coordinately regulated.

These findings also suggest that NK cells and mast cells are related in other ways. Clearly both are capable of granule exocytosis and cytokine production. Moreover, both appear poised to respond in the earliest phases of the immune response. Further characterization of their relationship may be rewarding.

Acknowledgements. This work was supported by funds from the Barnes-Jewish Hospital Research Foundation and grants from the NIH. We gratefully thank Paul LeBlanc, Indira Mehta, and Azza Idris for reagents; Eric Long for discussion of unpublished results; Matt Thomas and Dave Plas for helpful discussion, advice, and reagents; and Susan Yang and Dortha Chu for critical reading of this manuscript.

References

Arm JP, Gurish MF, Reynolds DS, Scott HC, Gartner CS, Austen KF, Katz HR (1991) Molecular cloning of gp49, a cell-surface antigen that is preferentially expressed by mouse mast cell progenitors and is a new member of the immunoglobulin superfamily. J Biol Chem 266:15966–15973

Brennan J, Takei F, Wong S, Mager DL (1995) Carbohydrate recognition by a natural killer cell receptor, Ly-49C. J Biol Chem 270:9691–9694

Brennan J, Lemieux S, Freeman JD, Mager DL, Takei F (1996a) Heterogeneity among Ly-49C natural killer (NK) cells: characterization of highly related receptors with differing functions and expression patterns. J Exp Med 184:2085–2090

Brennan J, Mahon G, Mager DL, Jefferies WA, Takei F (1996b) Recognition of class I major histocompatibility complex molecules by Ly-49: specificities and domain interactions. J Exp Med 183:1553–1559

Burshtyn DN, Scharenberg AM, Wagtmann N, Rajagopalan S, Berrada K, Yi T, Kinet J-P, Long EO (1996) Recruitment of tyrosine phosphatase HCP by the killer cell inhibitory receptor. Immunity 4:77–85

Campbell KS, Dessing M, Lopez-Botet M, Cella M, Colonna M (1996) Tyrosine phosphorylation of a human killer inhibitory receptor recruits protein tyrosine phosphatase 1C. J Exp Med 184:93–100

Castells MC, Wu X, Arm JP, Austen KF, Katz HR (1994) Cloning of the gp49B gene of the immunoglobulin superfamily and demonstration that one of its two products is an early-expressed mast cell surface protein originally described as gp49. J Biol Chem 269:8393–8401

Colonna M, Samaridis J (1995) Cloning of immunoglobulin-superfamily members associated with HLA-C and HLA-B recognition by human natural killer cells. Science 268:405–408

Colonna M, Brooks EG, Falco M, Ferrara GB, Strominger JL (1993) Generation of allospecific natural killer cells by stimulation across a polymorphism of HLA-C. Science 260:1121–1124

Correa I, Raulet DH (1995) Binding of diverse peptides to MHC class I molecules inhibits target cell lysis by activated natural killer cells. Immunity 2:61–71

D'Ambrosio D, Hippen KL, Minskoff SA, Mellman I, Pani G, Siminovitch KA, Cambier JC (1995) Recruitment and activation of PTP1C in negative regulation of antigen receptor signaling by FcγRIIB1. Science 268:293–297

D'Andrea A, Chang C, Franz-Bacon K, McClanahan T, Phillips JH, Lanier LL (1995) Molecular cloning of NKB1: a natural killer cell receptor for HLA-B allotypes. J Immunol 155:2306–2310

Daniels BF, Karlhofer FM, Seaman WE, Yokoyama WM (1994a) A natural killer cell receptor specific for a major histocompatibility complex class I molecule. J Exp Med 180:687–692

Daniels BF, Nakamura MC, Rosen SD, Yokoyama WM, Seaman WE (1994b) Ly-49A, a receptor for H-2D^{d}, has a functional carbohydrate recognition domain. Immunity 1:785–792

Döhring C, Samaridis J, Colonna M (1996) Alternatively spliced forms of human killer inhibitory receptors. Immunogenetics 44:227–230

Doody GM, Justement LB, Delibrias CC, Matthews RJ, Lin J, Thomas ML, Fearon DT (1995) A role in B cell activation for CD22 and the protein tyrosine phosphatase SHP. Science 269:242–244

Dorshkind K, Pollack SB, Bosma MJ, Phillips RA (1985) Natural killer (NK) cells are present in mice with severe combined immunodeficiency (scid). J Immunol 134:3798–3801

Fry AM, Lanier LL, Weiss A (1996) Phosphotyrosines in the killer cell inhibitory receptor motif of NKB1 are required for negative signaling and for association with protein tyrosine phosphatase 1C. J Exp Med 184:295–300

Gumperz JE, Parham P (1995) The enigma of the natural killer cell. Nature 378:245–248

Guthmann MD, Tal M, Pecht I (1995) A secretion inhibitory signal transduction molecule on mast cells is another C-type lectin. Proc Natl Acad Sci USA 92:9397–9401

Kane KP (1994) Ly-49 mediates EL4 lymphoma adhesion to isolated class I major histocompatibility complex molecules. J Exp Med 179:1011–1015

Karlhofer FM, Ribaudo RK, Yokoyama WM (1992) MHC class I alloantigen specificity of Ly-49$^+$ IL-2 activated natural killer cells. Nature 358:66–70

Karlhofer FM, Hunziker R, Reichlin A, Margulies DH, Yokoyama WM (1994) Host MHC class I molecules modulate in vivo expression of a NK cell receptor. J Immunol 153:2407–2416

Katz HR, Vivier E, Castells MC, McCormick MJ, Chambers JM, Austen KF (1996) Mouse mast cell gp49B1 contains two immunoreceptor tyrosine-based inhibition motifs and suppresses mast cell activation when coligated with the high-affinity Fc receptor for IgE. Proc Natl Acad Sci USA 93:10809–10814

Lazetic S, Chang C, Houchins JP, Lanier LL, Phillips JH (1996) Human natural killer cell receptors involved in MHC class I recognition are disulfide-linked heterodimers of CD94 and NKG2 subunits. J Immunol 157:4741–4745

LeBlanc PA, Russell SW, Chang S-MT (1982) Mouse mononuclear phagocyte antigenic heterogeneity detected by monoclonal antibodies. J Retic Soc 32:219–231

Ljunggren H-G, Kärre K (1985) Host resistance directed selectively against H-2-deficient lymphoma variants: analysis of the mechanism. J Exp Med 162:1745–1759

Ljunggren H-G, Kärre K (1990) In search of the "missing self": MHC molecules and NK cell recognition. Immunol Today 11:237–244

Malnati MS, Peruzzi M, Parker KC, Biddison WE, Ciccone E, Moretta A, Long EO (1995) Peptide specificity in the recognition of MHC class I by natural killer cell clones. Science 267:1016–1018

Mandelboim O, Reyburn HT, Valés-Gómez M, Pazmany L, Colonna M, Borsellino G, Strominger JL (1996) Protection from lysis by natural killer cells of group 1 and 2 specificity is mediated by residue 80 in human histocompatibility leukocyte antigen C alleles and also occurs with empty major histocompatibility complex molecules. J Exp Med 184:913–922

Mason LH, Ortaldo JR, Young HA, Kumar V, Bennett M, Anderson SK (1995) Cloning and functional characteristics of murine large granular lymphocyte-1: a member of the Ly-49 gene family (Ly-49G2). J Exp Med 182:293–303

Mason LH, Anderson SK, Yokoyama WM, Smith HRC, Winkler-Pickett R, Ortaldo JR (1996) The Ly-49D receptor activates murine natural killer cells. J Exp Med 184:2119–2128

Mombaerts P, Iacomini J, Johnson RS, Herrup K, Tonegawa S, Papaioannou VE (1992) RAG-1-deficient mice have no mature B and T lymphocytes. Cell 68:869–877

Moretta A, Sivori S, Vitale M, Pende D, Morelli L, Augugliaro R, Bottino C, Moretta L (1995) Existence of both inhibitory (p58) and activatory (p50) receptors for HLA-C molecules in human natural killer cells. J Exp Med 182:875–884

Muta T, Kurosaki T, Misulovin Z, Sanchez M, Nussenzweig MC, Ravetch JV (1994) A 13-amino-acid motif in the cytoplasmic domain of FcγRIIB modulates B-cell receptor signalling. Nature 368:70–73

Olcese L, Lang P, Vély F, Cambiaggi A, Marguet D, Bléry M, Hippen KL, Biassoni R, Moretta A, Moretta L, Cambier JC, Vivier E (1996) Human and mouse killer-cell inhibitory receptors recruit PTP1C and PTP1D protein tyrosine phosphatases. J Immunol 156:4531–4534

Orihuela M, Margulies DH, Yokoyama WM (1996) The natural killer cell receptor Ly-49A recognizes a peptide-induced conformational determinant on its major histocompatibility complex class I ligand. Proc Natl Acad Sci USA 93:11792–11797

Pei D, Lorenz U, Klingmüller U, Neel BG, Walsh CT (1994) Intramolecular regulation of protein tyrosine phosphatase SH-PTP1: a new function for Src homology 2 domains. Biochemistry 33:15483–15493

Pende D, Biassonni R, Cantoni C, Verdiani S, Falco M, Di Donato C, Accame L, Bottino C, Moretta A, Moretta L (1996) The natural killer cell receptor specific for HLA-A allotypes: a novel member of the p58/p70 family of inhibitory receptors that is characterized by three immunoglobulin-like domains and is expressed as a 140-kD disulphide-linked dimer. J Exp Med 184:505–518

Pérez-Villar JJ, Melero I, Rodriguez A, Carretero M, Aramburu J, Sivori S, Orengo AM, Moretta A, Lopez-Botet M (1995) Functional ambivalence of the Kp43 (CD94) NK cell-associated surface antigen. J Immunol 154:5779–5788

Phillips JH, Chang C, Mattson J, Gumperz JE, Parham P, Lanier LL (1996) CD94 and a novel associated protein (CD94AP) form a NK cell receptor involved in the recognition of HLA-A, HLA-B, and HLA-C allotypes. Immunity 5:163–172

Rojo S, Burshtyn DN, Long EO, Wagtmann N (1997) Type I transmembrane receptor with inhibitory function in mouse mast cells and NK cells. J Immunol 158:9–12

Shinkai Y, Rathbun G, Lam K-P, Oltz EM, Stewart V, Mendelsohn M, Charron J, Datta M, Young F, Stall AM, Alt FW (1992) RAG-2-deficient mice lack mature lymphocytes owing to inability to initiate V(D)J rearrangement. Cell 68:855–867

Smith HRC, Karlhofer FM, Yokoyama WM (1994) Ly-49 multigene family expressed by IL-2-activated NK cells. J Immunol 153:1068–1079

Smith HRC, Karlhofer FM, Yokoyama WM (1995) Expression of Ly-49 related molecules as heterodimers on IL-2 activated NK cells. 9th International Congress of Immunology, p 2844

Stoneman ER, Bennett M, An J, Chesnut KA, Wakeland EK, Scheerer JB, Siciliano MJ, Kumar V, Mathew PA (1995) Cloning and characterization of 5E6 (Ly-49C), a receptor molecule expressed on a subset of murine natural killer cells. J Exp Med 182:305–313

Wagtmann N, Biassoni R, Cantoni C, Verdiani S, Malnati MS, Vitale M, Bottino C, Moretta L, Moretta A, Long EO (1995a) Molecular clones of the p58 NK cell receptor reveal immunoglobulin-related molecules with diversity in both the extra-and intracellular domains. Immunity 2:439–449

Wagtmann N, Rajagopalan S, Winter CC, Peruzzi M, Long EO (1995b) Killer cell inhibitory receptors specific for HLA-C and HLA-B identified by direct binding and by functional transfer. Immunity 3:801–809

Wang LL, Mehta IK, LeBlanc PA, Yokoyama W (1997) Mouse natural killer cells express gp49B1, a structural homologue of human killer inhibitory receptors. J Immunol 158:13–17

Wong S, Freeman JD, Kelleher C, Mager D, Takei F (1991) Ly-49 multigene family: new members of a superfamily of type II membrane proteins with lectin-like domains. J Immunol 147:1417–1423

Yokoyama WM (1995) Right-side-up and up-side-down NK cell receptors. Curr Biol 5:982–985

Yokoyama WM, Seaman WE (1993) The Ly-49 and NKR-P1 gene families encoding lectin-like receptors on natural killer cells: the NK gene complex. Annu Rev Immunol 11:613–635

Yokoyama WM, Jacobs LB, Kanagawa O, Shevach EM, Cohen DI (1989) A murine T lymphocyte antigen belongs to a supergene family of type II integral membrane proteins. J Immunol 143:1379–1386

Yokoyama WM, Kehn PJ, Cohen DI, Shevach EM (1990) Chromosomal location of the Ly-49 (A1, YE1/48) multigene family: genetic association with the NK11 antigen. J Immunol 145:2353–2358

Yu YYL, George T, Dorfman JR, Roland J, Kumar V, Bennett M (1996) The role of Ly49A and 5E6 (Ly49C) molecules in hybrid resistance mediated by murine natural killer cells against normal T cell blasts. Immunity 4:67–76

Stimulatory Receptors in NK and T Cells

A. MORETTA[1], S. SIVORI[2], M. PONTE[3], M.C. MINGARI[4], and L. MORETTA[5]

1 Introduction

Although it has long been known that natural killer (NK) cells lyse certain tumor or virally infected cells (HERBERMAN et al. 1979; KIESSLING et al. 1979; TRINCHIERI 1989), the mechanism(s) by which they discriminate between these target cells and normal cells remained mysterious. More recently, important progress both in mice and in humans has allowed at least in part the clarification of the molecular mechanisms involved in NK cell function and in their ability to identify and lyse potentially dangerous target cells (YOKOYAMA and SEAMAN 1993; MORETTA L. et al. 1992, 1994; MORETTA A. et al. 1996). An inverse correlation has been established between the expression of surface MHC class I molecules on potential target cells and their susceptibility to NK cell mediated lysis (LJUNGGREN and KÄRRE 1990; KÄRRE 1992). This led to the hypothesis that the surface expression of MHC molecules in some way protects cells from NK cell mediated attack. Cells in which MHC molecules are not expressed (as may occur in tumor or virus-infected cells) are susceptible to NK cells (LJUNGGREN and KÄRRE 1985). Thus NK cells may play a unique role in immune defenses by selectively removing cells that have lost the ability to express MHC class I molecules.

[1]Dipartimento di Scienze Biomediche e Biotecnologie, Università di Brescia, Brescia, and Istituto di Istologia ed Embriologia Generale, Via G.B. Marsano 10, Università di Genova, 16132 Genoa, Italy

[2]Istituto di Istologia ed Embriologia Generale, Via G.B. Marsano 10, Università di Genova, 16132 Genoa, Italy

[3]Istituto Scientifico Tumori e Centro Biotecnologie Avanzate, Largo R. Benzi 10, 16132 Genoa, Italy

[4]Istituto Scientifico Tumori e Centro Biotecnologie Avanzate, Largo R. Benzi 10, and, Dipartimento di Oncologia Clinica e Sperimentale, and Istituto di Patologia Generale, Università di Genova, 16132 Genoa, Italy

[5]Istituto Scientifico Tumori e Centro Biotecnologie Avanzate, Largo R. Benzi 10, and Istituto di Patologia Generale, Università di Genova, 16132 Genoa, Italy

These concepts were proposed by LJUNGGREN and KÄRRE (1990) in the so-called "missing self" hypothesis. Important advances have been made in humans, in part because of the ability to clone human NK cells (FERRINI et al. 1987; PANTALEO et al. 1988). This made possible the demonstration that NK cells do not simply recognize HLA class I molecules but rather display a clonally distributed ability to specifically recognize given groups of HLA class I alleles (CICCONE et al. 1992; MORETTA A. et al. 1990a,b; LITWIN et al. 1993). This led to the discovery of various receptors capable of discriminating minor differences among class I alleles. These receptors have now been molecularly identified and cloned. The interest in NK cells and their receptors was further increased by the discovery that a subset of T lymphocytes express these receptors (MORETTA A. et al. 1990a,b; FERRINI et al. 1994), and that their engagement leads to downregulation of T cell receptor (TCR) mediated T cell function (MINGARI et al. 1995; PHILLIPS et al. 1995). Importantly, in normal individuals receptors are largely confined to $CD8^+$ subsets that have a memory phenotype and are oligoclonal or monoclonal in nature (MINGARI et al. 1996).

2 The HLA Class I Specific Inhibitory Receptors

The first identified receptors were those specific for two groups of HLA-C alleles (p58.1 and p58.2) (MORETTA A. et al. 1990a,b). These were found to belong to the Ig superfamily and to be characterized by two extracellular Ig-like domains (WAGTMANN et al. 1995; COLONNA and SAMARIDIS 1995). Monoclonal antibody (mAb) mediated masking of p58 molecules led to lysis of HLA-C "protected" cells (MORETTA A. et al. 1993). Interestingly, the HLA-C alleles recognized by p58.1 share the amino acid position 77 (Ser) and 80 (Asn), whereas those recognized by p58.2 are characterized by Asn-77 and by S-80 (COLONNA et al. 1992, 1993). These amino acid positions are crucial for the p58-mediated recognition, as shown by experiments of site-directed mutagenesis (BIASSONI et al. 1995). Although only a fraction of NK cells (different in different individuals) express p58 molecules, it became evident that the ability to recognize HLA class I molecules is a common property of all NK cells. Thus the use of $p58^-$ NK cell clones allowed the definition of additional HLA class I allele specificities and the receptors involved in their recognition. A p70 molecule characterized by three Ig-like domains was found to mediate recognition of HLA alleles belonging to the Bw4 supertypic specificity (LITWIN et al. 1994; COLONNA and SAMARIDIS 1995; VITALE et al. 1996); in addition, a 70-/140-kDa molecule (p140) mediated specific recognition of defined HLA-A alleles, including A11 and A3 (PENDE et al. 1996; Döhring et al. 1996). A role of the HLA class I bound peptides in the NK cell mediated recognition has been shown in HLA-Bw4 specific clones (MALNATI et al. 1995). However, the small proportion of HLA class I molecules which bind a given peptide suggests a limited role of peptides in altering the ability of NK cells to recognize a given class I allele. Perhaps this occurs only in particular situations in which few peptides dominate the set of MHC-bound peptides (for example, in some viral infections).

The various killer inhibitory receptors (KIRs) identified so far display a high degree of homology. For example, p58, p70, and p140 are characterized by a common motif in their intracytoplasmic tail. They share two (V/I)XYXXL sequences termed immunoreceptor tyrosine based inhibitory motif (ITIM). KIR crosslinking mediated by the natural ligand or by specific mAbs results in tyrosine phosphorylation and recruitment of the SH2 domain containing tyrosine phosphatases (SHP) (BURSHTYN et al. 1996; OLCESE et al. 1996; CAMPBELL et al. 1996). The effect of SHP is crucial in explaining why KIR/MHC interaction leads to inhibition of NK cell function. Indeed, SHP mediates dephosphorylation of adaptor/effector molecules that are part of the NK cell activating pathways.

In mice the inhibitory receptors for MHC class I molecules that have been characterized so far are represented by Ly49 molecules which do not belong to the Ig superfamily but are type II transmembrane proteins containing a C-type lectin domain (YOKOYAMA and SEAMAN 1993). Recently a previously identified type II protein CD94 (ARAMBURU et al. 1990) has been shown to be involved in MHC class I recognition.

In early studies CD94 was described as an inhibitory NK receptor able to recognize at least some HLA-Bw6 alleles but not Bw4 alleles (MORETTA A. et al. 1994). Subsequent studies showed that CD94 can function as a HLA class I specific inhibitory receptor characterized by a broad specificity as it recognizes various HLA-A, HLA-B, or HLA-C alleles (SIVORI et al. 1996; LAZETIC et al. 1996). CD94 has been found to be heterogeneous in function as both inhibitory and activating forms have been identified in different NK cell clones (PEREZ-VILLAR et al. 1995, 1996). More recently the inhibitory form of CD94 has been shown to be a heterodimeric complex, being associated with another type II protein characterized by intracytoplasmic ITIM motifs (CARRETERO et al. 1997; LAZETIC et al. 1996). This protein is identified with the molecular product of the NKG2A-encoding cDNA. The presence of a C-type lectin domain in CD94/NKG2A molecules suggests that a carbohydrate moiety common to different class I alleles plays at least a partial role in the binding of this receptor to class I molecules. The redundancy of class I specific inhibitory receptors may be important to sense different epitopes of MHC class I molecules. In addition, no KIRs belonging to the Ig superfamily that are specific for HLA-Bw6 alleles or for the majority of HLA-A alleles have been identified so far. Therefore the redundancy of NK receptors appears to be confined to the recognition of certain HLA class I allotypes, while CD94/NKG2A may represent the only receptor available for recognition of all the remaining HLA-B or HLA-A alleles. In this context, the CD94/NKG2A receptor may represent an important device to control the potential autoreactivity of a relevant proportion of NK cells.

3 Surface Molecules and Mechanisms Involved in NK Cell Activation

NK cells have evolved powerful mechanisms to exert an inhibitory control on their cytolytic function. The requirement for this safety device is clearly indicated by the effect of masking the inhibitory receptors or their MHC ligand (i.e., lysis of target cells). This implies that NK cells must constitutively express not only a powerful lytic machinery but also receptors which upon interaction with their ligands (expressed on most nucleated cells) lead to NK cell triggering and lysis of target cells. At present we know more about NK cell inactivation than about their activation. The triggering surface receptors which play a predominant role in target cell recognition and lysis have remained elusive. Several surface molecules which can mediate NK cell triggering have been identified; however, their actual role in natural cytotoxicity has not been clarified so far.

Adhesion Molecules. Adhesion molecules not only mediate NK cell adhesion to other cells but can also transduce triggering signals which may lead to cell activation and triggering of the cytolytic machinery. In this respect, NK cell triggering may result from a number of interactions between various adhesion molecules and their ligands (Lanier et al. 1997). De novo expression or upregulation of various adhesion molecules may be induced by inflammatory cytokines such as tumor necrosis factor α. It is possible that the expression of an appropriate pattern of adhesion molecules by NK cell and/or of high density of the corresponding ligands may be responsible for NK cell activation. NK cells constitutively express CD2, CD11a/CD18 (LFA-1), CD49/CD29 VLA-4. Moreover, expression of these molecules is upregulated upon NK cell activation.

CD69 Molecule. Another surface molecule which mediates potent NK cell triggering is CD69. CD69 is surface expressed upon NK cell activation (Moretta A. et al. 1991). The natural ligand has not been identified so far, and the possible involvement of the CD69/CD69-ligand interaction in triggering the NK cell cytotoxicity in natural immunity has not been elucidated. The finding that CD69 is expressed by NK cells only upon activation suggests a possible role in the ability of activated NK cells to lyse with higher efficiency a broader spectrum of tumor target cells than resting NK cells.

The Low-Affinity Receptor for the Fc Portion of IgG (FcγRIII or CD16). This is a well known NK cell marker which is expressed by most (but not all) peripheral blood NK cells. IgG-coated target cells trigger NK cells to lyse via an antibody-dependent cellular cytotoxicity mechanism and to produce cytokines (Trinchieri 1989). CD16 is associated with FcεRIγ and with CD3ζ chains that are involved in signal transduction. CD16 mediates a potent NK cell triggering; however, there is no evidence so far that it serves functions other than antibody-dependent cellular cytotoxicity, or that ligands different from IgG immune complexes may bind to and trigger CD16.

Cytokine Receptors. Efficient NK cell triggering also occurs in response to several cytokines, including interleukins 2, 12, and 15 and tumor necrosis factor-α. For example, the interleukin 2 mediated signaling results in the release of cytokines, primarily IFN-γ, which are likely to play an important role in the innate response of NK cells to pathogens. It is unlikely that cytokine receptors expressed by NK cells play any role in natural cytotoxicity.

p46 Molecule. A surface molecule has recently been characterized by the use of mAbs selected on the basis of the ability to mediate strong NK cell triggering and target cell lysis. This 46-kDa molecule, termed p46, unlike other NK cell surface molecules, is strictly NK cell specific (SIVORI et al. 1997). Thus p46 is expressed by all resting and activated NK cells, including the minor NK cell subset lacking CD16. Moreover, neither T or B cells or macrophages nor other cell lineages (either normal or neoplastic) have been found to express p46. It should be stressed that typical "NK cell markers" including CD16 and CD56 are also expressed by other cell types (e.g., T cell subsets). The same holds true for NKRP1 (POGGI et al. 1997) and for the various HLA class I specific inhibitory receptors (including p58, p70, p140, and CD94/NKG2A) (MINGARI et al. 1995, 1997) which are expressed by subsets of T cells. Neither fresh nor cultured T cell populations or clones expressing these markers express p46 molecules. Upon mAb-mediated crosslinking p46 molecules induce strong NK cell triggering, leading to $[Ca^{2+}]_i$ increases, lymphokine production, and cytolytic activity both in resting NK cells and in NK cell clones. The p46-mediated NK cell triggering is downregulated by the simultaneous engagement of inhibitory HLA class I specific receptors. In view of its unique cellular distribution and function, p46 may represent a relevant candidate for an activating receptor involved in the recognition of non-MHC ligand (recognition of MHC molecules has been directly ruled out) expressed on NK susceptible target cells (SIVORI et al. 1997).

As discussed above, a possible view of the mechanisms of NK cell triggering in the natural cytotoxicity is that multiple receptors are expressed on NK cells and may cooperate to induce optimal cell activation. It is not necessary to postulate that all triggering receptors function simultaneously since their engagement may depend on the presence and/or density of their specific ligands on target cells. In agreement with this view, anti-p46 mAb inhibit the cytolytic activity of NK cell clones against some (Fcγ receptor$^-$) target cells but not others. The finding that even in these cases only a partial inhibition occurs, suggests that p46 molecules cooperate with other triggering receptors to induce maximal NK cell triggering. In addition, the fact that T cells, including CD8$^+$ activated populations, or clones displaying NK-like activity, do not express p46 implies that these cells utilize different surface molecules to lyse HLA class I$^-$ target cells. The definition of possible correlations between p46 and other functional molecules expressed by NK cells and the identification of ligand(s) awaits cloning of the molecule and the use of soluble p46 molecules.

The Activating Form of HLA Class I Specific NK Receptors. mAbs directed to the HLA-C specific p58.1 and p58.2 have also been found to react with activating receptors displaying a lower molecular weight (p50) (MORETTA A. et al. 1995). Molecular cloning reveals a high degree of homology with the corresponding inhibitory receptors in the extracellular domains (Biassoni et al. 1996). In contrast, while the inhibitory forms (p58) have a transmembrane region formed by nonpolar amino acids, p50 contains the charged amino acid Lys (Biassoni et al. 1996). In addition, the cytoplasmic tail is short (39 amino acids) and does not contain ITIM. The activating p50 receptors display HLA-C specificity and are coexpressed with at least one inhibitory receptor specific for another class I allele (Moretta A. et al. 1995). The inhibitory receptors always predominate over the activating ones, thus preventing lysis of autologous cells (following the p50/HLA-C interaction).

The physiological role played by activating receptors is still undefined although they may represent yet another pathway involved in NK cell triggering (in the case of HLA class I^+ target cells). A measurable NK cell triggering via p50 receptors occurs only in the absence of inhibitory interactions, for example, in the case of HLA class I^- cells transfected with the relevant HLA-C allele recognized by p50 receptors. In vivo this situation may occur either following downregulation or peptide-induced alteration of the HLA class I allele interacting with the inhibitory receptors. Although the activating form of receptors appears to display the same allele specificity of the corresponding p58 receptor, it is possible to speculate that inhibitory and activating receptors sense different HLA-bound peptides. Regarding the mechanism of signal transduction, noteworthy is the presence in the transmembrane domain of a single charged amino acid residue (Lys). This occurs in several cell surface receptors (e.g., TCR α/β, FcεRI) that are associated with polypeptides containing immunoreceptor tyrosine-based activation motifs (ITAMs), including CD3γ, CD3δ, CD3ζ, and FcεRIγ. The single membrane charged amino acid residue is required for the assembly of ITAM-bearing polypeptides into multimeric receptors.

Interestingly, a novel set of phosphorylated polypeptides termed killer activating receptor-associated proteins (KARAPs) have recently been identified (Olcese et al. 1997). These proteins, which are phosphorylated upon receptor crosslinking, range from 12 to 16 kDa, depending on the origin of NK cells. It will be important to determine the KARAP molecular structure in order to define whether they contain ITAM(s), and whether they are distinct molecules or, rather, represent different isoforms of the same protein, possibly reflecting different levels of phosphorylation of the same protein. Both activating p50 receptors (Mandelboim et al. 1997) and activating receptors reacting with anti-p70 or anti-p140 mAbs (Ponte et al. manuscript in preparation) have also been detected in T cells.

Mandelboim et al. (1997) proposed a possible role for these molecules, showing a costimulatory activity in TCR-mediated responses. Indeed, $p50^+$ T lymphocytes were found to respond to a lower dose of superantigen, depending on the expression of the appropriate HLA-C ligand on target cells. Further studies in antigen-specific systems are clearly required to better define the role of HLA class I specific activating receptors in T lymphocytes.

Acknowledgements. This work was supported by grants from the Associazione Italiana per la Ricerca sul Cancro, Istituto Superiore di Sanità, Consiglio Nazionale delle Ricerche–Progetto Finalizzato A.C.R.O., and Ministero dell' Università e della Ricerca Scientifica e Tecnologica to L. Moretta, M.C. Mingari, and A. Moretta. We wish to thank Stefano Canu for typing the manuscript.

References

Aramburu J, Balboa MA, Ramirez A, Silva A, Acevedo A, Sanchez-Madrid F, de Landàzuri MO, López-Botet M (1990) A novel functional cell surface dimer (Kp43) expressed by natural killer cells and T cell receptor- /δ+ T lymphocytes. Inhibition of IL-2 dependent proliferation by anti-Kp43 monoclonal antibody. J Immunol 44:3238–3247

Biassoni R, Falco M, Cambiaggi A, Costa P, Verdiani S, Pende D, Conte R, Di Donato C, Parham P, Moretta L (1995) Amino acid substitutions can influence the NK-mediated recognition of HLA-C molecules. Role of Serine-77 and lysine-80 in the target cell protection from lysis mediated by "group 2" or "group 1" NK clones. J Exp Med 182:605–609

Biassoni R, Cantoni C, Falco M, Verdiani S, Bottino C, Vitale M, Conte R, Poggi A, Moretta A, Moretta L (1996) The HLA-C-specific "activatory" or "inhibitory" natural killer cell receptors display highly homologous extracellular domains but differ in their transmembrane and intracytoplasmic portions. J Exp Med 183:645–650

Burshtyn DN, Scharenberg AM, Wagtmann N, Rajagopalan S, Berrada K, Yi T, Kinet JP, Long EO (1996) Recruitment of tyrosine phosphatase HCP by the killer cell inhibitory receptor. Immunity 4:77–85

Campbell KS, Dessing M, Lopez-Botet, M, Cella M, Colonna M (1996) Tyrosine phosphorylation of a human killer inhibitory receptor recruits protein phosphatase 1 C. J Exp Med 184:93–100

Carretero M, Cantoni C, Bellón T, Bottino C, Biassoni R, Rodríguez A, Pérez-Villar JP, Moretta L, Moretta A, López-Botet M (1996) The CD94 and NKG2-A C-type lectins covalently assemble to form a natural killer cell inhibitory receptor for HLA class I molecules. Eur J Immunol 27:563–567

Ciccone E, Pende D, Viale O, Di Donato C, Tripodi G, Orengo AM, Guardiola J, Moretta A, Moretta L (1992) Evidence of a natural killer (NK) cell repertoire for (allo)antigen recognition: definition of five distinct NK-determined allospecificities in humans. J Exp Med 175:709–718

Colonna M, Spies T, Strominger JL, Ciccone E, Moretta A, Moretta L, Pende D, Viale O (1992) Alloantigen recognition by human natural killer cells is associated with HLA-C or a closely linked gene. Proc Natl Acad Sci USA 89:7983–7985

Colonna M, Borsellino G, Falco M, Ferrara GB, Strominger JL (1993) HLA-C is the inhibitory ligand that determines dominant resistance to lysis by NK1- and NK2-specific natural killer cells. Proc Natl Acad Sci USA 90:12000–12004

Colonna M, Samaridis J (1995) Cloning of immunoglobulin-superfamily members associated with HLA-C and HLA-B recognition by human natural killer cells. Science 268:405–408

Döhring C, Scheidegger D, Samaridis J, Cella M, Colonna M (1996) A human killer inhibitory receptor specific for HLA-A. J Immunol 156:3098–3101

Ferrini S, Miescher S, Zocchi MR, von Fliedner V, Moretta A (1987) Phenotypic and functional characterization of recombinant interleukin-2 (rIL-2)-induced activated killer cells. Analysis at the population and clonal levels. J Immunol 138:1297

Ferrini S, Cambiaggi A, Meazza R, Sforzini S, Marciano S, Mingari MC, Moretta L (1994) T cell clones expressing the NK-related p58 receptor molecule display heterogeneity in phenotypic properties and p58 function. Eur J Immunol 24:2294–2298

Herberman RB, Nunn ME, Lavrin DH (1975) Natural cytotoxic reactivity of mouse lymphoid cells against syngeneic and allogeneic tumours. I. Distribution of reactivity and specificity. Int J Cancer 16:216–229

Kärre K (1992) An unexpected petition for pardon. Curr Biol vol 2 11:613–616

Kiessling R, Klein E, Wigzell H (1975) "Natural killer" cells in the mouse I. Cytotoxic cells with specificity for mouse Moloney leukemia cells. Specificity and distribution according to genotype. Eur J Immunol 5:112–117

Lanier LL, Corliss B, Phillips JH (1997) Arousal and inhibition of human NK cells. Immunol Rev 155:145–154

Lazetic S, Chang C, Houchins JP, Lanier LL, Philips JH (1996) Human natural killer cell receptors involved in MHC class I recognition are disulphide-linked heterodimers of CD94 and NKG2 subunits. J Immunol 157:4741–4745

Litwin V, Gumperz J, Parham P, Phillips JH, Lanier LL (1993) Specificity of HLA class I antigen recognition by human NK clones: evidence for clonal heterogeneity, protection by self and non-self alleles, and influence of the target cell type. J Exp Med 178:1321–1336

Litwin V, Gumperz JE, Parham P, Phillips JH, Lanier LL (1994) NKB1: a natural killer cell receptor involved in the recognition of polymorphic HLA-B molecules. J Exp Med 180:537:543

Ljunggren HG, Kärre K (1985) Host resistance directed selectively against H-2-deficient lymphoma variants: analysis of the mechanism. J Exp Med 162:1745–1759

Ljunggren HG, Kärre K (1990) In search of the "missing self". MHC molecules and NK cell recognition. Immunol Today 11:237–244

Mandelboim O et al (1997) Enhancement of class II restricted-T cell responses by co-stimulatory class I NK receptors. Science (in press)

Malnati MS, Peruzzi M, Parker KC, Biddison WE, Ciccone E, Moretta A, Long EO (1995) Peptide specificity in the recognition of MHC class I by natural killer cell clones. Science 267:1016–1018

Mingari MC, Vitale C, Cambiaggi A, Schiavetti F, Melioli G, Ferrini S, Poggi A (1995) Cytolytic T lymphocytes displaying natural killer (NK)-like activity: expression of NK-related functional receptors for HLA class I molecules (p58 and CD94) and inhibitory effect on the TCR-mediated target cell lysis or lymphokine production. Int Immunol 7 4:697–703

Mingari MC, Schiavetti F, Ponte M, Vitale M, Maggi E, Romagnani S, Demarest J, Pantaleo G, Fauci AS, Moretta L (1996) Human CD8$^+$ T lymphocyte subsets that express HLA-class I specific inhibitory receptors represent oligoclonally or monoclonally expanded cell populations. Proc Natl Acad Sci USA 93:12433–12438

Mingari MC, Ponte M, Cantoni C, Vitale C, Schiavetti F, Bertone S, Bellomo R, Tradori Cappai A, Biassoni R (1997) HLA-class I-specific inhibitory receptors in human cytolytic T lymphocytes: molecular characterization, distribution in lymphoid tissues and co-expression by individual T cells. Int Immunol vol 9 4:485–491

Moretta A, Bottino C, Pende D, Tripodi G, Tambussi G, Viale O, Orengo A, Barbaresi M, Merli A, Ciccone E, Moretta L (1990a) Identification of four subsets of human CD3-CD16$^+$ NK cells by the expression of clonally distributed functional surface molecules. Correlation between subset assignment of NK clones and ability to mediate specific alloantigen recognition. J Exp Med 172:1589–1598

Moretta A, Tambussi G, Bottino C, Tripodi G, Merli A, Ciccone E, Pantaleo G, Moretta L (1990b) A novel surface antigen expressed by a subset of human CD3-CD16$^+$ natural killer cells. Role in cell activation and regulation of cytolytic function. J Exp Med 171:695–714

Moretta A, Poggi A, Pende D, Tripodi G, Orengo AM, Pella N, Augugliaro R, Bottino C, Ciccone E, Moretta L (1991) CD69-mediated pathway of lymphocyte activation. Anti-CD69 mAbs trigger the cytolytic activity of different lymphoid effector cells with the exception of cytolytic T lymphocytes expressing TCR α/β. J Exp Med 174:1393–1398

Moretta A, Vitale M, Bottino C, Orengo AM, Morelli L, Augugliaro, R, Barbaresi M, Ciccone E, Moretta L (1993) P58 molecules as putative receptors for MHC class I molecules in human natural killer (NK) cells. Anti-p58 antibodies reconstitute lysis of MHC class I-protected cells in NK clones displaying different specificities. J Exp Med 178:597–604

Moretta A, Vitale M, Sivori S, Bottino C, Morelli L, Augugliaro R, Barbaresi M, Pende D, Ciccone E, Lopez-Botet M, Moretta L (1994) Human natural killer cell receptors for HLA-class I molecules. Evidence that the Kp43 (CD94) molecule functions as receptor for HLA-B alleles. J Exp Med 180:545–555

Moretta A, Sivori S, Vitale M, Pende D, Morelli L, Augugliaro R, Bottino C, Moretta L (1995) Existence of both inhibitory (p58) and activatory (p50) receptors for HLA-C molecules in human natural killer cells J Exp Med 182:875–884

Moretta A, Bottino C, Vitale M, Pende D, Biassoni R, Mingari MC, Moretta L (1996) Receptors for HLA-class I-molecules in human natural killer cells. Annu Rev Immunol 14:619–648

Moretta L, Ciccone E, Moretta A, Höglund P, Öhlen C, Kärre K (1992) Allorecognition by NK cells: nonself or no self? Immunol Today 13:300–306

Moretta L, Ciccone E, Mingari MC, Biassoni R, Moretta A (1994) Human NK cells: origin, clonality, specificity and receptors. Adv Immunol vol 55:341–380

Olcese L, Lang P, Vély F, Cambiaggi A, Marguet D, Bléry M, Hippen KL, Biassoni R, Moretta A, Moretta L, Cambier JC, Vivier E (1996) Human and mouse natural killer cell inhibitory receptors recruit the PTP1 C and PTP1D protein tyrosine phosphatases. J Immunol 156:4531–4534

Olcese L, Cambiaggi A, Semenzato G, Bottino C, Moretta A, Vivier E (1997) Human killer cell activatory receptors for MHC class I molecules are induced in a multimeric complex expressed by natural killer cells. J Immunol 158:5083–5086

Pantaleo G, Zocchi MR, Ferrini S, Poggi A, Tambussi G, Bottino C, Moretta L, Moretta A (1988) Human cytolytic cell clones lacking surface expression of T cell receptor α/β or $/\delta$. Evidence that surface structures other than CD3 or CD2 molecules are required for signal transduction. J Exp Med 168:13–24

Pende D, Biassoni R, Cantoni C, Verdiani S, Falco M, Di Donato C, Accame L, Bottino C, Moretta A, Moretta L (1996) The natural killer cell receptor specific for HLA-A allotypes: a novel member of the p58/p70 family of inhibitory receptors which is characterized by three Ig-like domains and is expressed as a 140 kD disulphide-linked dimer. J Exp Med 184:505–518

Pérez-Villar JJ, Melero I, Rodríguez A, Carretero M, Aramburu J, Sivori S, Orengo AM, Moretta A, López-Botet M (1995) Functional ambivalence of the Kp43 (CD94) NK cell-associated surface antigen. J Immunol 154:5779–88

Pérez-Villar JJ, Carretero M, Navarro F, Melero I, Rodríguez A, Bottino C, Moretta A, Lopez-Botet M (1996) Biochemical and serological evidence for the existence of functionally distinct isoforms of the CD94 NK-cell receptor. J Immunol 157:5367–5374

Poggi A, Costa P, Zocchi MR, Moretta L (1997) Phenotypic and functional analysis of $CD4^{+}$ $NKRP1A^{+}$ human T lymphocytes. Direct evidence that NKRP1 A molecule is involved in transendothelial migration. Eur J Immunol 27:00–00

Sivori S, Vitale M, Bottino C, Marcenaro E, Sanseverino L, Parolini S, Moretta L, Moretta L (1996) CD94 functions as a natural killer cell inhibitory receptor for different HLA-class-I alleles. Identification of the inhibitory form of CD94 by the use of novel monoclonal antibodies. Eur J Immunol 26:2487–2492

Sivori S, Vitale M, Morelli L, Sanseverino L, Augugliaro R, Bottino C, Moretta L, Moretta A (1997) p46, a novel natural killer cell-specific surface molecule which mediates cell activation. J Exp Med (in press)

Trinchieri G (1989) Biology of natural killer cells. Adv Immunol 47:187–376

Vitale M, Sivori S, Pende D, Augugliaro R, Di Donato C, Amoroso A, Malnati M, Bottino C, Moretta L, Moretta A (1996) Physical and functional independency of p70 and p58 NK cell receptors for HLA-class I. Their role in the definition of different groups of alloreactive NK cell clones. Proc Natl Acad Sci USA 93:1453–1457

Wagtmann N, Rajagopalan S, Winter CC, Peruzzi M, Long EO (1995) Killer cell inhibitory receptors specific for HLA-C and HLA-B identified by direct binding and by functional transfer. Immunity 3:801–809

Yokoyama WM, Seaman WE (1993) The Ly49 and NKR-P1 gene families encoding lectin-like receptors on natural killer cells: the NK gene complex. Ann Rev Immunol 11:613–635

Killer Cell Inhibitory Receptor Expression by T Cells

A. D'ANDREA and L.L. LANIER

1 Introduction

The killer cell inhibitory receptors (KIR) are a family of immunoglobulin (Ig)-like cell surface receptors which are differentially expressed by cytotoxic lymphocyte populations and recognize subsets of human leukocyte antigen (HLA) class I molecules on potential target cells (LONG et al. 1996). Originally identified as inhibitory receptors of natural killer (NK) cells having discrete specificities for HLA class I allotypes, KIR are also expressed by a small but significant population of T cells (FERRINI et al. 1994; MINGARI et al. 1995; PHILLIPS et al. 1995). Importantly, KIR recognition of their complementary class I ligands can modulate T cell function in a manner comparable to that observed for NK cells. This contribution summarizes recent advances in understanding the functional significance of T cell expression of KIR family members.

DNAX Research Institute of Molecular and Cellular Biology, Department of Immunobiology, 901 California Avenue, Palo Alto, CA 94304, USA

2 Antigen-Specific Cytotoxicity and Natural Killing

The mechanisms of natural resistance, which are characterized by a low level of specificity, can be activated in response to infectious pathogens within minutes to hours after infection. Although in some instances these responses are sufficient to reduce the infection to clinically undetectable levels, they are usually not capable of complete clearance of the pathogens. It is only with the development of an antigen-specific adaptive immune response (occurring a few days after the initial infection) that the immune system completely eliminates foreign invaders of the host.

The two major populations of cytotoxic lymphocytes, $CD8^+$ cytotoxic T lymphocytes (CTL) and NK cells, provide the immune system with cells that mediate similar functions (elimination of diseased host cells and lymphokine production) but differ in the speed and specificity of their responses. NK cells as effectors of innate immunity are activated early following pathogenic insult and serve to reduce the load of infection, as well as promote conditions favorable for the subsequent generation of CTL (reviewed in SCOTT and TRINCHIERI 1995). Although NK cells express several membrane molecules that can activate their effector functions (e.g., NKR-P1, CD2, CD16), the role of these receptors in vivo in response to pathogens is not well understood (reviewed in LANIER et al. 1997). On the other hand, CTL recognize foreign antigens using a T cell antigen receptor (TcR); however, T cells require time to undergo clonal expansion after exposure to pathogens, but once generated these effectors are able to act with precision to eliminate infected cells and provide long-term specific immunity (reviewed in ZINKERNAGEL et al. 1996).

3 The Central Role of MHC Class I Molecules in CTL and NK Cell Responses

MHC class I molecules are expressed on the surface of most nucleated cells and are composed of a polymorphic heavy chain, a nonpolymorphic light chain (β_2-microglobulin, β_2m) and a variable peptide of eight to ten amino acids (reviewed in YORK and ROCK 1996). Elucidation of the structure of this trimolecular complex clearly demonstrated the role of class I molecules as peptide-binding transport and display proteins. The polymorphism found within the class I heavy chains is extensive, and variable positions cluster in and around the peptide binding groove. The effect of these amino acid substitutions allows different class I alleles to bind diverse arrays of peptides. Class I presented peptides can be of cellular origin (self) or from the proteins of intracellular pathogens (foreign) and are generated by proteosome degradation of cytosolic polypeptides. The peptides, usually composed of eight to ten amino acids, combine with class I heavy chains and β_2m in the endoplasmic reticulum (ER) after being delivered into the lumen of the ER by TAP transporter proteins (reviewed in YORK and ROCK 1996). The TcR binds to the MHC class I peptide complex (GARBOCZI et al. 1996; GARCIA et al. 1996).

It is now established that both CTL and NK cells recognize class I molecules, and that this interaction controls their functions (LJUNGGREN and KARRE 1990). Antigen-specific CTL recognition of class I complexed with a foreign peptide usually results in stimulation and ultimately the destruction of the presenting cell. Activation of the T cells is initiated by TcR recognition of the foreign peptide bound to some of the polymorphic residues within an autologous MHC molecule. The TcR appears to contact a portion of both the antigen peptide fragment and the MHC (GARBOCZI et al. 1996; GARCIA et al. 1996). In contrast, when NK cells encounter class I molecules their cytotoxic activity is often inhibited, and it appears that an inhibitory interaction with class I expressed on the surface of potential target cells is the primary mechanism governing NK cell responses (reviewed in LANIER 1997). NK cells recognize the trimeric MHC class I peptide complex. However, unlike T cells, the MHC receptors expressed on NK cells often recognize closely related class I alleles and are less influenced by the bound peptide (CORREA and RAULET 1995; MALNATI et al. 1995; ORIHUELA et al. 1996; PERUZZI et al. 1996).

Before a great deal was known about how NK cells recognize and are inhibited by class I expression on target cells, KARRE and coworkers (1986) introduced the "missing self" model to explain the divergent responses of NK cells and CTL following class I recognition. This model proposes that NK cells survey the cells of the body for expression of autologous class I alleles and eliminate those cells which have lost or downregulated their class I. This strategy would target for destruction by NK cells those cells that evade detection by class I restricted CTL. In recent years studies with mouse and human NK cells have defined families of genes which encode the molecules responsible for this unique mechanism of surveillance for cells that lack expression of MHC class I.

Three distinct types of inhibitory receptors for class I have been identified on the surface of NK cells from mice and humans. The first inhibitory receptor discovered was the murine Ly-49A molecule which exhibited specificity for the murine MHC class I alleles, H-2 D^d and K^d (KARLHOFER et al. 1992). This receptor belongs to a family of molecules that are homodimeric, type II integral membrane proteins having homology with C-type lectins (reviewed in YOKOYAMA 1995). The Ly-49 family members are preferentially expressed on subsets of NK cells, are inhibitory upon binding to their ligands and, where studied, different Ly-49 receptors have been shown to have unique specificities for murine H-2 alleles (BRENNAN et al. 1994, 1996; DANIELS et al. 1994; KARLHOFER et al. 1992; MASON et al. 1995; STONEMAN et al. 1995). More recently a structurally related but distinct receptor has also been identified on human NK cells. Similar to Ly-49 receptors, the CD94/NKG2A receptor is C-type lectin expressed by NK cells that recognizes broad groups of HLA-A, HLA-B, and HLA-C class I alleles (PHILLIPS et al. 1996; SIVORI et al. 1996). Unlike the Ly-49 receptors, the CD94/NKG2A receptor is a heterodimer composed of two disulfide-bonded glycoproteins (LAZETIC et al. 1996). CD94 is an invariant protein encoded by a single gene (CHANG et al. 1995) that associates with glycoprotein subunits encoded by a different family of C-type lectins (members of the NKG2 family (ADAMKIEWICZ et al. 1994; HOUCHINS et al. 1991; YABE et al. 1993). The disulfide-bonded heterodimers formed by CD94 and NKG2A subunits are able to inhibit NK cell activation (LAZETIC et al. 1996), and it is likely that this heterodimeric receptor specifically recognizes HLA class I ligands, although this has not been formally demonstrated (LAZETIC et al. 1996). The third type of NK cell receptor for MHC class I has a fundamentally different structure from Ly-49 and CD94, yet also recognizes class I alleles and can inhibit NK cell function following this interaction. These KIR were initially discovered on human NK cells but are also present on a subset of T lymphocytes (FERRINI et al. 1994; MINGARI et al. 1995; PHILLIPS et al. 1995). The unique properties of these molecules and their role in regulating T cell responses are discussed in detail in the remainder of this review.

4 Killer Cell Inhibitory Receptors

KIR are a family of closely related of molecules originally identified on human NK cells as specific receptors for polymorphic determinants of HLA class I heavy chains (COLONNA and SAMARIDIS 1995; D'ANDREA et al. 1995; WAGTMANN et al. 1995). Using monoclonal antibodies (mAbs) generated against NK clones, MORETTA and colleagues (1993) identified one set of KIR family members (the p58 family) which are receptors for HLA-C alleles and appear to distinguish a diallelism present in HLA-C molecules at positions 77 and 80 of the α_1 domain (COLONNA et al. 1993). Certain KIR molecules reactive with the mAb EB6 recognize HLA-Cw4 and related alleles, while the GL183 mAb defines KIR responsible for the recognition of HLA-Cw3 and related alleles (MORETTA et al. 1993). The first member of a different set of KIR (the p70 family) was identified using the mAb DX9 (LITWIN et al. 1994) that reacted with a 70-kDa glycoprotein (named NKB1) on a subset of NK cells specific for HLA-B allotypes possessing the Bw4 motif at residues 77–83 of the α_1-helix (GUMPERZ et al. 1995). Thus the p58 and p70 KIR molecules appear to recognize public epitopes formed by polymorphisms at the C-terminal portion of the α_1 helix of HLA-B and HLA-C alleles. It was not until the cDNAs encoding the different p58 and p70 cDNAs were cloned and sequenced that it became apparent that these molecules form a family of human NK cell surface receptors for HLA class I alleles.

4.1 KIR Family Members Are Ig-like

The determination of the original KIR nucleotide sequences indicated that the p58 and p70 forms are closely related, and these proteins are type I integral membrane proteins exhibiting homology with members of the Ig superfamily (COLONNA and SAMARIDIS 1995; D'ANDREA et al. 1995; WAGTMANN et al. 1995). The difference in molecular mass between the two types is a result of the p58 receptors having two extracellular Ig domains and the p70 receptors having three. Once it was established that KIR are the products of a multigene family, PCR-based approaches were used to identify new KIR sequences, and this strategy has greatly increased the number of unique KIR sequences. At present, more than 30 KIR family members have been isolated; however, except for those that react with the mAbs EB6 (p58.1), GL183 (p58.2), and DX9 (NKB1) little is known about the HLA class I specificity of these new KIR. One notable exception is the 3 Ig domain (p70) KIR, designated NKAT4, which has recently been shown to recognize HLA-A3 (DOHRING et al. 1996; PENDE et al. 1996). Although the functional significance of the expression of 2 or 3 Ig domains by KIR is unclear, there is a tendency of 2 Ig receptors to recognize HLA-C alleles, whereas, 3 Ig KIR appear restricted to HLA-A and HLA-B molecules. Further study of the class I specificity of new family members should determine whether this trend is applicable to all KIR.

4.2 KIR Can Have Diverse Cytoplasmic Tails

The cytoplasmic domains are another source of difference between the various members of the KIR family. Although they are highly conserved (more than 70% identity), they can be short (39 amino acids) or long (76, 84, or 95 amino acids). All of the KIRs with a long cytoplasmic tail possess two immune receptor tyrosine-based inhibitory motif (ITIM) sequences (YXXL) separated by 26–28 amino acids. These motifs, which are present in other inhibitory receptors (D'AMBROSIO et al. 1995; DAERON et al. 1995; GUTHMANN et al. 1995; HOUCHINS et al. 1997; KATZ et al. 1996; LAW et al. 1996; MUTA et al. 1994; PANI et al. 1995; SARKAR et al. 1996), have been shown to be critical for the inhibitory signals generated by KIR upon binding to a class I ligand. The ITIM of KIR and other inhibitory receptors generate a negative signal by recruiting and activating protein tyrosine phosphatases (SHP-1 and SHP-2; BINSTADT et al. 1996; BURSHTYN et al. 1996; CAMPBELL et al. 1996; FRY et al. 1996; OLCESE et al. 1996), which counter the stimulatory effects of protein tyrosine kinases associated with activation pathways. The KIR-possessing short cytoplasmic tails (p50) lack ITIM sequences and do not inhibit NK cell function following class I binding. Rather it appears that these receptors are actually stimulatory, and the characteristic presence of a charged amino acid (Lys) in their transmembrane domains suggests an ability to associate with other signal transducing polypeptides that have stimulatory capacity (BIASSONI et al. 1996).

5 KIR Expression by T Cells

Although originally identified and characterized as NK cell specific receptors, KIR, as with most other NK markers, are also expressed by small populations of T cells (FERRINI et al. 1994; MINGARI et al. 1995; PHILLIPS et al. 1995). Given their inhibitory and potentially stimulatory activities, the expression by T cells of KIR capable of recognizing autologous class I molecules likely adds subtlety to antigen-specific T cell responses. In this view, KIR function on T cells is analogous to that of costimulatory receptors, such as CD28 (stimulatory) and CTLA-4 (inhibitory; reviewed by LENSCHOW et al. 1996) and thus contrasts with KIR usage by NK cells in which these

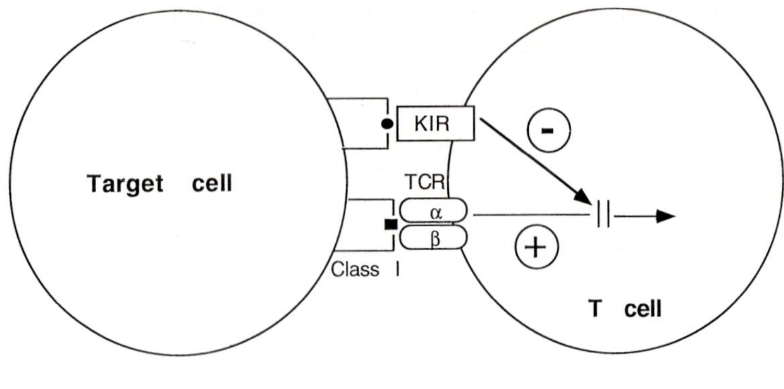

Fig. 1. Model of competition between positive and negative signaling pathways initiated by simultaneous recognition of class I by TcR and KIR on a potential target cell

receptors appear to dominate NK cell function. Thus, stimulatory or inhibitory KIR expression serves more to lower or raise the threshold of T cell activation through the TCR but under most circumstances probably does not completely alter whether a given KIR^+ T cell responds to antigen. A simple model for the effect of inhibitory KIR on T cell function is presented in Fig. 1.

5.1 Functional Implications of KIR Expression on T Cell Responses

The first evidence that KIR expression by T cells can lead to inhibition of T cell activity was provided by PHILLIPS and coworkers (1995). Using superantigen-stimulated T cells that express the KIR NKB1, it was shown that simultaneous ligation of the T cell receptor by superantigen/MHC class II complexes and NKB1 by its $Bw4^+$ class I ligand diminishes the ability of the T cells to mediate cytotoxicity (PHILLIPS et al. 1995). More recently this analysis has been extended to demonstrate that activation of antigen-specific T cells following recognition of a class II presented peptide is also subject to inhibition by concomitant binding of KIR to an inhibitory class I allele. Other forms of T cell recognition, including anti-CD3 redirected lysis and non-MHC restricted killing, have also been found to be sensitive to negative regulation by KIR (FERRINI et al. 1994; MINGARI et al. 1995). In addition, cell-mediated cytotoxicity is not the only T cell response that is sensitive to the inhibitory activities of KIR. We have found that KIR^+ T cells stimulated with superantigens are limited in their ability to produce lymphokines because of a constitutive negative regulatory pressure mediated by engagement of KIR with self class I alleles (D'ANDREA et al. 1996). If recognition of self class I alleles is blocked by addition of anti-KIR or anti-class I antibodies to the assays, the T cells are freed from inhibition and respond with substantially increased lymphokine production. These findings suggest that all T cell responses that are dependent on cell-cell contact are subject to inhibition if a responding T cell expresses KIR specific for self class I alleles. Finally, T cells also express functionally intact p50 (short cytoplasmic tail) KIR which can enhance T cell responses if they encounter their class I ligand (MANDELBOIM et al. 1996).

5.2 KIR Distribution on T Cell Subsets

Virtually every major subpopulation of T cells can express KIR, and analysis of T cell clones from any given donor reveals cells expressing no KIR, inhibitory KIR only, stimulatory KIR (p50) only, or various combinations of stimulatory and inhibitory receptors. Within the T cell compartment KIR are expressed predominantly on $CD8^+$, $\alpha\beta$ TCR expressing T cells, but detectable populations are found on $CD4^+$ and $\gamma\delta$ TCR^+ T cells as well (Figs. 2, 3).

Flow cytometric analyses of fresh peripheral blood T cells for KIR expression and a variety of cell surface markers has shown a surface phenotype typical of "memory" T cells. For instance, KIR^+ T cells are $CD28^-$, and in studies performed with $p58^+$ T cells they were $CD45RA^-$ but expressed high levels of CD44, CD29, and CD57, all indicative of a memory phenotype. These findings suggest that KIR expression is induced following antigenic stimulation. Consistent with this view, T cells obtained from the fetal thymus or cord blood (Fig. 4) do not express KIR. However, studies by GUMPERZ et al. (1996) performed on monozygotic twins show the same distribution of KIRs on T cells from peripheral blood, indicating that the exposure to different antigens does not have an effect on selecting or expanding a particular subset of KIR^+ T cells. Furthermore, efforts to induce KIR expression by a variety of in vitro stimulation protocols by our group have thus far been unsuccessful. Nevertheless, the recent report by ALBI and coworkers (1996) indicating a dramatic increase in $p58^+$ T cells in patients following bone marrow transplantation argues that under some conditions in vivo KIR^+ T cells undergo preferential expansion, or alternatively that KIR expression on T cells is inducible.

5.3 KIR and TCR Usage

In an effort to understand whether the memory phenotype of KIR^+ T cells is a result of antigenic stimulation, MINGARI and coworkers (1996) analyzed TCR Vβ usage by KIR^+ T cells from different individuals. Using KIR^+ cultured T cell lines they analyzed the expression of various Vβ families from each individual by flow cytometry and concluded that the KIR^+ T cells from these donors were using a restricted set of Vβ families. In addition, they also cloned and sequenced a number of Vβ transcripts from one of the cell lines and observed that the overwhelming majority of clones had identical VDJ rearrangements, indicating that the TCR obtained from this line were oligoclonal. From these studies they concluded that KIR^+

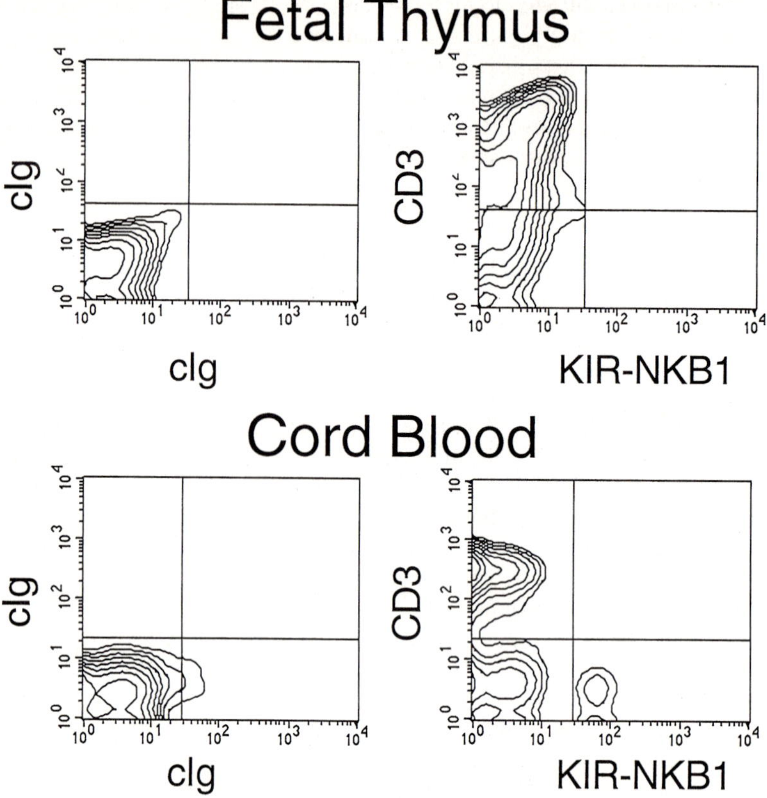

Fig. 2. T cells obtained from the fetal thymus or cord blood do not express the KIR NKB1. Lymphocytes from the fetal thymus and cord blood were analyzed by flow cytometry for the coexpression of CD3 and the KIR NKB1

T cells likely arise following chronic antigen stimulation, perhaps after prolonged exposure to superantigens. These findings are compelling and of potential importance for understanding the induction of KIR$^+$ T cells in an individual; however, we have obtained different results, examining KIR$^+$ T cells in fresh peripheral blood. Although in a few donors we have observed restricted Vβ usage by KIR$^+$ T cells, in others there was no skewing of the TCR repertoire in the KIR expressing T cells (Table 1). This apparent discrepancy might be explained by the use of in vitro cultured T cells by Mingari et al. (1996) which could have resulted in skewing of the Vβ repertoire during culture rather than in vivo. However, given the limited number of donors examined by both studies, further clarification of this issue requires more in-depth analysis.

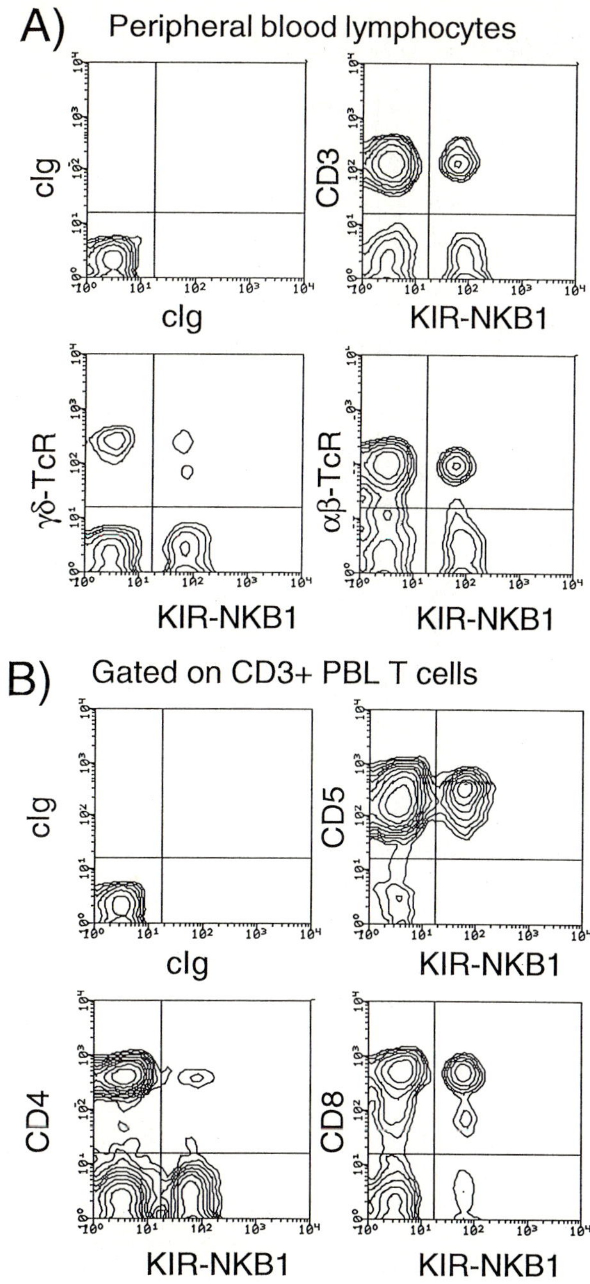

Fig. 3. A Expression of the KIR NKB1 by αβ and γδ T cells. Peripheral blood lymphocytes (*PBL*) were analyzed by flow cytometry for the coexpression of CD3, γδ TCR, and αβ TCR with the KIR NKB1. **B** Expression of the KIR NKB1 by $CD4^+$ and $CD8^+$ T cells. Three color immunofluorescence analyses were performed on peripheral blood lymphocytes (*PBL*) from a representative individual. $CD3^+$ T cells were gated and analyzed for their expression of the T cell markers CD5, CD4 and CD8 and the KIR NKB1

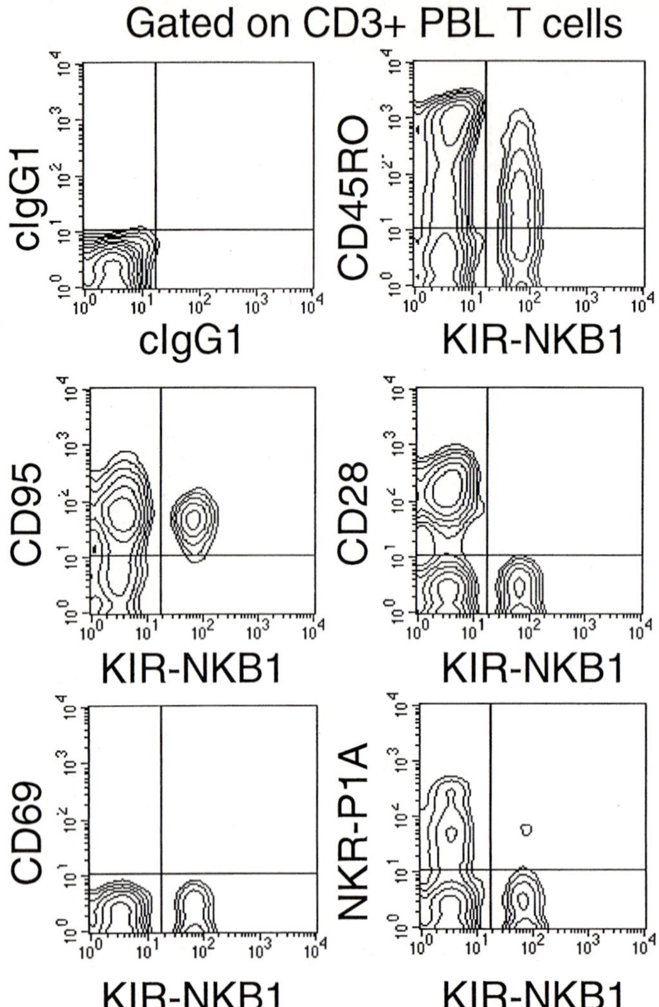

Fig. 4. Phenotype of KIR^+ peripheral blood T cells

Table 1. Vα/β-TcR on KIR+ and KIR- T cells

TCR chain	Donor 1 NKB1 (DX9) KIR +(%)	Donor 1 NKB1 (DX9) KIR –(%)	Donor 1 Ratio	Donor 2 NKB1 (DX9) KIR +(%)	Donor 2 NKB1 (DX9) KIR –(%)	Donor 2 Ratio	Donor 3 NKB1 (DX9) KIR +(%)	Donor 3 NKB1 (DX9) KIR –(%)	Donor 3 Ratio	Donor 4 p 58 (DX27) KIR +(%)	Donor 4 p 58 (DX27) KIR –(%)	Donor 4 Ratio	Donor 5 p 58 (DX27) KIR +(%)	Donor 5 p 58 (DX27) KIR –(%)	Donor 5 Ratio	Donor 6 p 58 (DX27) KIR +(%)	Donor 6 p 58 (DX27) KIR –(%)	Donor 6 Ratio
Vα24	0.22	0.25	0.88	0.34	0.25	1.36	0.53	0.16	3.31	0.57	0.25	2.28	0.45	0.23	1.96	0.00	0.17	0.00
Vβ2	1.07	7.17	0.15	0.65	6.08	0.11	2.63	5.54	0.47	0.54	6.52	0.08	0.29	6.48	0.04	4.41	7.84	0.56
Vβ3	5.01	1.37	3.66	2.92	2.51	1.16	3.70	1.59	2.33	2.22	2.52	0.88	5.53	2.29	2.41	2.71	1.90	1.43
Vβ8	2.76	2.79	0.99	1.95	4.02	0.49	1.05	1.86	0.56	1.39	2.07	0.67	0.68	3.03	0.22	1.56	3.17	0.49
Vβ11	1.25	0.32	3.91	0.23	0.24	0.96	0.58	0.25	2.32	0.52	0.38	1.37	0.47	0.32	1.47	0.28	0.31	0.90
Vβ14	1.50	1.74	0.86	0.58	1.56	0.37	2.79	1.37	2.04	0.00	1.57	0.00	0.52	1.94	0.27	2.42	1.63	1.48
Vβ16	2.36	0.53	4.45	1.21	0.19	6.37	26.26	8.58	3.06	22.44	9.21	2.44	0.86	1.08	0.80	0.14	0.56	0.25
Vβ17	0.88	3.72	0.24	5.83	4.53	1.19	3.45	2.73	1.26	0.80	3.53	0.23	1.31	4.68	0.28	0.79	3.07	0.26

Freshly isolated peripheral blood mononuclear cells of six unrelated healthy donors were analyzed by flow cytometry (LANIER and RECKTENWALD 1991) for the expression of Vα/β-TCR on KIR+ and KIR– T cells. Cells were stained with CyChrome conjugated anti-CD3 (Leu 4), phycoerythrin (PE)-conjugated anti-KIR NKB1 mAb (DX9) or PE-conjugated anti-KIR p58 mAb DX27 (similar to GL183) (LANIER et al. 1997), and FITC-conjugated mAbs specific for Vα24 or the indicated Vβ-TCR (obtained from Immunotech, Westbrook, ME). an electronic gate was placed to identify all KIR–, CD3+ T cells and KIR+, CD3+ T cells and then the frequency of KIR– T cells or KIR+ T cells expressing the indicated Vα-TcR or Vβ-TcR was determined. Data are expressed as the %Vα or Vβ-TcR+ cells present within the KIR– T cell or KIR+ T cell population. The ratio of the percentage of Vα-TcR or Vβ-TcR+ cells within the KIR– T cell and KIR+ T cell subsets is also shown (N.B. a ratio of 1.0 would indicate no skewing of TcR usage within the populations). Cells were also stained with CyChrome-conjugated, PE-conjugated, and FITC-conjugated control Ig to exclude non-specific staining (not shown).

6 Conclusions

The expression of KIR by T cells has provided yet another mechanism of modulating antigen-specific T cell responses by receptors other than the TCR. A number of important questions remain that need to be addressed before their role in the adaptive immune response is understood completely. These include: to what extent do KIR determine the nature, duration, and type of T cell responses, and how do KIR$^+$ T cells arise? Luckily, the molecular tools are now available and will likely aid in the elucidation of these questions and many others in the near future.

Acknowledgements. DNAX Research Institute is supported by Schering Plough Corporation.

References

Adamkiewicz TV, McSherry C, Bach FH, Houchins JP (1994) Natural killer lectin-like receptors have divergent carboxy-termini, distinct from C-type lectins. Immunogenetics 39:218

Albi N, Ruggeri L, Aversa F, Merigiola C, Tosti A, Tognellini R, Grossi CE, Martelli MF, Velardi A (1996) Natural killer (NK)-cell function and antileukemic activity of a large population of CD3+/CD8+ T cells expressing NK receptors for major histocompatibility complex class I after "three-loci" HLA-incompatible bone marrow transplantation. Blood 87:3993–4000

Biassoni R, Cantoni C, Falco M, Verdiani S, Bottino C, Vitale M, Conte R, Poggi A, Moretta A, Moretta L (1996) The human leukocyte antigen (HLA)-C-specific "activitory" or "inhibitory" natural killer cell receptors display highly homologous extracellular domains but differ in their transmembrane and intracytoplasmic portions. J Exp Med 183:645–650

Binstadt BA, Brumbaugh KM, Dick CJ, Scharenberg AM, Williams BL, Colonna M, Lanier LL, Kinet J-P, Abraham RT, Leibson PJ (1996) Sequential involvement of Lck and SHP-1 with MHC-recognizing receptors on NK cells inhibits FcR-initiated tyrosine kinase activation. Immunity 5:629–638

Brennan J, Mager D, Jefferies W, Takei F (1994) Expression of different members of the Ly-49 gene family defines distinct natural killer cell subsets and cell adhesion properties. J Exp Med 180:2287–2295

Brennan J, Mahon G, Mager DL, Jefferies WA, Takei F (1996) Recognition of class I major histocompatibility complex molecules by Ly-49: specificities and domain interactions. J Exp Med 183:1553–1559

Burshtyn DN, Scharenberg AM, Wagtmann N, Rajagopalan S, Berrada K, Yi T, Kinet J-P, Long EO (1996) Recruitment of tyrosine phosphatase HCP by the killer cell inhibitory receptor. Immunity 4:77–85

Campbell KS, Dessing M, Lopez-Botet M, Cella M, Colonna M (1996) Tyrosine phosphorylation of a human killer inhibitory receptor recruits protein tyrosine phosphatase 1C. J Exp Med 184:93–100

Chang C, Rodriguez A, Carretero M, Lopez-Botet M, Phillips JH, Lanier LL (1995) Molecular characterization of human CD94: a type II membrane glycoprotein related to the C-type lectin superfamily. Eur J Immunol 25:2433–2437

Colonna M, Samaridis J (1995) Cloning of Ig-superfamily members associated with HLA-C and HLA-B recognition by human NK cells. Science 268:405–408

Colonna M, Borsellino G, Falco M, Ferrara GB, Strominger JL (1993) HLA-C is the inhibitory ligand that determines dominant resistance to lysis by NK1- and NK2-specific natural killer cells. Proc Natl Acad Sci USA 90:12000–12004

Correa I, Raulet DH (1995) Binding of diverse peptides to MHC class I molecules inhibits target cell lysis by activated natural killer cells. Immunity 2:61–71

D'Ambrosio D, Hippen KL, Minskoff SA, Mellman I, Pani G, Siminovitch KA, Cambier JC (1995) Recruitment and activation of PTP1C in negative regulation of antigen receptor signaling by FcγRIIBI. Science 268:293–297

D'Andrea A, Chang C, Franz-Bacon K, McClanahan T, Phillips JH, Lanier LL (1995) Molecular cloning of NKB1: A natural killer cell receptor for HLA-B allotypes. J Immunol 155:2306–2310

D'Andrea A, Chang C, Phillips JH, Lanier LL (1996) Regulation of T cell lymphokine production by killer cell inhibitory receptor recognition of self HLA class I alleles. J Exp Med 184:789–794

Daeron M, Latour S, Malbec O, Espinosa E, Pina P, Pasmans S, Fridman WH (1995) The same tyrosine-based inhibition motif, in the intracytoplasmic domain of FcγRIIB, regulates negatively BCR-, TCR-, and FcR-dependent cell activation. Immunity 3:635–646

Daniels B, Karlhofer FM, Seaman WE, Yokoyama WM (1994) A natural killer cell receptor specific for a major histocompatibility complex class I molecule. J Exp Med 180:687–692

Dohring C, Scheidegger D, Samaridis J, Cella M, Colonna M (1996) A human killer inhibitory receptor specific for HLA-A. J Immunol 156:3098–3101

Ferrini S, Cambiaggi A, Meazza R, Sforzini S, Marciano S, Mingari MC, Moretta L (1994) T cell clones expressing the natural killer cell-related p58 receptor molecule display heterogeneity in phenotypic properties and p58 function. Eur J Immunol 24:2294–2298

Fry A, Lanier LL, Weiss A (1996) Phosphotyrosines in the KIR motif of NKB1 are required for negative signaling and for association with PTP1C. J Exp Med 184:295–300

Garboczi DN, Ghosh P, Utz U, Fan QR, Biddison WE, Wiley DC (1996) Structure of the complex between human T-cell receptor, viral peptide and HLA-A2. Nature 384:134–141

Garcia KC, Degano M, Stanfield RL, Brunmark A, Jackson MR, Peterson PA, Teyton L, Wilson IC (1996) A ab T cell receptor structure at 2.5 A and its orientation in the TCR-MHC complex. Science 274:209–221

Gumperz JE, Litwin V, Phillips JH, Lanier LL, Parham P (1995) The Bw4 public epitope of HLA-B molecules confers reactivity with NK cell clones that express NKB1, a putative HLA receptor. J Exp Med 181:1133–1144

Gumperz JE, Valiante NM, Parham P, Lanier LL, Tyan D (1996) Heterogeneous phenotypes of expression of the NKB1 natural killer cell class I receptor among individuals of different HLA types appear genetically regulated, but not linked to MHC haplotype. J Exp Med 183:1817–1827

Guthmann MD, Tal M, Pecht I (1995) A secretion inhibitory signal transduction molecule on mast cells is another C-type lectin. Proc Natl Acad Sci USA 92:9397–9401

Houchins JP, Yabe T, McSherry C, Bach FH (1991) DNA sequence analysis of NKG2, a family of related cDNA clones encoding type II integral membrane proteins on human natural killer cells. J Exp Med 173:1017–1020

Houchins JP, Lanier LL, Niemi E, Phillips JH, Ryan JC (1997) Natural killer cell cytolytic activity is inhibited by NKG2-A and activated by NKG2-C. J Immunol 158:3603–3609

Karlhofer FM, Ribuado RK, Yokoyama WM (1992) MHC class I alloantigen specificity of Ly-49^+ IL-2-activated natural killer cells. Nature 358:66–70

Karre K, Ljunggren HG, Piontek G, Kiessling R (1986) Selective rejection of H-2-deficient lymphoma variants suggests alternative immune defense strategy. Nature 319:675–678

Katz HR, Vivier E, Castells MC, McCormick MJ, Chambers JM, Austen KF (1996) Mouse mast cell gp49B1 contains two immunoreceptor tyrosine-based inhibition motifs and suppresses mast cell activation when coligated with the high-affinity Fc receptor for IgE. Proc Natl Acad Sci USA 93:10809–10814

Lanier LL (1997) NK cell receptors and MHC class I interactions. Curr Opin Immunol 9:126–131

Lanier LL, Corliss B, Phillips JH (1997) Arousal and inhibition of human NK cells. Immunol Rev 155:145–154

Law C-L, Sidorenko SP, Chandran KA, Zhao Z, Shen S-H, Fischer EH, Clark EA (1996) CD22 associates with protein tyrosine phosphatase 1C, Syk, and phospholipase Cg1 upon B cell activation. J Exp Med 184:547–560

Lazetic S, Chang C, Houchins JP, Lanier LL, Phillips JH (1996) Human NK cell receptors involved in MHC class I recognition are disulfide-linked heterodimers of CD94 and NKG2 subunits. J Immunol 157:4741–4745

Lenschow DJ, Walunas TL, Bluestone JA (1996) CD28/B7 system of T cell costimulation. Annu Rev Immunol 14:233–258

Litwin V, Gumperz J, Parham P, Phillips JH, Lanier LL (1994) NKB1: an NK cell receptor involved in the recognition of polymorphic HLA-B molecules. J Exp Med 180:537–543

Ljunggren H-G, Karre K (1990) In search of the 'missing self': MHC molecules and NK cell recognition. Immunol Today 11:237–244

Long EO, Colonna M, Lanier LL (1996) Inhibitory MHC class I receptors on NK and T cells: a standard nomenclature. Immunol Today 17:100

Malnati MS, Peruzzi M, Parker KC, Biddison WE, Ciccone E, Moretta A, Long EO (1995) Peptide specificity in the recognition of MHC class I by natural killer cell clones. Science 267:1016–1018

Mandelboim O, Davis DM, Reyburn HT, Vales-Gomez M, Sheu EG, Pazmany L, Strominger JL (1996) Enhancement of class II-restricted T cell responses by costimulatory NK receptors for class I MHC proteins. Science 274:2097–2100

Mason LH, Ortaldo JR, Young HA, Kumar K, Bennett M, Anderson SK (1995) Cloning and functional characteristics of murine LGL-1: a member of the Ly-49 gene family (Ly-49G2). J Exp Med 182:293–304

Mingari MC, Vitale C, Cambiaggi A, Schiavetti F, Melioli G, Ferrini S, Poggi A (1995) Cytotoxic T lymphocytes displaying natural killer (NK)-like activity: expression of NK-related functional receptors for HLA class I molecules (p58 and CD94) and inhibitory effect on the TCR-mediated target cell lysis of lymphokine production. Int Immunol 7:697–703

Mingari MC, Schiavetti F, Ponte M, Maggi E, Romagnani S, Demarest J, Pantaleo G, Fauci AS, Moretta L (1996) Human CD8+ T lymphocyte subsets that express HLA class I-specific inhibitory receptors represent oligoclonally or monoclonally expanded cell populations. Proc Natl Acad Sci USA 93:12433–12438

Moretta A, Vitale M, Bottino C, Orengo AM, Morelli L, Augugliaro R, Barbaresi M, Ciccone E, Moretta L (1993) p58 molecules as putative receptors for major histocompatibility complex (MHC) class I molecules in human natural killer (NK) cells. Anti-p58 antibodies reconstitute lysis of MHC class I-protected cells in NK clones displaying different specificities. J Exp Med 178:597–604

Muta T, Kurosaki T, Misulovin Z, Sanchez M, Nussenzweig MC, Ravetch RV (1994) A 13-amino acid motif in the cytoplasmic domain of FcgRIIB modulates B-cell receptor signalling. Nature 368:70–73

Olcese L, Lang P, Vely F, Cambiaggi A, Marguet D, Blery M, Hippen KL, Biassoni R, Moretta A, Moretta L, Cambier JC, Vivier E (1996) Human and mouse killer-cell inhibitory receptors recruit PTP1C and PTP1D protein tyrosine phosphatases. J Immunol 156:4531–4534

Orihuela M, Margulies DH, Yokoyama WM (1996) The NK cell receptor Ly-49A recognizes a peptide-induced conformational determinant on its MHC class I ligand. Proc Natl Acad Sci USA 93:11792–11797

Pani G, Kozlowski M, Cambier JC, Mills GB, Siminovitch KA (1995) Identification of the tyrosine phosphatase PTP1C as a B cell antigen receptor-associated protein involved in the regulation of B cell signaling. J Exp Med 181:2077–2084

Pende D, Biassoni R, Cantoni C, Verdiani S, Falco M, Di Donato C, Accame O, Bottino C, Moretta A, Moretta L (1996) The natural killer cell receptor specific for HLA-A allotypes: a novel member of the p58/p70 family of inhibitory receptors that is characterized by three immunoglobulin-like domains and is expressed as a 140-kD disulphide-linked dimer. J Exp Med 184:505–518

Peruzzi M, Parker KC, Long EO, Malnati MS (1996) Peptide sequence requirements for the recognition of HLA-B*2705 by specific natural killer cells. J Immunol 157:3350–3356

Phillips JH, Gumperz JE, Parham P, Lanier LL (1995) Superantigen-dependent, cell-mediated cytotoxicity inhibited by MHC class I receptors on T lymphocytes. Science 268:403–405

Phillips JH, Chang C, Mattson J, Gumperz JE, Parham P, Lanier LL (1996) CD94 and a novel associated protein (94AP) form a NK cell receptor involved in the recognition of HLA-A, -B, and -C allotypes. Immunity 5:163–172

Sarkar S, Schlottmann K, Cooney D, Coggeshall KM (1996) Negative signaling via FcgammaRIIB1 in B cells blocks phospholipase Cgamma2 tyrosine phosphorylation but not Syk or Lyn activation. J Biol Chem 271:20182–20186

Scott P, Trinchieri G (1995) The role of natural killer cells in host-parasite interactions. Curr Opin Immunol 7:34–40

Sivori S, Vitale M, Bottino C, Marcenaro E, Parolini S, Moretta L, Moretta A (1996) CD94 functions as a natural killer cell inhibitory receptor for different HLA class I alleles: identification of the inhibitory form of CD94 by the use of novel monoclonal antibodies. Eur J Immunol 26:2487–2492

Spits H, Lanier LL, Phillips JH (1995) Development of human T and natural killer cells. Blood 85:2654–2670

Stoneman ER, Bennett M, An J, Chesnut KA, Scheerer JB, Siciliano MJ, Kumar V, Mathew PA (1995) Cloning and characterization of 5E6 (Ly-49C), a receptor molecule expressed on a subset of murine natural killer cells. J Exp Med 182:305–314

Wagtmann N, Biassoni R, Cantoni C, Verdiani S, Malnati MS, Vitale M, Bottino C, Moretta L, Moretta A, Long EO (1995) Molecular clones of the p58 natural killer cell receptor reveal Ig-related molecules with diversity in both the extra- and intracellular domains. Immunity 2:439–449

Yabe T, McSherry C, Bach FH, Fisch P, Schall RP, Sondel PM, Houchins JP (1993) A multigene family on human chromosome 12 encodes natural killer-cell lectins. Immunogenetics 37:455–460

Yokoyama WM (1995) Natural killer cell receptors. Curr Opin Immunol 7:110–120

York IA, Rock KL (1996) Antigen processing and presentation by the class I major histocompatibility complex. Annu Rev Immunol 14:369–396

Zinkernagel RM, Bachmann MF, Kundig TM, Oehen S, Pirchet H, Hengartner H (1996) On immunological memory. Annu Rev Immunol 14:333–367

The CD94/NKG2 C-Type Lectin Receptor Complex

M. LÓPEZ-BOTET, M. CARRETERO, T. BELLÓN, J.J. PÉREZ-VILLAR, M. LLANO, and F. NAVARRO

1 Introduction

NK cell mediated cytotoxicity is suppressed upon specific recognition of target MHC class I molecules (LJUNGGREN and KÄRRE 1990). It is currently thought that the control of NK cell activity depends on a subtle balance between inhibitory and activating signals; accordingly, every mature NK cell should bear at least one type of dominant inhibitory receptor for a self MHC class I product, thus preventing autoreactivity against normal cells. Recognition of H-2 products is mediated by members of the Ly-49 C-type lectin family (YOKOYAMA 1995). In humans several inhibitory NK cell receptors (NKR) encoded by an immunoglobulin (Ig)-related multigene family specifically interact with different HLA class I allotypes (COLONNA and SAMARIDIS 1995; WAGTMANN et al. 1995; LANIER and PHILLIPS 1995; MORETTA et al. 1996), and the term killer inhibitory receptors (KIRs) has been proposed. A common structural feature of the inhibitory NKR is the presence of cytoplasmic "immunoreceptor tyrosine-based inhibitory motifs" (ITIMs, V/IxYxxL sequences) which upon their tyrosine phosphorylation recruit protein tyrosine phosphatases (SHP-1 and SHP-2) involved in the downregulation of NK cell activity (BURSHTYN et al. 1996; CAMPBELL et al. 1996; FRY et al. 1996; OLCESE et al. 1996). Remarkably, other members of the Ig superfamily (Ig-SF) NKR trigger NK cell mediated lysis upon their ligation by specific monoclonal antibodies (mAbs). These activating receptors (p50) are closely homologous to inhibitory molecules (p58) but contain shorter intracytoplasmic domains lacking ITIMs and display a different transmembrane region (MORETTA et al. 1996).

Servicio de Inmunología, Hospital de la Princesa. Universidad Autónoma de Madrid, Diego de León 62, 28006 Madrid, Spain. E-mail: mlbotet/princesa@hup.es

Multiple combinations of these structures may be coexpressed by individual NK clones/subsets, thus rendering difficult the dissection of their individual role in conventional cellular assays. The expression of each receptor is variable among different individuals, and there are indications that the NKR repertoire is influenced by genetic factors (GUMPERZ et al. 1996). Remarkably, all known NKR are detected on αβ and γδ T lymphocyte subsets, regulating T-cell receptor (TCR)-mediated and NK-like cytotoxicity (MORETTA et al. 1996; LANIER and PHILLIPS 1995).

The question as to whether human members of the C-type lectin superfamily constitute NKR specific for HLA class I molecules has been debated (LÓPEZ-BOTET et al. 1996). Several type II integral membrane glycoproteins (CD94, NKG2, and hNKR-P1A), that contain an extracellular C-type carbohydrate recognition domain (CRD) and display partial homology with the murine NK gene complex (NKC) families (NKR-P1 and Ly-49), have been identified in human NK cells (LANIER et al. 1994; HOUCHINS et al. 1991; YABE et al. 1993; ADAMKIEWICZ et al. 1994; DÜCHLER et al. 1995; CHANG et al. 1995; LÓPEZ-BOTET 1995). All the corresponding genes, together with that encoding for the CD69 C-type lectin, have been localized in chromosome 12, the syntenic of murine chromosome 6 where the NKC genes are clustered (RENEDO et al. 1997). Recently it has been shown that the CD94 molecule covalently assembles with glycoproteins of the NKG2 family to form different heterodimers (LAZETIC et al. 1996; CARRETERO et al. 1997). Moreover, functional data have been reported indirectly supporting the CD94/NKG2 C-type lectin receptor complex as being involved in NK cell mediated recognition of different HLA allotypes (MORETTA et al. 1994; SIVORI et al. 1996; PHILLIPS et al. 1996; PÉREZ-VILLAR et al. 1997).

2 Structure of the CD94/NKG2 Receptor Complex

The CD94 surface antigen was originally described to be selectively expressed as a disulfide-linked dimer on NK cells and a minor subset of T lymphocytes that includes $CD8^+$ $TcR\text{-}\alpha\beta^+$, and $TcR\text{-}\gamma\delta^+$ (ARAMBURU et al. 1990, 1991; RUBIO et al. 1993; LÓPEZ-BOTET 1995). Ligation with CD94-specific mAbs was shown to induce divergent functional effects (i.e., triggering or inhibition) by distinct subsets of NK clones (termed A and B, respectively), in which CD94 molecules appeared to be differently coupled to signaling pathways (PÉREZ-VILLAR et al. 1995; BRUMBAUGH et al. 1996). Early biochemical studies carried out in polyclonal NK cells indicated that CD94 is assembled as a 70-kDa dimer, and a ^{125}I-labeled 43 kDa molecule (kp43) was detected under reducing conditions. We reported (PÉREZ-VILLAR et al. 1996) that CD94 precipitates from group A clones displayed a lower molecular weight (39 kDa) than the homologous product of group B clones (43 kDa); coexpression of both forms by some cells was also observed. Moreover, a novel reagent (Z199) that reacts selectively with the inhibitory kp43 glycoprotein has been characterized (PÉREZ-VILLAR et al. 1996; SIVORI et al. 1996). The ability to distinguish kp43 and p39 serologically indicated that they differ in the conformation of the extracellular region, and depending on their divergent functions it was predicted that the structure of the cytoplasmic regions could also vary.

In contrast to such complexity, expression cloning with an anti-CD94 mAb revealed the existence of a 180 amino acid type II glycoprotein with a short cytoplasmic tail, encoded by a single-copy gene of the C-type lectin superfamily (CHANG et al. 1995; RODRIGUEZ et al. 1998). Immunoprecipitates obtained from ^{125}I-labeled CD94 transfectants were hardly detectable; consequently, the relationship of CD94 with the kp43/p39 molecules could not be precisely established. Nevertheless, the electrophoretic mobility of the cloned CD94 molecule clearly differed from kp43; moreover, the CD94-transfectants were not recognized by the Z199 mAb (PÉREZ-VILLAR et al. 1996). Strategies seeking to determine whether the kp43 and p39 proteins were encoded by differentially spliced transcripts of the cloned CD94 gene were unsuccessful.

PHILLIPS et al. (1996) reported that a polyclonal antiserum raised against the cloned CD94 protein did not react in western blotting with kp43, termed CD94-associated protein (CD94AP), thus supporting the notion that they were very different. These authors proposed that the inhibitory receptor is formed by the covalent assembly of the cloned CD94 molecule (inefficiently labeled with ^{125}I) with an unrelated 43-kDa subunit, tyrosine phosphorylated upon pervanadate treatment of NK cells. This could explain why our attempts to approach expression cloning of kp43 with the Z199 mAb also failed (T. Bellón, unpublished). Thus we considered the possibility that the kp43 glycoprotein is encoded by other known genes of the C-type lectin superfamily; NKG2-A and NKG2-B (generated by alternative splicing) display cytoplasmic ITIMs and are predicted to mediate an inhibitory function. Based on the current knowledge, cotransfection of CD94 and NKG2-A cDNAs was carried out (CARRETERO et al. 1997). Anti-CD94 mAbs bound to both CD94$^+$ and CD94/NKG2-A$^+$ COS cells, while the Z199 mAb selectively reacted with CD94/NKG2-A$^+$ COS cells. Both anti-CD94 and Z199 mAbs immunoprecipitated a strongly ^{125}I-labeled glycoprotein from CD94/NKG2-A$^+$ transfectants. A comparative peptide mapping analysis of the kp43 molecule from NK cells and the NKG2-A protein obtained from CD94/NKG2-A$^+$ COS cells unequivocally confirmed their identity. Similar conclusions have been reached by LAZETIC et al. (1996) and BROOKS et al. (1997) using different approaches. The NKG2-B sequence, generated by alternative splicing of the NKG2-A gene, lacks 18 residues between the transmembrane region and the CRD but conserves cytoplasmic ITIMs. Cotransfection experiments have shown that Z199$^+$ CD94/NKG2-B dimers are formed in COS cells (LAZETIC et al. 1996; CARRETERO et al. 1997). The expression of CD94/NKG2-B inhibitory receptors by normal NK cells is indirectly supported by the occasional immunoprecipitation with Z199 of a 38- to 39-kDa band together with the major 43-kDa molecule (Pérez-Villar, unpublished). The structural differences between NKG2-A and NKG2-B may have functional consequences and warrant attention. Recent results suggest that CD94/NKG2-A (-B) couples to SHP phosphatases, as previously demonstrated for p58/p70 NKR (G. Palmieri and M. Carretero, unpublished; Fig. 1).

Additional members of the NKG2 multigene family have been identified (HOUCHINS et al. 1991; ADAMKIEWICZ et al. 1994), and may assemble with CD94 in transfectants (LAZETIC et al. 1996; CARRETERO et al. 1997). NKG2-C and NKG2-E

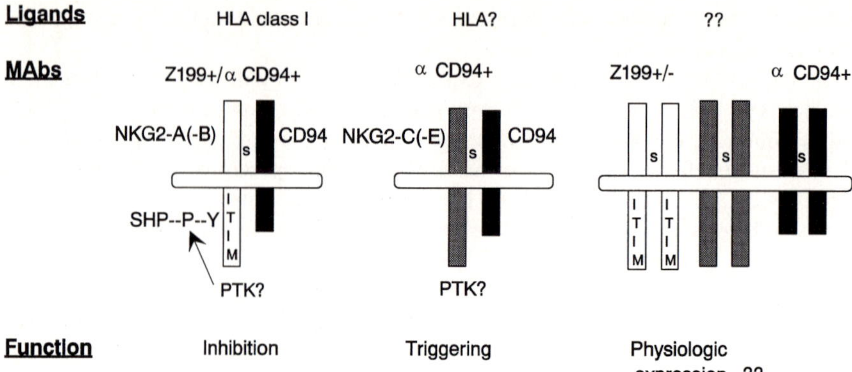

Fig. 1. Structure of the CD94/NKG2 C-type lectin receptor complex

are homologous to NKG2-A but lack cytoplasmic ITIMs (Fig. 2); consequently, the CD94/NKG2-C and CD94/NKG2-E dimers are not expected to exert an inhibitory function and likely correspond to the activating receptors (CD94/p39; Fig. 1). The signaling properties of NKG2-A and NKG2-C cytoplasmic domains coupled to murine NKR-P1 extracellular region have been recently reported (HOUCHINS et al. 1997). By reverse-transcriptase polymerase chain reaction analysis in a limited number of NK clones we have confirmed that Z199$^+$ group B cells express NKG2-A and p39$^+$ group A cells express NKG2-C/E. However, several NKG2 sequences are amplified in some clones, further suggesting that the expression of the various CD94/NKG2 dimers is not mutually exclusive (PÉREZ-VILLAR et al. 1996). Specific mAbs are required to assess precisely the physiological distribution and function of every CD94/NKG2 receptor in NK/T cells. The putative activating role of CD94/NKG2-C (-E) dimers points out a remarkable resemblance between Ig-SF (p58/p50) (MORETTA et al. 1996) and C-type lectin (CD94/NKG2) NKR. In both instances pairs of molecules closely homologous in the extracellular region can fulfill divergent functions.

NKG2-D is distantly related to the other NKG2 molecules and should be regarded separately; in fact, the formation of CD94/NKG2-D dimers has not been detected in transfectants (LAZETIC et al. 1996; Carretero et al., unpublished). Nevertheless, the existence of additional members of the NKG2 family and/or allelic variants is not ruled out. A further potential level of complexity is related to the fact that CD94 and NKG2 molecules assemble as homodimers in transfectants; to what extent this also takes place in some normal NK/T cells, and the functional implications, need to be explored. In this line, data supporting the interaction of a soluble NKG2-C fusion protein with the HLA-negative K562 tumor cell line have been documented (DÜCHLER et al. 1995).

```
NKG2A   MDNQGVTYSDLNLPPNPKRQQRKPKGNKSSILATEQEITYAELNLQKASQDFQGNDKTYHCKDLPSAPEKLIVGILGIICLILMASVVTIVVIPSTLIQRHNNSSLNIRTQKARHC
NKG2C   -SK-RGTF-EVS-AQD----------------SG-----FQV-----NP-LNH--I--I-D-QG-LPP-----TAEV------IV---T-LKTI-LIPF-E-   ----P----------
NKG2E   -NK-RGTF-EVS-AQD--P-------------SG-----FQV-----N--LNH--I--I-D-QG-LPP-----TAEV------IV---T-LKTI-LIPF-E-   ----P--------P-

NKG2A   GHCPEEWITYSNSCYYIGKERRIWEESLLACTSKNSS LLSIDNEEEMKFLSIISPSSWIGVFRNSSHHPWVTMNGLAFKHEIKDSDNAELNCAVLQVNRLKSAQCGSSIIYHCKHKL
NKG2C   ------------------------------------- ---------I---AS-L-----------------I-------K--------------------------M--------
NKG2E   ---------------------------Q--A-----S-------------AS-L-----------------I-------------H--R---M-H-RG-I-D-----R-IRRGFIMLTRLVLNS
```

Fig. 2. Sequences of the NKG2 C-typ**e lectins.** *Underlined*, the transmembrane region. The lower block corresponds to the CRD

3 The CD94/NKG2 Receptor Complex Is Involved in Recognition of HLA Class I Molecules

Conventional experimental systems analyze the activity of NK clones/subsets against HLA class I defective tumor cell lines of hematopoietic origin transfected with individual class I allotypes. Specific recognition leads to the inhibition of cytotoxicity, which can be reconstituted by the antagonistic effect of mAbs directed against either MHC molecules or their putative NKR. More formal proofs for the role of Ig-SF NKR in recognition of HLA molecules have been obtained. Transfer of individual KIRs with a vaccinia expression system conferred the predicted specificity to NK clones; moreover, specific binding of KIR fusion proteins to the HLA-transfected cells has been demonstrated (WAGTMANN et al. 1995; DÖHRING and COLONNA 1996).

MORETTA et al. (1994) reported that a subset of NK clones, mainly p58-negative, were inhibited by the expression on targets of certain $Bw6^+$ HLA-B molecules, and, moreover, that their cytolytic activity was similarly reconstituted by either anti-CD94 or HLA class I mAbs. Anti-CD94 mAbs have recently been shown to restore NK cell cytolysis against HLA-defective cell lines transfected with a wider variety of HLA allotypes (PHILLIPS et al. 1996; SIVORI et al. 1996). However, there is no evidence for CD94-mediated recognition of other HLA molecules including $Bw4^+$ and certain $Bw6^+$ HLA-B allotypes (Table 1). By similar indirect functional criteria we and others have observed that the CD94/NKG2-A receptor is involved in recognition of the 721.221 HLA-defective cell line transfected with the class Ib HLA-G1 molecule, normally detected on the cytotrophoblast (PÉREZ-VILLAR et al. 1997; PENDE et al. 1997; SODERSTRÖM et al. 1997). It is noteworthy that most decidual NK cells are stained by both conventional anti-CD94 mAbs (GUDELJ et al. 1996) and the Z199 mAb (A. King, personal communication), thus indicating that they express the CD94/NKG2-A (-B) inhibitory receptor. In discrepancy with another report (PAZMANY et al. 1996), we and others have been unable to substantiate any role of the serologically identifiable p58/p70 KIRs in recognition of 721.221 cells expressing HLA-G1. By contrast, we have shown the interaction of HLA-GI with a novel in hibitory receptor (ILT2/LIR1) (COLONNA et al. 1997).

The participation of CD94 in recognition of HLA class I transfectants was reported in NK cells expressing the inhibitory CD94/NKG2-A receptor ($Z199^+$) and, according to our experience, in the subset inhibited in rADCC assays upon ligation by CD94-specific mAbs (group B). It is of note that some NK clones which did not respond to conventional anti-CD94 mAbs in rADCC were inhibited by the Z199 mAb, suggesting that they express functional CD94/NKG2-A (-B) receptors; however, their ability to recognize HLA class I transfectants was not clearly substantiated (F. Navarro, unpublished). It is possible that the function of CD94/NKG2-A in these clones may be counterbalanced by their coexpression of activating CD94/NKG2 dimers. Considering the high homology between NKG2-C (-E) and the inhibitory NKG2-A molecule, it can be speculated that the triggering receptors somehow sense alterations in the expression of HLA/peptide complexes induced during infections by intracellular pathogens.

Table 1. CD94-mediated recognition of HLA class I transfectants

Allotype[a]	77–83 sequence	CD94-mediated recognition[a]	Transfected target
Cw*0102	SLRNLRG	Yes	721.221
Cw*0302	SLRNLRG	Yes	721.221
B*0702 (Bw6)	SLRNLRG	Yes	721.221/C1R
B*1401 (Bw6)	SLRNLRG	Yes	C1R
B*1501 (Bw6)	SLRNLRG	No	721.221
Cw*0401	NLRKLRG	Yes	721.221
Cw*1503	NLRKLRG	No	721.221
B*2705 (Bw4)	DLRTLLR	No	721.221/C1R
B*5101 (Bw4)	NLRNALR	No	721.221
B*5801 (Bw4)	NLRIALR	No	721.221
A*2403	NLRIALR	Yes	721.221
A*0101	NLGTLRG	Yes	C1R
A*3601	NLGTLRG	Yes	721.221

[a] Based on: MORETTA et al. 1994; PHILLIPS et al. 1996; SIVORI et al. 1996. For further information on other allotypes studied see references
[b] Specific inhibition of cytotoxicity reconstituted by anti-CD94 mAbs.

When CD94/NKG2-A$^+$ NK clones coexpress KIRs specific for the same HLA allotype expressed on the target cells, either anti-CD94 or Z199 mAbs fail to completely restore lysis unless the appropriate KIR-specific mAb is present (Phillips et al. 1996; Sivori et al. 1996; Pérez-Villar et al. 1997). These observations indirectly support a complementary/redundant role of both receptor systems; however, there is no formal confirmation that they indeed interact with the same structure on transfected cells. To interpret the apparent broad reactivity of the CD94/NKG2-A receptor it has been proposed that it recognizes a structural motif shared by different HLA class I allotypes (Sivori et al. 1996; Moretta et al. 1996). Several studies on KIR-mediated interaction with HLA molecules point out the influence of a defined region of the α_1 domain (positions 77–83); nevertheless, a comparison of that sequence from various HLA class I allotypes does not reveal any clear relation with the apparent susceptibility to CD94/NKG2-mediated recognition (Table 1). Others (Lazetic et al. 1996; Lanier et al. 1997) have hypothesized that the CD94/NKG2-A complex may constitute a coreceptor; as applied to T cells (i.e., CD4 and CD8), this concept implies also an interaction with a conserved region of the same ligand recognized by the specific receptor (i.e., MHC). According to this view, CD94/NKG2-A$^+$ NK clones which lack serologically identified KIRs and are inhibited by different HLA class I transfectants, should bear other unidentified receptor(s) responsible for the specific recognition. This hypothesis does not clearly explain the fact that anti-CD94 mAbs often suffice to reconstitute cytotoxicity, comparably to anti-HLA class I mAbs. We are currently exploring (in collaboration with D.E. Geraghty, Fred Hutchinson Cancer Research Center, Seattle) the possibility that CD94/NKG2 may interact with the HLA-E non-classical class I molecule, whose surface expression has been shown to be secondarily induced in 721.221 cells upon transfection with certain HLA allotypes (Lee et al. 1998). In addition, the CD94/NKG2 inhibitory receptor has been proposed to be involved in recognition of the UL18 glycoprotein, a human cytomegalovirus homologue of HLA class I (Reyburn et al. 1997); yet, it is of note that the evidence provided was indirect and further experimental support is warranted.

The unexpected patterns of reactivity against HLA transfectants occasionally noted in some CD94/NKG2-A$^+$ NK clones may be interpreted by the random distribution of other unidentified receptors and/or by the putative coexpression of different CD94/NKG2 dimers. Hence appropriate experimental systems in which the function of individual receptors is analyzed are essential to overcome the limitations of conventional cellular assays. Our preliminary studies to assess specific binding of HLA transfectants to CHO cells stably expressing the CD94/NKG2-A receptor complex have been unsuccessful. This system was previously employed to demonstrate the Ly-49/H2-D interaction (Yokoyama 1995). It is likely that a relatively low affinity/avidity of CD94/NKG2-A for HLA molecules may be masked by the influence of other cell adhesion receptors. The development of more sensitive functional assays is in progress to address precisely the ligand specificity of the individual CD94/NKG2 dimers.

The CD94/NKG2-A receptor appears to be functionally similar to the rodent Ly-49 dimers. Neither murine CD94/NKG2 nor human Ly-49 homologs have yet been reported but they likely exist (Brown et al. 1997). Taking into account the structural conservation of MHC class I molecules (i.e., 65% homology between HLA-B7 and H-2D), the evolutionary divergence of the identified human and rodent C-type lectin receptor families involved in MHC recognition is striking. Whether the glycosylation site of HLA class I molecules contributes to the interaction, as shown for Ly-49 (Daniels et al. 1995), and the influence of HLA-bound peptides in CD94/NKG2-mediated recognition should be considered.

4 Regulation of Cell Adhesion Mechanisms by the CD94/NKG2-A Inhibitory Receptor

Early experiments on the function of CD94 were carried out in polyclonal interleukin-2 activated NK cell populations, prior to the knowledge on the structural and functional complexity of the receptor. Soluble F(ab')2 fragments of anti-CD94 mAbs were reported to induce homotypic cell aggregation, NK-cell mediated killing of normal T cell blasts, autocytotoxicity (inhibition of proliferation), and induction of TNF production (Aramburu et al. 1990, 1991, 1993). All these effects required intercellular contact, as they were prevented by anti-LFA-1 mAbs or in the absence of divalent cations. The induction of cytotoxicity by soluble anti-CD94 mAbs against either autologous or allogeneic cells is clearly observed in KIR^- $CD94/kp43^+$ NK cells (Pérez-Villar et al., unpublished), consistent with the idea that the CD94/NKG2-A complex prevents autoreactivity by NK cells that lack other inhibitory receptors.

On the other hand, the ability of anti-CD94 mAbs to induce rapidly integrin-mediated homotypic adhesion is reminiscent of the effects mediated by mAbs directed against other lymphocyte receptors, generally considered to involve active mechanisms (Collins et al. 1994). Indeed we have observed that ligation by soluble bivalent mAbs of the CD94/NKG2-A inhibitory receptor complex rapidly enhance the avidity for different β_1- and β_2-integrin ligands (Pérez-Villar, unpublished). These data suggest that ligation with soluble F(ab')2 anti-CD94 mAbs not only prevent the interaction of CD94/NKG2-A with self HLA class I molecules but also actively upregulate NK cell adhesion mechanisms. Moreover, signaling via CD94/NKG2 may promote proliferation of the $CD56^{bright}$ NK cell subset (M. Robertson, personal communication) and exert with anti-CD3 mAbs costimulatory effects in γ/δ T cells (P. Aparicio, personal communication). A similar costimulation of B cell function has been reported to be inducible with mAbs specific for CD22, an ITIM-bearing receptor (Thomas 1995). Tyrosine phosphorylation of KIRs has been detected upon their ligation, suggesting the involvement of as yet unidentified PTK(s) (Burshtyn et al. 1996); preliminary results support that similar events take place in the CD94/NKG2-A pathway (G. Palmieri and M. Carretero, unpublished) and may contribute to explain the positive induction of cell adhesion mechanisms. We have hypothesized (López-Botet et al. 1997) that a reduced avidity of the interaction between CD94/NKG2-A and HLA class I molecules not only abolishes the receptor-mediated negative signaling but concomitantly promotes NK cell integrin-mediated adhesion, thereby costimulating the function of triggering receptors.

Acknowledgements. The authors are supported by grants from the European Commission (BIO4-CT95-0062), Spanish Ministry of Health (FIS 94/0105), and Plan Nacional I+D (SAF96/0335).

References

Adamkiewicz TV, McSherry C, Bach FH, Houchins JP (1994) Natural killer lectin-like receptors have divergent carboxy-termini distinct from C-type lectins. Immunogenetics 39:218

Aramburu J, Balboa MA, Ramírez A, Silva A, Acevedo A, Sánchez-Madrid F, de Landázuri MO, López-Botet M (1990) A novel functional cell surface dimer (Kp43) expressed by natural killer cells and T cell receptor-γ/δ+ T lymphocytes. Inhibition of IL-2 dependent proliferation by anti-Kp43 monoclonal antibody. J Immunol 144:3238–3247

Aramburu J, Balboa MA, Izquierdo M, López-Botet M (1991) A novel functional cell surface dimer (Kp43) expressed by natural killer cells and γ/δ+ T lymphocytes. Modulation of natural killer cytotoxicity by anti Kp43 monoclonal antibody. J Immunol 147:714–721

Aramburu J, Balboa MA, Rodríguez A, Melero I, Alonso M, Alonso JL, López-Botet M (1993) Stimulation of IL-2-activated natural killer cells through the Kp43 surface antigen up-regulates TNF-α production involving the LFA-1 integrin. J Immunol 151:3420–3429

Brooks AG, Posch PE, Scorzelli CJ, Borrego F, Coligan JE (1977) NKG2A complexed with CD94 defines a novel inhibitory natural killer cell receptor. J Exp Med 185:795–800

Brown MG, Fulmek S, Matsumoto K, Cho R, Lyons PA, Levy ER, Scalzo AA, Yokoyama WM (1977) A 2-Mb YAC contig and physical map of the natural killer gene complex on mouse chromosome 6. Genomics 42:18–25

Brumbaugh KM, Pérez-Villar JJ, Dick CJ, Schoon R, López-Botet M, Leibson PJ (1996) Clonotypic differences in signaling from CD94 (Kp43) on NK cells lead to divergent cellular responses. J Immunol 157:2804–2812

Burshtyn DN, Scharenberg AM, Wagtmann N, Rajagopalan S, Berrada K, Yi T, Kinet J-P, Long EO (1996) Recruitment of tyrosine phosphatase HCP by the killer cell inhibitory receptor. Immunity 4:77–85

Campbell KS, Dessing M, López-Botet M, Cella M, Colonna M (1996) Tyrosine phosphorylation of a human killer inhibitory receptor recruits protein tyrosine phosphatase 1C. J Exp Med 184:93–100

Carretero M, Cantoni C, Bellón T, Bottino C, Biassoni R, Rodríguez A, Pérez-Villar JJ, Moretta L, Moretta A, López-Botet M (1997) The CD94 and NKG2-A C-type lectins covalently assemble to form an NK cell inhibitory receptor for HLA class I molecules. Eur J Immunol

Chang C, Rodríguez A, Carretero M, López-Botet M, Phillips J, Lanier LL (1995) Molecular characterization of human CD94: a type II membrane glycoprotein related to the C-type lectin superfamily. Eur J Immunol 25:2433–2437

Collins TL, Kassner PD, Bierer B, Burakoff SJ (1994) Adhesion receptors in lymphocyte activation. Curr Opin Immunol 6:385–393

Colonna M, Samaridis J (1995) Cloning of immunoglobulin-superfamily members associated with HLA-C and HLA-B recognition of human Natural Killer cells. Science 268:405–408

Colonna M, Navarro F, Bellón T, Llano M, García P, Samaridis J, Angmann L, Cella M, López-BotetM (1977) A common inhibitory receptor for major histocompatibility complex class I molecules on human lymphoid and myelomonocytic cells. J Exp Med 186:1809–1818

Daniels BF, Nakamura MC, Rosen SD, Yokoyama WM, Seaman WE (1995) Ly-49A, a receptor for H-2D^d, has a functional carbohydrate recognition domain. Immunity 1:785–792

Döhring C, Colonna M (1996) Human natural killer cell inhibitory receptors bind to HLA class I molecules. Eur J Immunol 26:365–369

Düchler M, Offterdinger M, Holzmüller H, Lipp J, Chu C-T, Aschauer B, Bach FH, Hofer E (1995) NKG2-C is a receptor on human natural killer cells that recognizes structures on K562 target cells. Eur J Immunol 25:2923–2931

Fry A, Lanier LL, Weiss A (1996) Phosphotyrosines in the KIR motif of NKB1 are required for negative signaling and for association with PTP1C. J Exp Med 184:295–300

Gudelj L, Deniz G, Rukavina D, Johnson PM, Christmas SE (1996) Expression of functional molecules by human CD3-decidual granular leucocyte clones. Immunology 87:609–615

Gumperz JE, Valiante NM, Parham P, Lanier LL, Tyan D (1996) Heterogeneous phenotypes of expression of the NKB1 natural killer cell class I receptor among individuals of different human histocompatibility leukocyte antigens types appear genetically regulated, but not linked to major histocompatibility complex haplotype. J Exp Med 183:1817–1827

Houchins JP, Yabe T, McSherry C, Bach FH (1991) DNA sequence analysis of NKG2, a family of related cDNA clones encoding type II integral membrane proteins on human natural killer cells. J Exp Med 173:1017–1020

Houchins JP, Lanier LL, Niemi EC, Phillips JH, Ryan JC (1977) Natural killer cell cytolytic activity is inhibited by NKG2-A and activated by NKG2-C. J Immunol 158:3603–3609

Lanier LL (1977) Natural killer cells: from no receptors to too many. Immunity 6:371–378

Lanier LL, Phillips JH (1995) Inhibitory MHC class I receptors on NK cells and T cells. Immunol Today 17:86–91

Lanier LL, Chang C, Phillips JH (1994) Human NKR-P1A: a disulfide-linked homodimer of the C-type lectin superfamily expressed by a subset of NK and T lymphocytes. J Immunol 153:2417–2428

Lazetic S, Chang C, Houchins JP, Lanier LL, Phillips JH (1996) Human Natural Killer cell receptors involved in MHC class I recognition are disulfide-linked heterodimers of CD94 and NKG2 subunits. J Immunol 157:4741–45

Lee N, Goodlett DR, Ishitani A, Marquardt H, Geraghty DE (1988) HLA-E surface expression depends on binding of TAP-dependent peptides derived from certain HLA class I signal sequences. J Immunol (in press)

Ljunggren H-G, Kärre K (1990) In search of the missing self: MHC molecules and NK cell recognition. Immunol Today 11:237–244

López-Botet M (1995) CD94 cluster report: overview of the characterization of the Kp43 NK-cell-associated surface antigen. In: Schlossman SF et al (eds) Leucocyte typing V. Oxford University Press, Oxford

López-Botet M, Moretta L, Strominger JL (1996) NK cell-receptors and recognition of MHC class-I molecules. Immunol Today 17:212–214

López-Botet M, Pérez-Villar JJ, Carretero M, Rodríguez A, Melero A, Bellón T, Llano M, Navarro F (1997) Structure and function of the CD94 C-type lectin receptor complex involved in recognition of HLA class I molecules. Immunol Rev 155 (in press)

Moretta A, Vitale M, Sivori S, Bottino C, Morelli L, Augugliaro R, Barbaresi M, Pende D, Ciccone E, López-Botet M, Moretta L (1994) Human natural killer cell receptors for HLA-class I molecules: evidence that the Kp43 (CD94) molecule functions as receptor for HLA-B alleles. J Exp Med 180:545–555

Moretta A, Bottino C, Vitale M, Pende D, Biassoni R, Mingari MC, Moretta L (1996) Receptors for HLA class I molecules in human natural killer cells. Annu Rev Immunol 14:619–648

Olcese L, Lang P, Vely F, Cambiaggi A, Marguet D, Blery M, Hippen KL, Biassoni R, Moretta A, Moretta L, Cambier JC, Vivier E (1996) Human and mouse killer-cell inhibitory receptors recruit PTP1-C and PTP1-D protein tyrosine phosphatases. J Immunol 156:4531–4534

Pazmany L, Mandelboim O, Valés-Gomez M, Davis DM, Reyburn HT, and Strominger JL (1996) Protection from natural killer cell-mediated lysis by HLA-G expression on target cells. Science 274:792–794

Pende D, Sivori S, Accame L, Pareti L, Falco M, Geraghty DE, Le Bouteiller P, Moretta L, Moretta A (1997) HLA-G recognition by human natural killer cells. Involvement of CD94 both as inhibitory and activating receptor complex. Eur J Immunol 27:1875–1880

Pérez-Villar JJ, Melero I, Rodríguez A, Carretero M, Aramburu J, Sivori S, Orengo AM, Moretta A, López-Botet M (1995) Functional ambivalence of the Kp43 (CD94) NK cell-associated surface antigen. J Immunol 154:5779–5788

Pérez-Villar JJ, Carretero M, Navarro F, Melero I, Rodríguez A, Bottino C, Moretta A, López-Botet M (1996) Biochemical and serologic evidence for the existence of functionally distinct forms of the CD94 NK cell receptor. J Immunol 157:5367–5374

Pérez-Villar JJ, Melero I, Navarro F, Carretero M, Bellón T, Llano M, Colonna M, Geraghty DE, López-Botet M (1997) The CD94/NKG2-A inhibitory receptor complex is involved in natural killer cell-mediated recognition of cells expressing HLA-G1. J Immunol 158:5736–5743

Phillips JH, Chang C, Mattson J, Gumperz JE, Parham P, Lanier LL (1996) CD94 and a novel associated protein (94AP) form a NK cell receptor involved in the recognition of HLA-A, -B, and -C allotypes. Immunity 5:163–172

Renedo M, Arce I, Rodríguez A, Carretero M, Lanier LL, López-Botet M, Fernández-Ruiz E (1997) The human natural killer gene complex is located on chromosome 12p12-p13. Immunogenetics 46:307–311

Reyburn HT, Mandelboim O, Vales-Gómez M, Davis DM, Pazmany L, Strominger JL (1997) The class I MHC homologue of human cytomegalovirus inhibits attack by natural killer cells. Nature 386:514–517

Rodríguez A, Carretero M, Glienke , Bellón T, Ramírez A, Lehrach H, Francis F, López-Botet M (1998) Structure of the human CD94 C-type lectin gene. Immunogenetics (in press)

Rubio G, Aramburu J, Ontañón J, López-Botet M, Aparicio P (1993) A novel functional cell surface dimer (Kp43) serves as accessory molecule for the activation of a subset of human γ/δ+ T cells. J Immunol 151:1312–1321

Sivori S, Vitale M, Bottino C, Marcenato E, Sanseverino L, Parolini S, Moretta L, Moretta A (1996) CD94 functions as a natural killer cell inhibitory receptor for different HLA class I alelles: identification of the inhibitory form of CD94 by the use of novel monoclonal antibodies. Eur J Immunol 26:2487–2492

Soderström K, Corliss B, Lanier LL, Phillips JH (1997) CD94/NKG2 is the predominant inhibitory receptor involved in recognition of HLA-G by decidual and peripheral blood NK cells. J Immunol 159:1072–1075

Thomas ML (1995) Of ITAMs and ITIMs. Turning on and off the B cell antigen receptor. J Exp Med 181:1953–1956

Wagtmann N, Rajagopalan S, Winter CC, Peruzzi M, Long EO (1995) Killer cell inhibitory receptors specific for HLA-C and HLA-B identified by direct binding and by functional transfer. Immunity 3:801–809

Yabe T, McSherry C, Bach FH, Fisch P, Schall RP, Sondel PM, Houchins JP (1993) A multigene family on human chromosome 12 encodes natural killer cell-lectins. Immunogenetics 37:455–460
Yokoyama WM (1995) Natural killer cell receptors. Curr Opin Immunol 7:110–120

Triggering of Natural Killer Cell Mediated Cytotoxicity by Costimulatory Molecules

B.J. CHAMBERS, J.L. WILSON, M. SALCEDO, K. MARKOVIC, M.T. BEJARANO, and H.G. LJUNGGREN

1 Introduction

Natural killer (NK) cell mediated cytotoxicity is affected by both triggering and inhibitory signals (see e.g., GUMPERZ and PARHAM 1995; LANIER and PHILIPS 1996; RAULET 1996). In several models target cell major histocompatibility complex (MHC) class I molecules have been demonstrated to be able to turn off NK cells (LJUNGGREN and KÄRRE 1990; KÄRRE 1995) by delivering inhibitory signals to MHC class I binding receptors (KARLHOFER et al. 1992; YOKOYAMA and SEAMAN 1993). The latter include members of the Ly-49 receptors in mouse and the killer-cell inhibitor receptors (KIR) in man (GUMPERZ and PARHAM 1995; LANIER and PHILIPS 1996; RAULET 1996). While much attention has been focused on the role of MHC class I inhibition of NK cell mediated cytotoxicity in recent years, significantly less attention has been devoted to receptor-ligand interactions that may trigger cytotoxicity. This review discusses new insights into the ability of costimulatory molecules to trigger NK cell mediated cytotoxicity.

Microbiology and Tumor Biology Center, Karolinska Institute, Box 280, 171 77 Stockholm, Sweden

2 NK Cell Activation

The current notion holds that NK cell mediated cytotoxicity is controlled by an interplay between stimulatory and inhibitory signals. Although the receptors and ligands that transduce inhibitory signals are being identified, the cell surface receptors and ligands that transduce activation signals to NK cells remain relatively unexplored (YOKOYAMA 1995; IMBODEN 1996; RAULET 1996). A few candidate receptors for NK cell mediated triggering have been suggested, but none of these has emerged as a "consensus candidate" for being *the* NK cell triggering receptor(s). The latter include CD16, CD2, NKRP-1, and CD69. Ligation of CD16, the receptor for the for the constant region of IgG molecules, or antibody-mediated stimulation of a number of surface molecules including CD2, NKRP-1, and CD69 triggers NK cell mediated cytotoxicity. Signals transmitted via these receptors are similar to those used by the antigen receptors of T and B cells, involving the stimulation of protein tyrosine kinases and the consequent activation signal cascades, including the phospholipase C pathway (LEIBSON 1995; IMBODEN 1996). However, other receptors capable of transmitting triggering signals to NK cells may exist, although little is known about their nature or about their ligands on susceptible targets. The present review focuses on some recent studies indicating a role for the costimulatory molecules in acting as ligands for triggering receptors on NK cells.

3 Costimulatory Molecules and Their Role in T Cell Activation

B7-1 (CD80) and B7-2 (CD86) are members of the Ig superfamily and are expressed on the majority of activated antigen-presenting cells (APC) such as dendritic cells, macrophages, and B-cells. These molecules and their counterreceptors CD28 and CTLA-4 on T cells have been extensively characterized in recent years in their ability to deliver costimulatory signals (LINSLEY and LEDBETTER 1993; ALLISON 1994; SHARPE 1995). Briefly, it is understood that the activation of T cells requires two signals from APC. The first signal, the engagement of the T cell receptor (TCR) to its cognate peptide-MHC ligand, provides specificity. The second signal is provided by costimulatory molecules expressed on APC binding to their counter receptors on the T lymphocyte (ALLISON and KRUMMEL 1995). Binding of the TCR with peptide-MHC complexes in the absence of costimulation results in T cell inactivation or "anergy," which is associated with a block of interleukin (IL) 2 gene transcription. Both B7-1 and B7-2 can interact with their counterreceptors, CD28 and CTLA-4, on T cells. On naive T cells CD28 appears to be expressed in the absence of CTLA-4. Once T cells are activated, however, they express CTLA-4. While interactions between B7-1/B7-2 and CD28 seem to be crucial for T cell activation (including proliferation and differentiation) CTLA-4 appears to play a negative role in the activation of the T cell expressing it (TIVOL et al. 1995; WATERHOUSE et al. 1995).

This may help to limit the early proliferative response of the T cells after initial activation.

4 NK Cell Interactions with Costimulatory Molecules

While human fetal NK cells are $CD28^+$, adult NK cells have been claimed to be $CD28^-$ (Azuma et al. 1992; L. Lanier, personal communication). In contrast to this notion, we have observed low levels of CD28 on human $CD56^+CD3^-$ NK cell lines (unpublished observations). In the murine system Nandi et al. (1994) have described that $NK1.1^+$ splenocytes and IL-2 activated splenocytes express CD28, but at lower levels than T cells. A similar observation has been made in our own laboratory (unpublished observations). CD28 expression has also been described on intraperitoneal NK cells from mice infected with *Toxoplasma gondii* (Hunter et al. 1997). We are unaware of any study to date describing expression of CTLA-4 on NK cells. FACS analyses of murine IL-2 activated NK cells have failed to demonstrate any expression of CTLA-4 on the cell surface (unpublished observations).

The first indication of interactions between NK cells and costimulatory molecules came from studies by Lanier and colleagues with a human NK leukemia cell line YT (Azuma et al. 1992). This cell line (or variants of this line) has been reported spontaneously to lyse both human and mouse cell lines expressing B7-1. This effect was mediated at least in part by a direct interaction between B7-1 and CD28 as blocking studies inhibited B7-1 mediated killing. Subsequent studies by Allison and colleagues in a murine model demonstrated that CD28-mediated costimulation plays an important role in regulating NK cell mediated proliferation and cytokine production (Nandi et al. 1994). However, this study failed to reveal any role for a B7-1 mediated triggering of cytotoxicity. Similar conclusions were reached by Chen et al. (1994) studying the NK cell sensitivity of EL-4 cells transfected with B7-1. In light of our present results (see below), these results might be explained by the level of activation of the NK cell used, although other explanations are not excluded. More recently rejection responses against murine B7-1 transfected tumor cell lines have been reported to involve an NK cell component (Cavallo et al. 1995; Geldhof et al. 1995; Wu et al. 1995; Yeh et al. 1995). Furthermore, in two of these studies B7-1 transfected tumor cell lines studied were killed by splenocytes (most likely NK cells although this was not demonstrated directly) in vitro at higher levels than the corresponding wild-type cell lines (Geldhof et al. 1995; Yeh et al. 1995). In the latter study the killing was blocked by CTLA-4 Ig, indicating that B7-1 is indeed the triggering molecule (Yeh et al. 1995).

5 Triggering of NK Cell Mediated Cytotoxicity by the Costimulatory Molecule B7-1

We discuss below our own studies assessing NK cell mediated cytotoxicity against murine lymphoma cells transfected with costimulatory molecules. Unless otherwise noted, the experiments were performed with murine effector cells, stimulated in vitro with IL-2. These effectors are referred to either as lymphokine-activated killer (LAK) cells or only as NK cells. Since most of our current experience derives from studies of the costimulatory molecule B7-1, the discussion focuses on this molecule, but we also discuss to some extent the role of other costimulatory molecules.

B6-derived LAK cells do not efficiently kill MHC class I positive EL-4 cells. In contrast, similar effector cells readily kill EL-4 cells transfected with B7-1 (EL-4 B7-1). These results are not a specific property of EL-4 B7-1 cells. The MHC class I positive RMA B7-1 and P815 B7-1 cell lines are also sensitive to LAK cell lysis. The lysis of EL-4 B7-1 and RMA B7-1 can be inhibited by addition of CTLA-4 Ig, demonstrating that B7-1 is the triggering signal for target cell lysis, and that the effect is not an indirect consequence of B7-1 expression (Chambers et al. 1996). To verify that the effector cells within the LAK population triggered by B7-1 expression on the tumor cell lines fulfill the criteria of being phenotypically normal NK cells, LAK cell cultures were sorted into NK1.1$^+$ and CD8$^+$ populations. It was observed that all cytotoxic activity towards EL-4 B7-1 resided in the NK1.1$^+$ population of the LAK cells. Similar effectors also preferentially killed the MHC class I deficient EL-4 subline C4.4-25$^-$ and the standard NK target cell line YAC-1.

A theoretical possibility is that all killing of B7-1 transfected target cells was mediated by a small fraction of NK1.1$^+$ T cells. However, NK1.1$^+$/TCR $\alpha\beta^-$ cells were found to lyse EL-4 B7-1 but not EL-4. We also subfractionated the NK1.1$^+$ population of LAK cells into NK1.1$^+$/Ly-49A$^+$, NK1.1$^+$/Ly-49A$^-$, NK1.1$^+$/Ly-49C$^+$, and NK1.1$^+$/Ly-49C$^-$ subpopulations. All four subpopulations of NK cells preferentially killed the B7-1 transfected EL-4 target cells over control EL-4 cells. Taken together these results indicate that the ability to be triggered by B7-1 molecules is a property of NK cells. This may be a property of all NK1.1$^+$/CD3$^-$ NK cells but it cannot be excluded that it is a property of only a subset of these cells (Chambers et al. 1996). Furthermore, the triggering of NK cells by costimulatory molecules may depend critically on the stage of activation of the NK cells, a matter that is currently under investigation.

One general notion has been that NK cells must be triggered by any of a distinct set of target cell ligands, but that all of these signals can be overruled by MHC class I mediated inhibition (see e.g., Correa et al. 1994). However, the lysis observed against MHC class I positive B7-1 transfectants of RMA and EL-4 seems to indicate that certain triggering signals have such strength that they readily overcome the MHC class I mediated protection. Controlled experiments reveal that transfection of the B7-1 gene into these cell lines does not alter their levels of MHC class I expression. A comparative analysis has revealed that B7-1 transfected EL-4 and RMA cells are rendered as sensitive to NK cell mediated lysis as MHC class I deficient variants of the EL-4 and RMA cell lines, respectively. Furthermore, transfection of MHC class

I deficient RMA-S cells with B7-1 further potentiate the NK sensitivity of this cell line. This indicates that although the expression of B7-1 can override the protection imposed by MHC class I expression, MHC class I molecules are still able to offer some degree of protection (CHAMBERS et al. 1996). In line with these observations we have observed that both the EL-4 and EL-4 B7-1 cell lines are killed at lower levels by NK1.1$^+$/Ly-49C$^+$ effector cells than the levels of lysis observed for the NK1.1$^+$/Ly-49C$^-$ subpopulation. This result is interesting in relation to the notion of Ly-49C being an inhibitory receptor for H-2K^b (YU et al. 1996), since, on the one hand, it provides additional support for the notion of B7-1 being able to override the protection mediated by MHC class I expression. However, on the other hand, it also indicates that MHC class I molecules confer some level of protection from NK cell mediated lysis despite B7-1 expression on the target cell (CHAMBERS et al. 1996).

CD28 and CTLA-4 are both receptors expressed by T cells that are able to recognize and interact with B7-1 molecules (LINSLEY and LEDBETTER 1993; ALLISON 1994; SHARPE 1995). To address the role of CD28 on NK cells with respect to the triggering effects imposed by B7-1 expressed on tumor targets we generated LAK effectors from CD28$^{-/-}$ mice. Effector cells from such mice killed EL-4 B7-1 targets equivalent to effectors from wild-type (B6) mice. Although this result did not exclude a role for CD28 on NK cells from wild-type mice, it suggested that receptors other than CD28 on NK cells are capable of interacting with B7-1. To further address the roles of both CD28 and CTLA-4 on B7-1 recognition by NK cells, LAK cells from B6 mice were preincubated with anti-CD28 or anti-CTLA-4 antibodies. These experiments failed to reveal any significant effects by either anti-CD28 or anti-CTLA-4 antibodies on the recognition of B7-1 on the transfected tumors, suggesting (or at least not excluding) that NK cells use receptors other than CD28 and CTLA-4 in interactions with B7-1 molecules.

To address whether in vitro killing of murine B7-1 expressing lymphoma targets depends on the perforin pathway or on pathways other than perforin-mediated killing LAK cells were prepared from perforin$^{-/-}$ mice. Using such effectors abolished all killing capacity, strongly suggesting that NK cell triggering by B7-1 in the mouse leads to cytotoxicity being mediated by or dependent upon perforin.

6 Rapid Elimination of B7-1 Expressing Tumor Cells In Vivo

Previous studies have implicated a role for NK cells in the clearance of B7-1 transfected tumors in vivo (CAVALLO et al. 1995; GELDHOF et al. 1995; WU et al. 1995; YEH et al. 1995). To address this issue more directly we performed rapid elimination studies of radiolabeled B7-1 transfected RMA and EL-4 cells. We have previously demonstrated that radiolabeled MHC class I deficient RMA or EL-4 cell mutants are rapidly eliminated in normal B6 mice, and that this elimination is abrogated by depleting the mice of NK cells. Recent results indicate a similar NK cell dependent mode of elimination of MHC class I expressing B7-1 transfected RMA or EL-4 cells. Elimination rapid elimination of B7-1 transfected cells is observed in normal as well as in RAG-1 deficient mice but not in NK cell depleted mice. However, it should be noted that at present these findings are preliminary, and additional control experiments are needed to firmly establish this notion.

7 NK Cell Mediated Killing of Macrophages and Dendritic Cells

Earlier observations indicated the ability of NK cells to interfere with lymphocyte proliferation in mixed lymphocyte cultures. In those studies it was speculated that NK cells exert this mechanism of action by interfering with APC such as dendritic cells (GILBERTSON et al. 1986). NK cell mediated recognition of target cells expressing costimulatory molecules implies that cells normally expressing such molecules are targeted by NK cells. Indeed, both autologous bone marrow derived macrophages and dendritic cells have been found to be highly susceptible to NK cell mediated lysis. In these studies CTLA-4 Ig failed to block killing of the bone marrow derived macrophages or dendritic cells, suggesting that molecules other than B7-1 and B7-2 are involved in NK cell triggering, although a role for these molecules cannot be excluded (CHAMBERS et al. 1996). The present findings implicate, but do not confirm, a role for NK cells in the control of immune responses involving activated APC. It can be speculated that NK cells control macrophages or dendritic cells in their stimulation of naive T cells in lymphoid organs, or ensure that these cells do not end up in the periphery and cause inflammatory or other unwanted responses. However, further studies are clearly needed to reveal insights into the physiological role of NK cell interaction with APC.

8 NK Cell Triggering by Costimulatory Molecules: Significance and Implications

This review discusses some recent insights into NK cell triggering by costimulatory molecules. A number of observations have indicated extensive similarities between NK cells and T cells (recently reviewed by VALIENTE and PARHAM 1996). The present observations of NK cell interaction with costimulatory molecules adds to this notion. Another similarity is the expression of class I binding inhibitory receptors which are now also being observed on many T cells (CICCONE et al. 1996; LANIER and PHILIPS 1996). Taken together, it is not unlikely that both NK and T cell mediated responses will be found to be controlled by a delicate balance of triggering and inhibitory stimuli, some of which may be shared by these two types of lymphocytes. Coincidentally, it may be that triggering molecules (costimulatory molecules as well as the MHC/peptide complex) were simply discovered first on T cells and that their control by inhibitory molecules is only now being uncovered. In contrast, for NK cells it was the inhibitory receptors and their ligands that were first discovered while we are now beginning to uncover their corresponding triggering molecules.

From an evolutionary point of view NK cells are considered to be old. It has been speculated that their ancestors were cytotoxic cells capable of mediating graft rejection responses in invertebrates (SCOFIELD et al. 1982). Likewise, costimulatory molecules have been speculated to be evolutionarily old, and JANEWAY (1992) has suggested that this type of molecule arose very early to trigger innate or nonclonal responses and to signal to lymphocytes that a particular antigen is associated with a micro-organism. We hypothesize that the NK cell triggering by costimulatory molecules such as B7-1 is an inherent property of NK cells that was propagated through the evolution of the cells.

The physiological relevance of NK cell triggering via costimulatory molecules is not clear. We have speculated on the possibility that NK cells control APC, but this clearly needs to be documented experimentally. The possibility of costimulatory molecules being triggering ligands for NK cells is also interesting from another point of view. These molecules are expressed preferentially on hematopoietic cells. Likewise, it has been demonstrated that NK cells kill target cells of a rather restricted nature. While hematopoietic cells often are good targets for NK cell mediated lysis, other nonhematopoietic cells are seldom killed. A few exceptions to the latter notion exist, however, such as in the case of melanomas. Nonetheless, we do believe that the target cell specificity of NK cells can very well be explained at a molecular level on the basis of their expressing of ligand capable of transmitting signals to triggering receptors.

The transfection of B7-1 into tumor cell lines has become an attractive means for antitumor immunotherapy to induce strong antitumor cytotoxic T cells. The notion holds that B7-1 expressing tumor cells function directly as professional APC, being capable of activating naive T cells. The present data, as well as previous indications (CAVALLO et al. 1995; GELDHOF et al. 1995; WU et al. 1995; YEH et al. 1995), suggest that B7-1 transfected tumor cells serve as targets for NK cells. These observations have led to a reinterpretation of the role of costimulatory molecules in antitumor immunity (CAVALLO et al. 1995; WU et al. 1995). The present results argue that cells transfected with costimulatory molecules are at least in part destroyed by NK cells. If this is indeed the case, cellular debris from tumor cells destroyed by NK cells could be processed by professional APC that then present tumor antigen on MHC molecules. This event in turn activates naive T cells, which leads to the antitumor specific responses.

The present studies demonstrate a delicate balance between triggering and inhibitory signals. The exploration of interactions between pathways transmitting triggering and inhibitory signals will most likely represent an exciting area of research. Future studies must also focus on costimulatory molecules other than B7-1 (CD80) in both the murine and human systems, their corresponding receptors on NK cells, the mechanisms of action upon interactions of these receptors with each other in an experimental, and an physiological context.

Acknowledgements. These studies were supported by the Swedish Medical Research Council, Swedish Cancer Society, Swedish Society for Medical Research, Åke Wiberg Foundation, Magnus Bergvall Foundation, and Karolinska Institute. We thank Jehad Charo, Rolf Kiessling, Alexander McAdam, Arlene

Sharpe, Christina Olsson, Mikael Dohlsten, Alfonso Martin Fontecha, Paolo Dellabona, Giulia Casorati, Tao Wen, Elisabeth Wolpert, Ennio Carbone, Klas Kärre, and members of our group for kind gifts of reagents, discussions, and support.

References

Allison JP (1994) CD28-B7 interactions in T cell activation. Curr Opin Immunol 6:414–419

Allison JP, Krummel MF (1995) The yin and yang of T cell costimulation. Nature 270:932–933

Azuma M, Cayabyab M, Buck D, Phillips JH, Lanier LL (1992). Involvement of CD28 in MHC-unrestricted cytotoxicity mediated by a human natural killer leukemia cell line. J Immunol 149:1115–1123

Cavallo F, Martin-Fontecha A, Bellone M, Heltai S, Gatti E, Tornaghi P, Freschi M, Forni G, Dellabona P, Casorati G (1995) Co-expression of B7-1 and ICAM-1 on tumors is required for rejection and the establishment of a memory response. Eur J Immunol 25:1154–1162

Chambers BJ, Salcedo M, Ljunggren HG (1996) Triggering of natural killer cells by the costimulatory molecule CD80 (B7-1). Immunity 5:311–317

Chen L, McGowan P, Ashe S, Johnston J, Li Y, Hellstršm I, Hellstršm, KE (1994) Tumor immunogenicity determines the effect of B7 costimulation on T cell-mediated tumor immunity. J Exp Med 179:523–532

Ciccone E, Grossi CE, Velardi A (1996) Opposing functions of activatory T-cell receptors and inhibitory NK-cell receptors on cytotoxic T cells. Immunol Today 17:450–453

Correa I, Corral L, Raulet DH (1994) Multiple natural killer cell-activating signals are inhibited by major histocompatibility complex class I expression in target cells. Eur J Immunol 24:1323–1331

Geldhof AB, Raes G, Bakkus M, Devos S, Thielmans K, De Baetselier P (1995) Expression of B7-1 by highly metastatic mouse T lymphomas induces optimal natural killer cell-mediated cytotoxicity. Cancer Res 55:2730–2733

Gilbertson SM, Shah PD, Rowley DA (1986) NK cells suppress the generation of Lyt-2^+ cytolytic T cells by suppressing or eliminating dendritic cells. J Immunol 136:3567–3571

Gumperz JE, Parham P (1995) The enigma of the natural killer cell. Nature 378:245–248

Hunter CA, Ellis-Neyer L, Gabriel KE, Kennedy MK, Grabstein KH, Linsley PS, Remington JS (1997) The role of the CD28/B7 interaction in the regulation of NK cell responses during infection with Toxoplasma gondii. J Immunol 158:2285–2293

Imboden J (1996) Innate immunity – turning off natural killers. Curr Biol 6:1070–1072

Janeway, CA (1992) The immune system evolved to discriminate infectious nonself from noninfectious self. Immunol Today 13:11–16

Kärre K (1995) Express yourself or die: peptides, MHC molecules and NK cells. Science 267:978–979

Karlhofer FM, Ribaudo RK, Yokoyama WM (1992) MHC class I alloantigen specificity of Ly-49^+ IL-2-activated natural killer cells. Nature 358:66–70

Lanier LL, Philips JH (1996) Inhibitory MHC class I receptors on NK cells and T cells. Immunol Today 17:86–91

Leibson PJ (1995) MHC-recognizing receptors: they're not just for T cells anymore. Immunity 3:5–8

Linsley PS, Ledbetter JA (1993) The role of the CD28 receptor during T cell responses to antigen. Annu Rev Immunol 11:191–212

Ljunggren HG, Kärre K (1990) In search of the "missing self": MHC molecules and NK cell recognition. Immunol Today 11:237–244

Nandi D, Gross JA, Allison JP (1994) CD28-mediated co-stimulation is necessary for optimal proliferation of murine NK cells. J Immunol 152:3361–3369

Raulet, DH (1996) Recognition events that inhibit and activate natural killer cells. Curr Opin Immunol 8:372–377

Scofield VL, Schlumpberger JM, West LA, Weissman IL (1982) Protochordate allo-recognition is controlled by a MHC-like gene system. Nature 295:499–502

Sharpe AS (1995) Analysis of lymphocyte co-stimulation in vivo using transgenic and "knockout" mice. Curr Opin Immunol 7:389–395

Tivol EA, Boriello F, Schweitzer AN, Lynch WP, Bluestone JA, Sharpe AH (1995) Loss of CTLA-4 leads to massive lymphoproliferation and fatal multiorgan tissue destruction, revealing a critical negative regulatory role of CTLA-4. Immunity 3:541–547

Valiante NM, Parham P (1996) NK cells and CTL: opposite sides of the same coin. In: Moretta L (ed) Molecular basis of NK cell recognition and function. Karger, Basel

Waterhouse P, Penninger JM, Timms E, Wakeham A, Shahinian A, Lee KP, Thompson CB, Griesser H, Mak TW (1995) Lymphoproliferative disorders with early lethality in mice deficient in CTLA-4. Science 270:985–988

Wu TC, Huang AYC, Jaffee EM, Levitsky HI, Pardoll DM (1995) A reassessment of the role of B7-1 expression in tumor rejection. J Exp Med 182:1415–1421

Yeh KY, Pulaski BA, Woods ML, McAdam AJ, Gaspari AA, Frelinger JG, Lord EM (1995) B7-1 enhances natural killer cell-mediated cytotoxicity and inhibits tumor growth of a poorly immunogenic murine carcinoma. Cell Immunol 165:217–224

Yokoyama WM (1995) Natural killer cell receptors. Curr Opin Immunol 7:110–120

Yokoyama WM, Seaman WE (1993) The Ly-49 and NKR-P1 gene families encoding lectin-like receptors on natural killer cells: the NK gene complex. Annu Rev Immunol 11:613–635

Yu YY, George T, Dorfman J, Roland J, Kumar V, Bennett M (1996) The role of Ly49A and 5E6 (Ly49C) molecules in hybrid resistance mediated by murine natural killer cells against normal T cell blasts. Immunity 4:67–76

Fc Receptors on Natural Killer Cells

B. PERUSSIA

1 Introduction

Cytotoxicity and cytokine production represent the two major functional effects that follow interaction of natural killer (NK) cells with a variety of target cells (reviewed in TRINCHIERI 1989). The receptor(s) involved in binding/recognition of target cells sensitive to spontaneous cytotoxicity (i.e., that mediated by NK cells from healthy nonimmunized individuals against nonsensitized targets) remain elusive. Target cells not bound spontaneously by NK cells can be recognized if coated with intact IgG antibodies, and NK cell recognition of these particulate immune complexes triggers antibody-dependent cell-mediated cytotoxicity (ADCC), following binding to receptors for the Fc portion of Ig (FcR) expressed on these cells. In these conditions, analogous to what is observed upon target cell recognition, cytokine expression and

Jefferson Medical College, Kimmel Cancer Institute, BLSB 750, 233 S. 10th Street, Philadelphia, PA 19107, USA

production are also induced with fast kinetics, and the same effects are elicited with monoclonal antibodies (mAb) to these molecules. Recognition of target cells that express major histocompatibility complex (MHC) class I antigens can modulate both FcR-dependent and FcR-independent NK cell activation, indicating that common biochemical events are elicited in both cases.

Several distinct molecules possibly participate in the spontaneous NK cell recognition process that triggers NK cell functions and, in different combinations, these may transduce signals activating one or more of the pathways responsible for the net result of the stimulation. It therefore remains difficult in these conditions to dissect the relative participation of specific molecules and biochemical pathways to induce activation of NK cell functions. Study of the role of FcR in activation/inhibition of NK cell functions has provided a more defined model system in which to dissect the mechanisms by which functions of these cells can be mediated and regulated by external stimuli. Here the knowledge on the type(s) of FcR expressed on NK cells is reviewed, as well as the mechanisms of signal transduction operating upon ligand interaction and their modulation, and the possible role of these receptors on NK cells in vivo. Several reviews have addressed the genetic characterization of these molecules, and the reader is referred to these for more details (HULETT and HOGARTH 1997; RAVETCH and KINET 1991).

2 FcR Types Expressed in NK Cells

Receptors for each Ig class exist on human and rodent leukocytes (reviewed in HULETT and HOGARTH 1997; RAVETCH and KINET 1991). Only the low-affinity receptor for IgG defined as CD16, or FcγRIIIA, has been identified unambiguously, and characterized biochemically and genetically, on the majority of NK cells from several species: humans (SCALLON et al. 1989; SELVARAJ et al. 1989; LANIER et al. 1988, 1989; RAVETCH and PERUSSIA 1989), mouse (QIU et al. 1990; PERUSSIA et al. 1989), rat (FARBER et al. 1993), and pig (HALLORAN et al. 1994; DATO et al. 1992; ALLER et al. 1995; SWEENEY et al. 1996). In each of these its expression, concomitant with that of CD56 and with lack of expression of T cell [T cell receptor (TCR)/CD3 complex], B cell (sIg), and myeloid-specific differentiation antigens, serves to define NK cells, and reagents to it can be used to purify them to homogeneity. The existence of a minor NK cell subset not expressing the receptor has also been reported in humans (NAGLER et al. 1989). This subset, characteristically expressing the high-affinity receptor for interleukin (IL)-2 (CD25) constitutively, differs from the majority of NK cells in its greater proliferative response to this cytokine and lack of interferon (IFN)-γ expression. Although it had been proposed that this FcγR$^-$ subset corresponds to NK cells at an immature stage of (functional) differentiation, no definitive evidence for this has been reported.

The possibility that a minor subset of NK cells expresses FcγR types other than FcγRIIIA has been suggested by data indicating coexpression of CD32, detected with mAb IV.3 and 41H16, on about 5% of the CD16$^+$ or the CD56$^+$/CD3$^-$ cells in highly enriched NK cell populations, and by the ability of these mAb to mediate redirected ADCC in the same populations and to transduce signals resulting in the activation of biochemical pathway(s) that lead to Ca^{2+} mobilization (MATES et al. 1994). In humans at least three distinct genes encode this type of low-affinity FcγR (reviewed in HULETT and HOGARTH 1997) in myeloid and B cells. Those encoding them in NK cells await definition and, in the absence of data confirming these finding in NK cell clones and additional preparations of NK cells purified to homogeneity, the possibility is not excluded yet that the cells recognized by the mAb are cell types copurifying with NK cells and possibly expressing both CD16 at low density and CD56.

Functional data also indicate that treatment of resting NK cells and of plastic-adherent IL-2-activated, homogeneous NK cell preparations with IgM induces signal transduction events that, similar to those discussed below for the FcγRIIIA, result in Ca^{2+} mobilization (RABINOWICH et al. 1996), association of the IgM binding molecule with additional chains, and activation of protein tyrosine kinases (PRICOP et al. 1993). Unlike IgG binding, however, IgM binding induces downregulation of IFN-γ expression in NK cells (RABINOWICH et al. 1996). It has therefore been suggested that a receptor for the Fc portion of IgM is also expressed constitutively on the majority of NK cells, where in striking contrast with FcγR it would serve to inhibit rather than to activate at least one NK cell function. Biochemical and/or molecular identification of this receptor on either NK cells or other leukocyte types is lacking, and additional studies are required to define the possible significance of these finding.

No indication exists for the presence of receptors for other Ig isotypes (i.e., FcαR, FcεR, or FcδR), and because FcγRIIIA remains at present the only FcR type surely expressed on NK cells, only data on this receptor are discussed here.

3 FcγRIIIA

3.1 Distribution and Molecular Characterization

Although the FcγRIIIA is not a distinctive marker of NK cells, being present also in macrophages (PERUSSIA and RAVETCH 1991; KINDT et al. 1991; RAVETCH and PERUSSIA 1989), and a minor T cell subset (ZUPO et al. 1993; LANIER et al. 1985; UCIECHOWSKI et al. 1992), its expression in the absence of markers of other cell types serves to identify NK cells unambiguously within mononuclear cells from healthy individuals. FcγRIIIA are expressed at the cell membrane as hetero-oligomeric complexes in which distinct chains serve different functions. The ligand (IgG) binding α chain is an integral type I single membrane spanning glycoprotein of about 50–70 kDa (SELVARAJ et al. 1989; LANIER et al. 1988; FLEIT et al. 1982; PERUSSIA et al. 1983a,b; RAVETCH and PERUSSIA 1989) with a peptide backbone of about 33–34 kDa (LANIER et al. 1988; RAVETCH and PERUSSIA 1989) and molecular heterogeneity due primarily to N-linked glycosylation, as indicated also for the murine receptor (MELLMAN and UNKELESS 1980). The FcγRIIIA α chain belongs to the Ig superfamily of proteins and, as the other low-affinity FcγRII on myeloid and B cells, presents two Ig-like domains in its extracytoplasmic region (reviewed in HULETT and HOGARTH 1997; RAVETCH and KINET 1991). It comprises a 191 amino acid extracellular domain, a 21 amino acid transmembrane region, and a small (25 amino acid) intracytoplasmic domain. The extracellular domain of this chain is responsible for low affinity (approx. 2×10^7 M^{-1}) (VANCE et al. 1992) IgG binding. Its transmembrane domain contains a stretch of 8 amino acids (LFAVDTGL) that includes a negatively charged aspartic acid residue conserved not only between human and mouse, but also between the α chains of both FcγRIIIA and the high-affinity FcεRI (RA et al. 1989).

This has been shown necessary for the association of the α chain with disulfide dimers (see below) that are indispensable to allow the surface expression and signal transduction function of the receptor complex (ORLOFF et al. 1990). Although the α chain cytoplasmic tail is required neither for its membrane expression nor for its association with the dimers, its most membrane-proximal domain (the four amino acids at position 230–233) has been reported to participate, via a mechanism still to be elucidated, in the signal transduction mediated by the complex (HOU et al. 1996). Deletion of this domain results in significant inhibition of the earliest event that follows receptor occupancy, i.e., tyrosine phosphorylation of several substrates, including the two kinases ZAP-70 and syk that associate to the receptor complex upon IgG binding to NK cells (VIVIER et al. 1993; STAHLS et al. 1994) and macrophages (DARBY et al. 1994) and the increase in intracellular Ca^{2+} concentration ($[Ca^{2+}]_i$) induced upon receptor occupancy by either the ligand or specific mAb (CASSATELLA et al. 1989).

The two disulfide-linked single membrane spanning chains, associated to the α-chain noncovalently as homo- or heterodimers and indispensable for receptor expression and signal transduction, are represented by the ζ chain (VIVIER et al. 1992) and the γ chain (ALTIN et al. 1994; BONNEROT et al. 1992; MOINGEON et al. 1992), originally described as part of the TCR/CD3 and the FcεRI complexes on T and on mast cells and basophils, respectively (ORLOFF et al. 1990; BLANK et al. 1989). Also, the β subunit of rat FcεRI has been shown capable of associating with the transmembrane domain of murine FcγRIIIA (KUROSAKI et al. 1992). Receptors comprised of the three possible combinations of ζ and γ chain dimers, with prevalence of those containing γ-γ homodimers, are expressed on human NK cells (LETOURNEUR et al. 1991), whereas the FcγRIIIA complexes in mouse (RA et al. 1989; KUROSAKI and RAVETCH 1989), rat (FARBER et al. 1993), and pig (SWEENEY et al. 1996) have been demonstrated to contain only γ chain homodimers. This is unlike the glycosil-phosphatidyl-inositol linked FcγRIIIB isoform of the receptor, constituted only of the α-chain and described only in humans (QIU et al. 1990). However, a characteristic of the receptor on NK cells, shared with its glycosil-phosphatidyl-inositol anchored isoform on polymorphonuclear neutrophils (PMN), is the easiness with which it is cleaved from the cell membrane by endogenous metalloproteases (HARRISON et al. 1991; RAVETCH and PERUSSIA 1989). The significance of this and the possible function of the soluble receptor remain unclear.

A single mRNA species encodes FcγRIIIA in human and mouse NK cells (RAVETCH and PERUSSIA 1989; QIU et al. 1990). Instead, several isoforms of the FcγRIIIA α-chain have been described in rat (FARBER et al. 1993), the biological significance of which remains to be determined. The gene encoding the human (hu) and murine (mu) FcγRIIIA includes 5 exons, of approximately 8 kb: two exons encode the 5' UTR and leader sequence, and one exon each encode the transmembrane, the cytoplasmic domain, and the 3' UTR (QIU et al. 1990). This gene has been mapped to the human chromosome 1, region q23–24, which contains also the genes encoding the ligand binding chains for the other low-affinity FcγR type (FcγRII) and the high-affinity FcεRI (PELTZ et al. 1989; QIU et al. 1990). Using transgenic mice carrying a 5.8-kb stretch of the 5' flanking sequences of the IIIA and the IIIB genes, it has been shown that this region contains elements that confer the cell type specific expression of the two receptor types in NK cells/macrophages and PMN, respectively (LI et al. 1996). Two distinct promoters have been identified that control the initiation of the transcripts (GESSNER et al. 1996).

3.2 Ligand Binding Specificity

Human FcγRIIIA on NK cells bind IgG of several species. As with the hu FcγRIIIB on PMN, and likely due to the high degree of homology between the two receptors in their extracellular domain, the binding hierarchy of human IgG isotypes is IgG1=3>2=4 (DEHAAS et al. 1996). The same is true for murine IgG, among which IgG3 are preferentially bound (ANASETTI et al. 1987; KIPPS et al. 1985). Additionally, mouse FcγRIIIA bind mu IgE with low affinity (TAKIZAWA et al. 1992), possibly due to the high homology (95%) in the extracellular domains of the two molecules. FcγRIIIA complexes in which the ligand binding chain is associated with the β chain of FcεRI have been demonstrated only in mouse mast cells (KUROSAKI et al. 1992), but it is unknown whether these complexes can bind different IgG isotypes or mediate functions different from those of the predominant FcγRIIIA. The characteristic low binding affinity of the receptor is likely to result in the possibility of its triggering primarily upon immune complexes binding. However, specific and saturable binding of monomeric human IgG1 and IgG3 to the receptors on NK cells, but not on PMN, has been demonstrated (VANCE et al. 1993) as well as an expression polymorphism at this functional level corresponding to the ability of the NK cells to mediate ADCC to nonnucleated target cells (erythrocytes) (VANCE et al. 1993). This observation seems supported by additional functional data indicating the possibility that monomeric IgG binding to FcγRIIIA results in inhibition of spontaneous cytotoxicity (SULICA et al. 1993). The significance of this, however, remains difficult to determine because NK cells freshly separated from peripheral blood retain cytotoxic capability.

Several mAb (prototypes of which are 3G8, B73.1, VEP13, Leu11A and B) (PERUSSIA and TRINCHIERI 1984; PERUSSIA et al. 1983a,b, 1984; FLEIT et al. 1982) recognize CD16, and most inhibit IgG binding to the receptor. mAb specific for the FcγRIIIA isoform are not available, likely because antigenically dominant epitopes are present in the highly conserved sequences shared by the extracellular domains of the two isoforms of the molecule (FLEIT et al. 1992). The only reagent available for the mouse receptor (2.4G2) (UNKELESS 1979) cross-reacts with murine FcγRII. Those available in human cross-react with the α-chain extracellular domains of FcγRIIIB (FLEIT et al. 1992). The differential reactivity of one mAb, CLBGranII (WERNER et al. 1988) with PMN but not NK cells depends on the existence of a polymorphism (NA-1/NA2), present in the α-chain of the FcγRIIIB, that results in the expression of two differentially glycosylated molecules, both of which are expressed in PMN, and only one (NA2, recognized by mAb GRM-1 (HUIZINGA et al. 1997) in the NK cell FcγRIIIA (TROUNSTINE et al. 1990; RAVETCH and PERUSSIA 1989). An additional polymorphism, reported more recently at the level of the first Ig-like domain in the FcγRIIIA α-chain in the sequence encoding the epitope recognized by the mAb B73.1, depends on a leucine to histidine substitution at amino acid 48 (DEHAAS et al. 1996). These substitutions have been shown to affect the ligand binding function of the receptor. Receptors expressing 48H have been demonstrated to have a greater binding ability for human IgG1, G3, and G4 than those expressing the 48L substitution (DEHAAS et al. 1996). These data not only suggest the possibility of distinct functional effects of FcγR triggering upon binding of distinct IgG isotypes in NK cells from different donors but also imply that the first Ig-like domain influences IgG binding.

The exact position of the Ig-binding sequence of the FcγRIIIA is still to be determined precisely. A strongly hydrophobic region in the second Ig-like domain (the F-G loop) has been shown to be involved in binding, based on lack of IgG binding ability by receptors in which seven of the eight amino acids in this loop are substituted, and on the results of IgG binding studies performed with chimeric molecules lacking this domain (HIBBS et al. 1994). However, the same report demonstrates that amino acid substitutions in adjacent regions in the B-C loop also affect the binding, suggesting that, although the second Ig-like domain is critical for this function, sequences outside this domain are also likely to be involved. This conclusion is also supported by results of cross-competition experiments using mAb that inhibit IgG binding. Several of these mAb have been determined to react with sequences in the proximity of the F-G loop (likely the B-C or C'E loops) or of the putative C' β sheet of the proximal Ig-like domain, suggesting the involvement of additional residues (TAMM and SCHMIDT 1996).

3.3 Signal Transduction

The earliest event following FcγRIIIA occupancy is represented by the induced phosphorylation on tyrosine residues of several molecules, analogous to what is observed upon occupancy of other immune cell receptors that have a molecular structure similar to that of the FcγRIIIA (i.e., TCD/CD3, sIg/B cell complex, FcεR) (for reviews see CHAN et al. 1994; HULETT and HOGARTH 1997), and most of the defined pathways of activation for these types of receptors are similar (for a review, see WEISS and LITTMAN 1994). Neither the α ligand binding chain of the receptor nor the associated dimers have intrinsic tyrosine kinase activity, and the intracytoplasmic domain of the ligand binding chain itself does not contain sequences with signal transduction motifs. Instead, conserved YXXL sequences defined as immune receptor tyrosine-based associated motifs (ITAM) (reviewed in RETH 1989; CAMBIER 1995), are present, regularly spaced, in the intracytoplasmic domain of the associated ζ and γ chain dimers, which contain, respectively, 3 and 1 of these motifs. These serve to dock to the receptor complex a protein tyrosine kinase (PTK) of the *src* family ($p56^{lck}$ in NK cells) (CONE et al. 1993; SALCEDO et al. 1993a,b). This kinase is constitutively associated in an inactive form to the receptor, and coprecipitates with the FcγRIIIA complex independently of its stimulation (SALCEDO et al. 1993b). Following ligand binding and receptor dimerization, phosphorylation occurs of the tyrosines in the ITAM in the ζ and γ chains (VIVIER et al. 1992; O'SHEA et al. 1991). This leads to phosphorylation on tyrosine residues and consequent enzymatic activation of $p56^{lck}$ (BONNEROT et al. 1992; PIGNATA et al. 1993; SALCEDO et al. 1993a,b; AZZONI et al. 1992) and to the recruitment to the receptor complex and activation of the syk family kinases ZAP-70 (VIVIER et al. 1993) and syk (STAHLS et al. 1994).

In addition to the associated dimers, several molecules are detected in NK cells after FcγRIIIA stimulation with immune complexes or anti-CD16 mAb that mimic the ligand that are either phosphorylated on tyrosine residues and as a consequence become activated in their enzymatic activity and/or are associated to the phosphotyrosine immunoprecipitates from the same but not from control nonstimulated cells. Among the former are both isoforms of phospholipase (PL) C γ1 and γ2 expressed in NK cells (AZZONI et al. 1992; TING et al. 1992a,b). Their activation has been shown to depend on activation of PTK independently of G protein activation (TING et al. 1991), supporting the notion that FcγRIIIA are not G protein coupled receptors. PLC-γ is responsible for the hydrolysis of phosphoinositides and the consequent increases in the $[Ca^{2+}]_i$. Transient $[Ca^{2+}]_i$ increases depend on Ca^{2+} mobilization from intracellular stores, but sustained intracellular Ca^{2+} levels are maintained for long periods of time following receptor stimulation depending on Ca^{2+} entrance from the extracellular compartment (CASSATELLA et al. 1989). It is interesting to note that most of the early biochemical events described above are also induced in the case of NK cell interaction with antibody-nonsensitized target cells. However, the kinases involved in this case have not been identified, and ζ phosphorylation is not detectable (VIVIER et al. 1991), excluding association of this chain to the putative receptor(s)/molecules involved.

Following IgG immune complexes binding to NK cells, and similar to what happens upon stimulation of the other two transmembrane FcγR types on myeloid cells (FcγRI and FcγRII), MAP kinases are detected phosphorylated and activated in their enzymatic activity in intact cells (TROTTA et al. 1996). The possibility that their activation is related, as in other receptor systems, to activation of the GTP/GDP exchange protein encoded by the *ras* proto-oncogene is supported by the observation that accumulation of the GTP-bound form of *ras* occurs transiently in NK cells under the same conditions of stimulation (GALANDRINI et al. 1996). Additionally, data in the same report indicate that both the p52 and the p46 forms of the oncoprotein Shc are phosphorylated upon FcγRIIIA occupancy, and that Shc immunoprecipitates from the FcγRIIIA-stimulated NK cells also contain the src homology (SH) 2/SH3 domain-containing Grb2 and an undefined 145-kDa phosphoprotein. Conversely, in addition to Shc, a tyrosine phosphoprotein of 36 kDa (p36) possibly constituting the intermediary allowing Grb2/Shc association, is associated, to the Grb2 SH2 domain, as demonstrated in in vitro binding assays performed with GST-Shc fusion proteins. Although a direct link between *ras* activation and activation of these proteins has not been established, it is well known that the same types of complexes participate to the activation of *ras*.

To further support this notion, the proto-oncogene Vav has also been reported to become phosphorylated upon FcγRIIIA stimulation and to be associated with a 70-kDa protein, the identity of which is unknown (Xu and Chong 1996). Based on the appearance of a 58-kDa molecule phosphorylated on serine and threonine residues in kinase assays performed on Vav immunoprecipitates from stimulated cells, it has also been proposed that an unidentified serine/threonine kinase is associated with the complex. The activity of this kinase, however, is not increased upon receptor occupancy (Xu and Chong 1996). The ability of FcγRIIIA to induce biochemical pathways resulting in Vav phosphorylation has been confirmed in macrophages (Darby et al. 1994). By analogy with this system, in which the 70-kDa syk non-src kinase becomes activated upon receptor occupancy, it may be proposed that the unidentified p70 protein discussed above corresponds to this kinase.

Within the phosphotyrosine immune precipitates from FcγRIIIA-stimulated NK cells, but not in those from control cells, is included also the phosphoinositide 3 (PI-3) kinase (Kanakaraj et al. 1994), whose enzymatic activity is also activated (Bonnema et al. 1994; Kanakaraj et al. 1994). Unlike the case of the molecules described above, neither of the two chains composing PI-3 kinase is phosphorylated upon FcγRIIIA stimulation; therefore association of the kinase to other proteins phosphorylated upon receptor occupancy is sufficient in this receptor system to activate its kinase activity. The specific PI-3 kinase-induced phosphoinositide products, i.e., inositol species phosphorylated in the D3 position of the inositol ring, have not been detected at significantly increased levels in primary NK cells after FcγRIIIA stimulation (Kanakaraj et al. 1994). However, it is possible that these results depend on insufficient sensitivity of the available techniques to detect transient increases of these products in primary cells, and such products have been clearly documented in T cell lines expressing a transfected FcγRIIIA α chain in association with either γ or ζ homodimers (Kanakaraj et al. 1994), confirming that FcγRIIIA stimulation is capable of inducing PI-3 kinase activation, and indicating that both types of receptor complexes expressed in NK cells can mediate it.

The observations discussed above clearly point to a primary role of PTK activation in the signals originated from FcγRIIIA but also indicate that the downstream signaling events regulated by these kinases are complex and involve yet unidentified serine/threonine kinases. Whether each of the proteins detected phosphorylated upon receptor occupancy is actually recruited to the complex and plays a significant role in signal transduction, or whether phosphorylation of at least some of them depends on some bystander effect remains to be resolved. However, the role of some of the different pathways described above in eliciting specific NK cell functions has been elucidated at least in part, and the data available are reviewed in the next section.

4 Functional Effects of Immune Complex–FcγRIIIA Interaction

4.1 FcγRIIIA Expression and Modulation

Binding of immune complexes (PERUSSIA et al. 1979) and anti-FcγRIIIA mAb (PERUSSIA et al. 1983a) and direct activation of protein kinase C (PKC) as that induced with TPA (TRINCHIERI et al. 1984) result in downmodulation of the receptor from the NK cell membrane. This may play a role in releasing the target cells from the receptor and in terminating the signal transduction events that follow receptor occupancy. Studies performed on the supernatants from NK cells treated with radiolabeled anti-FcγRIII mAb have demonstrated that the mAb can be recovered intact in the supernatants from cells treated with monomeric mAb, but that its molecular mass in those from cells on which the mAb has been cross-linked with a second anti-mouse reagent is indicative of its digestion (PERUSSIA and TRINCHIERI 1988). This supports likely internalization and subsequent intracellular digestion of the mAb, and it strongly suggests that the receptor becomes internalized and possibly degraded rather than recycled directly and intact to the cell membrane. In support of this contention, the kinetics of reappearance of the receptor at the cell membrane following downmodulation induced upon immune complexes binding is extremely slow (PERUSSIA et al. 1979).

The above data indicate the possibility that the fate of the receptor depends on the type of ligands and predominant pathways elicited by them and possibly on the time of duration or involvement of different receptor numbers in the receptor-ligand interaction. This is also supported by the observations that inhibitors of Zn^{2+}-dependent metalloproteases can inhibit the spontaneous and the TPA-induced shedding of the receptors, induced in a PKC-dependent fashion (BORREGO et al. 1994), but not the ligand-induced receptor downmodulation, and that both inhibitors of PTK and an inhibitor of PKC that inhibits TPA-induced downmodulation behave similarly (BORREGO et al. 1994). Therefore only downmodulation of the receptor resulting from its shedding (as the spontaneous or the TPA-induced) occur in a PKC-dependent way whereas other undefined, but neither PTK- nor PKC-dependent, pathways are responsible for the downmodulation related to receptor internalization following ligand binding. As indicated below, this is in contrast with the essential role played by PTK to trigger other functional effects.

Increased or induced expression of the receptor has been documented following IFN-γ (WEISHANK et al. 1988) or platelet-derived growth factor stimulation on macrophages (PHILLIPS et al. 1991), but neither effect has been observed in NK cells, and it remains to be determined whether increased receptor expression corresponds to increased function.

4.2 NK Cell Mediated Cytotoxicity

It has been suggested that IgG ligands and antibodies to the receptor exert either inhibitory or stimulatory effects on cytotoxicity, and it has been proposed that IgG inhibit spontaneous cytotoxicity when bound to the receptor in monomeric form, whereas bivalent soluble mAb is able not only to induce it but also to reverse the inhibitory effect of the IgG in some individuals (defined as responders) (GALATIUC et al. 1995). The molecular basis for this are unknown. Based on data indicating activation of distinct biochemical pathways or distinct kinetics of activation of the same pathways in NK cells stimulated with monomeric or dimeric IgG depending on whether they are cross-linked at the cell membrane, it has been proposed that various agonists induce distinct substrates that in turn mediate distinct functional effects. Specifically, a particularly strong phosphorylation of $p56^{lck}$ has been associated with the inhibitory effect of monomeric IgG upon cross-linking (MANCIULEA et al. 1996). These data, however, are very difficult to reconcile with the lack of definite indication that FcγRIII is involved in spontaneous cytotoxicity, based on the observation that antibodies to the receptor do not inhibit it.

Although the exact sequence of events leading to ADCC or to FcγR-dependent modulation of spontaneous cytotoxicity is still unclear, a better understanding of the involvement of FcγRIII in cytotoxicity derives from studies performed to determine how its stimulation affects known modes of cell-mediated cytotoxicity and the expression of its mediators. Analogous to the interaction with nonsensitized target cells, interaction of NK cells with IgG immune complexes induces exocytosis/degranulation (TING et al. 1992b). The "granule exocytosis model" has been proposed as one of the modes of lymphocyte-mediated cytolysis (reviewed in YOUNG and COHN 1986; HENKART 1985). According to this model, preformed cytotoxic molecules contained in the cytoplasmic granules (e.g., perforin and granzymes) are discharged in the area of contact between the target and the effector cells and variably participate to mediate NK cell dependent cytotoxicity. The model implies a Ca^{2+}-dependent step needed in order for perforin to insert pores in the target cell membrane and allow intracellular discharge of other cytotoxic molecules (PODACK et al. 1985). FcγRIIIA stimulation induces degranulation, as indicated by the induced secretion of serine esterases (BONNEMA et al. 1994).

The observation that NK cells are unable to mediate spontaneous cytotoxicity after binding of immune complexes (PERUSSIA et al. 1979; SULICA et al. 1993) likely depends at least in part on induced depletion of these proteins, as also suggested by the reverse observation that the cells are unable of mediating ADCC despite conserved functional FcγR expression after interaction with NK-sensitive target cells (PERUSSIA and TRINCHIERI 1981). Degranulation occurs also upon stimulation of NK cells with phorbol-diesters (TPA) (BONNEMA et al. 1994), and triggering of both spontaneous cytotoxicity and degranulation follows PKC activation induced by this chemical, which instead inhibits ADCC due at least in part to the induced shedding of FcγRIIIA (TRINCHIERI et al. 1984).

The role played in this type of cytotoxicity by the different biochemical pathways induced upon FcγRIIIA stimulation has been analyzed using chemical inhibitors. When NK cells are pretreated with PTK inhibitors, both ADCC and spontaneous cytotoxicity are abolished (O'SHEA et al. 1992). This observation confirms the essential role of receptor-mediated tyrosine phosphorylation as a proximal signal-transducing event not only needed for cytotoxicity/degranulation to occur but also shared by FcγR and the other undefined receptor molecules involved in target cell recognition. However, using inhibitors that affect events specifically related to activation of distinct second messengers without inhibiting this initial activation step, it has been possible to determine that the pathways responsible for triggering cytotoxicity in the two conditions are distinct. Wortmannin is a fungal metabolite that specifically inhibits PI-3 kinase activity (YANO et al. 1993). Pretreatment of NK cells with this compound does not prevent the more proximal events in FcγRIIIA-dependent signal transduction (i.e., tyrosine phosphorylation and increased $[Ca^{2+}]_i$) and does not result in nonspecific toxicity to NK cells (Kanakaraj et al., unpublished observation). Both degranulation and cytotoxicity triggered via FcγRIIIA, but not those triggered upon binding-recognition of target cells or TPA stimulation, are inhibited by wortmannin (BONNEMA et al. 1994), indicating that the PI-3 kinase dependent and PKC-independent pathways are predominant in ADCC, and that distinct pathways, PI-3 kinase independent and PKC-dependent, are predominant in triggering spontaneous cytotoxicity. PI-3 kinase has been shown to regulate degranulation in other cell systems, and it is likely that its participation in ADCC reflects this function. How this occurs upon FcγRIIIA occupancy, and which events are instead triggered to allow FcγRIIIA-independent degranulation remain to be investigated. Wortmannin has been used extensively in other systems to inhibit PLD activation induced by several stimuli, and PLD is one of the enzymes activated upon stimulation via FcγRIIIA and via another molecule (CD94) (BALBOA et al. 1992) also reported to trigger cytotoxicity. If activation of PLD in these conditions is sensitive to wortmannin, one may envisage that this enzyme represents one of the substrates utilized by PI-3 kinase in the NK cell degranulation events induced upon immune complexes binding.

Because granzymes and perforin play a role in the exocytosis-dependent cytotoxicity, several studies have also addressed the question of whether expression of these proteins is regulated by stimuli, including IgG immune complexes, that trigger it. Most data indicate that expression of the mRNA encoding these molecules is not decreased upon receptor occupancy, excluding that the decreased spontaneous cytotoxicity observed in immune complex pretreated NK cells (PERUSSIA et al. 1979) depends on receptor-induced suppression of their production. Rather, FcγRIIIA stimulation has been shown to induce accumulation of mRNA encoding some of these cytotoxic molecules, specifically perforin and granzyme B (SALCEDO et al. 1993a). Given that the kinetics of cell-mediated cytotoxicity is faster than that with which mRNA accumulation for these molecules is induced upon receptor occupancy, it is unlikely that the latter effect participates in the immediate cytotoxicity that follows receptor occupancy. Rather, induced production of these molecules may be important to restore efficient levels of these mediators after depletion, thus allowing a faster regeneration of NK cell cytotoxic functions. Although this may not be the sole mechanism operating, the observation that incomplete downmodulation of these functions follows stimulation of the cells with CD16 ligands and cytokines (e.g., IL-2, unpublished data) that synergize in this effect (SALCEDO et al. 1993a) supports the possibility that this effect may be involved, at least in part.

In addition to the Ca^{2+}-dependent degranulation process described above, spontaneous cytotoxicity and ADCC can be mediated via a mechanism involving Fas/Fas ligand interaction, when Fas-sensitive target cells are recognized by human (MONTEL et al. 1995) or murine NK cells (ARASE et al. 1995). This has been clearly confirmed by the observation that NK cells from perforin (WALSH et al. 1994; KAGI et al. 1994) and granzyme A (EBNET et al. 1995) deficient mice can induce DNA fragmentation (indicative of apoptotic cell death) in tumor targets. In order to mediate Fas-dependent cytotoxicity the effector cells need to express Fas ligand. Although murine NK cells have been reported to express Fas ligand constitutively (ARASE et al. 1995), human NK cells do not, strongly suggesting target-inducible but not constitutive expression. Clearly supporting this possibility is the demonstration that Fas ligand is induced on human NK cells upon FcγRIIIA stimulation, and that killing of Fas^+ target cells can be inhibited by anti-Fas mAb only when FcγR-stimulated NK cells are used as effectors (EISCHEN et al. 1996). The biochemical mechanisms responsible for the FcγRIIIA-induced Fas ligand expression are unknown at present, and it remains to be established whether all or only specific NK cell subsets are capable of mediating this type of cytotoxicity.

4.3 Activation of Non-cytotoxic Functions

Concomitant with the proximal signal transduction events triggering immediate functions that depend at least in part on induced exocytosis of preformed molecules, second messengers are activated upon FcγRIIIA occupancy, which control later functional effects regulating at both transcriptional and posttranscriptional levels the expression of genes encoding cytokines (ANEGON et al. 1988), proto-oncogenes (c-*fos*) (TROTTA et al. 1996), or receptor molecules such as IL-2Rα, CD25 (CASSATELLA et al. 1989; ANEGON et al. 1988), CD69 (BORREGO et al. 1993), Fas ligand (EISCHEN et al. 1996), VLA-6 (GISMONDI et al. 1992) relevant to the biology of NK cells.

Several cytokines, the best characterized of which are IFN-γ, tumor necrosis factor (TNF)-α, and granulocyte-macrophage colony-stimulating factor (GM-CSF) (CUTURI et al. 1989; ANEGON et al. 1988), are produced within 12–18 h after stimulation of peripheral blood NK cells with FcγR ligands, and with faster kinetics in cultured NK cells, and distinct cytokines (IL-2 and IL-12) synergize with the ligands to induce this effect (ANEGON et al. 1988). None of the produced cytokines has been shown to be released from preformed stores in NK cells, and it is clear that actual transcription of both IFN-γ and TNF-α mRNA occurs within 20 min after stimulation of FcγRIIIA (ANEGON et al. 1988). Although FcγRIIIA and the stimulatory cytokines have no significant synergistic effect at the transcriptional level (CASSATELLA et al. 1989; ANEGON et al. 1988), signals transduced by FcγRIIIA and IL-2R synergize to stabilize the mRNA of both produced cytokines, explaining at least in part the observed synergy at the protein level, which likely depends on the induction of distinct mechanisms by the two stimuli.

Only FcγRIIIA stimulation results in increased $[Ca^{2+}]_i$ (ANEGON et al. 1988), and only the FcγRIIIA -induced transcription of both cytokines strictly depends on the increased $[Ca^{2+}]_i$ following extracellular Ca^{2+} entrance in the cells, whereas extracellular Ca^{2+} chelation does not prevent cytokine transcription induced by IL-2 or IL-12 (CASSATELLA et al. 1989). Because in these conditions both $[Ca^{2+}]_i$ increases from mobilization of intracellular stores and phosphoinositide hydrolysis are preserved (unpublished data), it is likely that the signal transduction pathways involving FcγRIIIA-induced PLC-γ activation per se are insufficient to mediate this effect, and that for most part receptor-induced cytokine expression depends on sustained increases of $[Ca^{2+}]_i$. The participation of a PTK-dependent mechanism in the FcγRIIIA-induced cytokine production has been documented, and lack of IFN-γ production is observed in NK cells pretreated with PTK inhibitors (O'SHEA et al. 1992), underscoring that tyrosine-induced phosphorylation is the earliest event following FcγR occupancy and is essential to most NK cell functions.

The observation that FcγRIIIA-induced cytokine production is independent of de novo protein synthesis (ARAMBURU et al. 1995; ANEGON et al. 1988) and is inhibited by cyclosporin A (ARAMBURU et al. 1995), suggested that Ca^{2+}-sensitive preformed elements in NK cells arc activated upon receptor stimulation to allow gene transcription, as it is the case for CD3/TCR-induced transcription of IL-2 in T cells. Evidence has been presented that the nuclear factor of activated T cells (NFATp) (MCCAFFREY et al. 1993) is constitutively expressed in NK cells and translocates to the nucleus upon FcγRIIIA but not upon IL-2 treatment (ARAMBURU et al. 1995). Nuclear extracts from NK cells stimulated with immune complexes bind oligonucleotide sequences corresponding to NFAT-binding sequences in the TNF-α and GM-CSF/IL-3 promoters, and NFATp can be detected with specific antibody in the complexes. This study demonstrated expression of a second NFAT (NFATc) inducible later (within 2 h), but no indication was obtained that this form is used by NK cells, unlike the case in CD3-stimulated T cell lines. These data support the notion that NFATp is utilized by NK cells as a transcription factor in the FcγRIIIA-induced transcription of TNF-α and GM-CSF. Information on the regulation of other cytokines is limited.

Of the kinases activated upon FcγRIIIA occupancy, PI-3 kinase plays a major role in the induced cytokine production, as indicated by the almost complete inhibition of IFN-γ production in NK cells pretreated with inhibitors of this kinase (KANAKARAJ et al., submitted). The participation of other molecules has also been analyzed. TROTTA et al. (1996) have shown that inhibition of MAP kinase, induced upon ligand binding to any of the three transmembrane activatory FcγR on leukocytes, results in the inhibition of TNF-α induced production in NK cells, and more recent evidence indicates that in FcγRIIIA-stimulated NK cells a predominant PI-3 kinase dependent pathway is responsible for the MAP kinase-dependent induction of cytokine production (including IFN-γ). FcγRIIIA-induced MAP kinase activation is almost completely abolished in wortmannin-pretreated cells, and cytokine production is inhibited to the same extent by either PI-3 kinase or MAP kinase inhibitors, with no additional inhibition observed in cells pretreated with either type of inhibitors. Whether the minimal residual cytokine expression in these conditions actually depends on alternative and yet undefined pathways remains to be investigated.

Unlike the case for cytokines, the mechanisms leading to receptor-induced expression of surface activation antigens or of proto-oncogenes have been elucidated only in part. As in the case for cytokines, FcγRIIIA-induced c-*fos* expression is abolished completely in NK cells pretreated with either MAP-kinase kinase inhibitors or wortmannin (P. KANAKARAJ et al., submitted), indicating that the PI-3 kinase dependent MAP kinase activation represents the predominant pathway involved also in receptor-induced expression of proto-oncogenes, and that in the signal transduction pathway activated upon FcγRIIIA occupancy MAP kinases act downstream of PI-3 kinase and may participate in the activation of DNA binding factors in the promoter for the genes discussed above. However, our preliminary data indicate that wortmannin is ineffective in preventing FcγRIIIA-dependent MAP kinase activation and c-*fos* expression in T cell lines expressing the transfected ligand binding α-chain of the receptor. Therefore it is likely that, although both PI-3 kinase dependent and independent pathways can be induced upon receptor occupancy, additional NK cell specific factors operate to regulate expression of the same genes in NK and T cells.

4.4 NK Cell Survival and Proliferation

In T cells TCR/CD3 engagement results in proliferation as a consequence at least in part of induced IL-2 production and membrane expression of IL-2R (reviewed in CHAN et al. 1994). In NK cells FcγRIIIA occupancy induces transcription of the α-chain of the IL-2R, resulting in membrane expression of CD25 (ANEGON et al. 1988). Unlike cytokine transcription and production, this is not prevented in cells pretreated with Ca^{2+} chelators (CASSATELLA et al. 1989), reflecting the existence of distinct requirements for the FcγRIIIA-dependent expression of this gene and possibly the participation of biochemical pathways different, at least in part, from those involved in cytokine production. Data from several laboratories have excluded that FcγR stimulation results in proliferation of NK cells. This is likely because within the cytokines produced by NK cells none is included that can sustain their survival or proliferation in an autocrine fashion.

Rather, evidence has accumulated that FcγR ligand binding induces NK cell death by apoptosis, provided the cells have been preactivated by cytokines, primarily IL-2, IL-12 (ORTALDO et al. 1995; AZZONI et al. 1995), and IL-15 (ORTALDO et al. 1997, and our unpublished data). The mechanisms leading to this effect are poorly understood. An indirect effect due to induced production of inhibitory cytokines upon receptor occupancy has been excluded, based on lack of inhibition of receptor-induced apoptosis in the presence of neutralizing antibodies to IFN-γ and TNF-α (AZZONI et al. 1995) or to TNF-receptor or Fas (ORTALDO et al. 1997) and on the independence of this phenomenon from RNA synthesis (AZZONI et al. 1995), which instead is needed for cytokine production (ARAMBURU et al. 1995; ANEGON et al. 1988). As discussed above, FcγRIIIA occupancy induces Fas ligand expression on NK cells (EISCHEN et al. 1996), and interaction of Fas ligand with their Fas receptor constitutively expressed on the same cells can result in autocrine or paracrine cell death (EISCHEN et al. 1996). Whether the Fas ligand is functional in all or only a subset of NK cells, and whether the same subset(s) can undergo both FcγRIII-A and Fas-dependent apoptosis is still to be elucidated.

The reasons why only previously activated NK cells undergo FcγR-induced apoptosis remains unresolved. Based on the inhibition of receptor-induced apoptosis in cells treated with c-*myc* antisense oligodeoxynucleotides, it is proposed that the sustained c-*myc* expression (AZZONI et al. 1995), as observed in cytokine-treated NK cells, represents one prerequisite (of possibly several). The possible significance of this observation to the biology of NK cells remains hypothetical. Given the need for preactivation and presence of immune complexes to stimulate FcR, FcγRIIIA-induced apoptosis is not expected to affect NK cells at the beginning of an immune response, but it may play a role in controlling NK cell proliferation later during a humoral immune response, in which proliferation of activated NK cells may be detrimental.

5 Stimuli Affecting FcγRIIIA-Dependent NK Cell Activation

The level of NK cells' response to their targets depends on the effects of a combination of stimuli, some of which are activatory, such as those discussed above resulting from FcγRIIIA stimulation or spontaneous recognition of target cells lacking MHC class I antigens, while others are inhibitory. Signals resulting in inhibition of both spontaneous cytotoxicity and ADCC can be elicited in NK cells, provided they express surface receptors, defined as killer inhibitory receptors (KIR), capable of recognizing MHC class I antigens (reviewed in LEIBSON 1995; RAULET and HELD 1995; LANIER and PHILLIPS 1995; LJUNGGREN and KARRE 1990; MORETTA et al. 1994). This occurs either when target cells expressing the appropriate MHC are recognized, or when the NK cells are simultaneously stimulated with anti-KIR mAb. Although the nature of the inhibitory signals transduced by the KIR are not well defined, it has been reported that the cytoplasmic domain of these molecules contain the amino acid sequence D/E(x2)YxxL(x)26YxxL which, based on its similarity with the ITAM discussed above, has been defined as the immune receptor tyrosine-based inhibitory motif (ITIM) (MUTA et al. 1994; AMIGORENA et al. 1992). Phosphorylation of the tyrosine residues of this motif both in KIR (FRY et al. 1996) and in other receptors, namely the FcγRIIB on B cells, results in association in vitro with Src homology 2 (SH2) domain containing proteins. The possibility of the association of the FcγRIIB ITIM with both the SHP-1 (PTP-1C) tyrosine phosphatase (D'AMBROSIO et al. 1995) and the inositol phosphatase SHIP (ONO et al. 1996) has been reported. At present only SHP-1 has been shown to be recruited to the KIR ITIM (FRY et al. 1996; BURSHTYN et al. 1996; CAMPBELL et al. 1996).

KIR engagement has been demonstrated to prevent target cell-induced phosphatidyl inositol hydrolysis and increased $[Ca^{2+}]_i$ (KAUFMAN et al. 1993), suggesting that the mechanisms involved in inhibition may affect the earliest events transduced upon target cell recognition. In a recent report BINSTADT et al. (1996) have analyzed the effect of KIR ligation on FcγRIIIA stimulation. They demonstrate conclusively that (a) upon cross-linking of the molecule itself phosphorylation of KIR is neither induced nor abolished upon FcγRIIIA stimulation, (b) overexpression of the *src* family kinase *lck* but not of *fyn* results in increased phosphorylation of the KIR, indicating that the catalytic activity of this kinase is necessary for KIR tyrosine phosphorylation, (c) KIR engagement reduces without abolishing the number of tyrosine-phosphorylated proteins detectable in FcγRIIIA-stimulated NK cells, specifically inhibiting tyrosine-induced phosphorylation of the receptor-associated ζ chain, ZAP-70 kinase, and PLC-γ and also resulting in inhibition of the FcR-induced phosphatidyl inositol hydrolysis and Ca^{2+} mobilization, and (d) overexpression of the SHP-1 phosphatase enhances the KIR-induced inhibition of ADCC. This, together with the tyrosine phosphorylation of ZAP-70, ζ chain, and PLC-γ, was reversed in the same NK cell clones overexpressing a catalytically inactive variant of the kinase. These data clearly indicate that very early signal transduction events in the FcγRIIIA pathway are interrupted via mechanisms that are still to be elucidated when interaction of FcγRIIIA with its specific ligand occurs simultaneously to the interaction between KIR and their MHC targets. The data support a model in which $p56^{lck}$-dependent phosphorylation of KIR results in recruitment of SHP-1 and consequent SHP-1-mediated inhibition of very proximal PTK-dependent signals originated from receptor occupancy.

The basis for the inhibition of ADCC therefore seems to involve the same phosphatase responsible for the KIR-dependent inhibition of the pathways elicited upon triggering spontaneous cytotoxicity (CAMPBELL et al. 1996). The specific substrates involved remain to be determined. It is also interesting to note that the molecule responsible for the KIR-dependent inhibition of both ADCC and spontaneous cytotoxicity is distinct from the SHIP inositol phosphatase shown to be involved in intact cells in the FcγRIIB-dependent inhibition of functions of several other cell types upon engagement of receptors that have a molecular structure similar to that of FcγRIIIA (ONO et al. 1996). Specifically, simultaneous stimulation of FcγRIIB results in SHIP-dependent inhibition of the sIg-induced stimulation of B cells or the release of pharmacological mediators from mast cells upon FcεRI engagement (ONO et al. 1996). In these cases more distal or distinct signaling events are inhibited, and only extracellular Ca^{2+} entrance, but neither Ca^{2+} mobilization from intracellular stores nor phosphatidyl inositol hydrolysis, is abolished (for a recent review on this topic see SCHARENBERG and KINET 1996). Given the similarities in the molecular complexes constituting the immune receptor family of which FcγRIIIA is a member and those in the signal transduction pathways elicited by them, and notwithstanding the differences discussed here between the mechanisms involved in spontaneous and FcγRIIIA-triggered NK cell activation, it is reasonable to speculate that the distinct (ITIM or other undefined) sequences in the KIR and FcγRIIB play a role in preferentially associating SHP-1 and SHIP or are involved in inhibition of distinct functions. Also, the additional possibility is not excluded that molecules are expressed in NK cells that influence the intermolecular interactions of the KIR. In this respect it will be interesting to analyze whether FcγRIIB artificially introduced in NK cells can inhibit FcγRIIIA-dependent functions, and if so, by which mechanism, and whether yet undefined molecules with KIR activity can interact with SHIP in NK cells. KIR-dependent modulation of FcγRIIIA-induced noncytotoxic functions of NK cells also remains to be analyzed.

6 Expression and Role of FcγRIIIA During NK Cell Differentiation

By analogy with the myeloid system, in which the FcγRIIIB has been demonstrated to appear at late stages of differentiation (FLEIT et al. 1984), and with the monocyte lineage, where FcγRIIIA appears to be expressed at significant detectable levels only at the stage of differentiated or activated macrophages, it is likely that also in NK cells this receptor represents a late differentiation marker. In vitro data in the human system seem to support this possibility. Unlike the majority of peripheral blood mature NK cells, only a minor proportion of those generated in any of the culture conditions analyzed for the differentiation of human NK cell progenitors from bone marrow or cord blood express FcγRIIIA at low density (BENNETT et al. 1996). However, it cannot be excluded that the lack of expression depends on in vitro artifacts (e.g., lack of supportive factors in the culture conditions analyzed) and does not reflect the in vivo situation, and a better definition of the process of NK cell differentiation is needed to determine definitely the stage of differentiation at which the receptors appear on NK cells.

Whether FcγRIIIA expression plays any role in NK cell development is also matter of speculation. Data in the mouse have indicated that a population of 14.5-day fetal thymocytes (RODEWALD et al. 1992) and fetal liver (MOINGEON et al. 1993), the majority of which express FcγRII/III, contains progenitors for both T cells and NK cells, but definitive confirmation that the $FcγRIII^+$ cells can differentiate to NK cells has not been presented. Recent evidence that in FcεRI γ chain transgenic mice the NK cell compartment is defective (FLAMAND et al. 1996) suggests the possibility that molecules which associate with this chain in NK cells play a role in their development. Although FcγRIIIA may be included among these, functional NK cells develop normally, as defined based on the ability of peripheral NK cells to mediate spontaneous cytotoxicity and to proliferate in response to cytokines. This is the case both in mice unable to express this receptor due to lack of the associated γ chain necessary for membrane expression (TAKAI et al. 1994) and in those lacking its ligand binding α chain (HAZENBOS et al. 1996), making this possibility unlikely. Additionally, Ig are not present under physiological conditions in primary lymphoid organs, including the bone marrow, likely site of NK cell differentiation. Therefore the nature of the ligand that would interact with a putative FcγRIII on NK cell progenitors to affect their differentiation remains unclear, and it can be assumed that, if present on immature progenitors, FcγRIIIA should bind yet to be identified molecules different from Ig.

No clinical conditions have been demonstrated in which NK cell functions are impaired because of specific lack of FcγRIIIA expression. However, cases have been reported of patients in which inefficient NK cell cytotoxic functions are correlated with normal numbers of NK cells expressing antigenically altered FcγRIIIA, suggesting the possibility that altered FcR expression in vivo influences NK cell activity/functional development. One patient presented with decreased numbers of $CD56^+$ cells and lack of expression of the FcγRIIIA epitope recognized by mAb B73.1 (JAWAR et al. 1996). The NK cells had reduced spontaneous cytotoxicity but normal levels of ADCC in vitro, and the clinical manifestations included recurrent herpes virus infections. Another patient suffered recurrent viral infections of the respiratory tract, and severe clinical manifestations following Epstein-Barr virus and varicella zoster infections (DeVries et al. 1996), similar to those reported in cases of NK cell deficiency (Biron et al. 1989). In this case the absolute number of ($CD7^+/CD3^-$) NK cells was within the normal range but, as in the former case, their NK cells FcγRIIIA did not react with the anti-CD16 mAb B73.1, being instead FcγRIIIB expressed and functional on PMN.

Based on the combined observations in mouse and humans, it is questionable that expression of FcγRIIIA plays a critical role for NK cell development/functions in vivo. However, this does not exclude the possibility that absence or abnormality of FcγRIIIA on NK cells (or other leukocyte subsets), although compatible with life under physiological conditions, influences the ability of NK cells to mediate antiviral functions in vivo.

7 Therapeutic Approaches Targeting NK Cell FcγRIIIA

NK cells have been proposed to play a role in immunosurveillance (see for a review Trinchieri 1989). Since the identification of the KIR molecules on these cells, the hypothesis that NK cells participate in controlling metastatic tumor growth has become appealing, and it can be proposed that tumor cells expressing significantly decreased MHC class I antigens are targets for NK cell recognition and cytotoxicity. Although adoptive immunotherapy with lymphokine-activated killer cells, comprising for the most part NK cells, has failed to produce significant therapeutic effects (reviewed in Trinchieri 1989), the possibility of exploiting the activatory role of FcγRIIIA on these cells specifically to redirect their killing activity to tumor targets has met with some success. The development of bispecific monoclonal antibodies recognizing simultaneously both FcγRIIIA on NK cells and tumor-associated antigens on their targets has led to the proposal of utilizing these reagents in immune therapy of cancer, with or without adoptive transfer of cytokine-activated NK cells.

A CD16/CD30 bispecific mAb has been shown capable both in vivo and in vitro of inducing lysis of Hodgkin-derived target cell lines by NK cells from healthy donors, and treatment of SCID mice injected with heterotransplantable tumors produced by the hybrid cell line expressing the mAb has been shown to induce tumor regression in the majority of the animals (Hombach et al. 1993). Chemical conjugation of mAb to CD3 and CD16 has been utilized to produce reagents that can direct the cytotoxicity of lymphocytes, and of purified NK cells stimulated or not with IL-2, against NK-resistant acute myeloid leukemia cells (Silla et al. 1995). The bispecific mAb 2B1, targeting HER-2/neu on a number of tumor cell types (Weiner et al. 1995) has been used to target tumor xenografts in immunodeficient SCID mice with or without additional administration of IL-2 to boost NK cell cytotoxic activity. The primary adverse side effects observed in the phase I clinical trial with this reagent included thrombocytopenia (by a still undefined mechanisms) and systemic production of cytokines, including TNF-α. Similar undesired effects (also defined as first-dose cytokine release syndrome) has been shown in other studies to depend directly on the systemic activation of NK cells, likely induced upon FcγRIIIA occupancy by the antibody-sensitized target cells. WING et al. (1996) have demonstrated that the effect of in vivo injection of the CAMPATH 1-H mAb to induce systemic release of TNF-α, IFN-γ, and IL-6 depends on the immunoglobulin isotype, which corresponds to those best bound by the FcγRIIIA, and can be inhibited by anti-CD16 mAb. Although NK cells likely contribute to the production of IFN-γ, a (possibly major) involvement of macrophages in the production of the other cytokines cannot be excluded.

Although these studies are promising, therapies directed to activating NK cell cytotoxic functions targeting their FcγRIIIA need to consider, together with the possible side effects, the possibility that in tumor-bearing patients the functions of NK cells, related or not to FcγRIIIA expression and triggering capability, may be altered by tumor-produced factors. Indeed a study has reported that NK cells from lymphocytes infiltrating tumor masses as well as T cells from the same infiltrates express decreased levels of the FcγRIIIA-associated ζ chain (NAKAGOMI et al. 1993).

8 Conclusions

FcγRIIIA are functionally important receptors on NK cells, capable of transducing activatory signals to trigger their functions. Although in spite of the knowledge accumulated no hint yet allows clear definition of the relevance of its expression to NK cell function/activation in vivo, studies on the receptor have provided a very useful model system in which to analyze with minor complications the biology of NK cells and have been instrumental in beginning to dissect the molecular bases of NK cell activation. Historically the recognition of distinct FcγR type expression on NK cells resulted in confirmation of the existence of NK cells as a discrete lymphocyte subset, and reagents to these receptors have been instrumental in allowing purification of these cells to homogeneity and production of long-term NK cell clones essential not only for biochemical and molecular studies but also for those related to the basis of target cell recognition. Given the commonality in the molecular composition of the receptor complex with that of other hematopoietic cell receptors, namely the antigen-specific receptors, it was to be expected that, as experimentally demonstrated, the molecular basis for the signal transduction events elicited upon occupancy of FcγRIIIA would for most part be shared. Definition of these pathways, their role in specific NK cell functions, and the mechanisms by which additional external stimuli influence the biochemical events transduced by them is now expected to provide more firm bases for understanding how functions of these cells are regulated. The promising preliminary reports on the possibility of targeting this receptor to specifically activate NK cell tumoricidal functions and possibly, via induced IFN-γ production, to facilitate the establishment of cell-mediated immunity represent additional steps for the possible translation to the clinical settings of the basic knowledge accumulated.

Acknowledgement. I wish to thank all the past and present collaborators in my laboratory who have contributed experimental work discussed here. The autor's research discussed here was supported in part by grants CA 37155 and CA45284 from NIH.

References

Aller SC, Cho D, Kim YB (1995) Characterization of the cytolytic trigger molecules G7/PNK-E as a molecular complex on the surface of porcine phagocytes. Cell Immunol 161:270–278

Altin JG, Pagler EB, Kinnear BF, Warren HS (1994) Molecular associations involving CD16, CD45 and zeta and gamma chains on human Natural Killer cells. Immunol Cell Biol 72:87–96

Amigorena S, Bonnerot C, Drake JR, Choquet D, Hunziker W, Guilet JG, Webster P, Sautes C, Mellman I, Fridman WH (1992) Cytoplasmic domain heterogeneity and functions of IgG Fc receptors in B lymphocytes. Science 256:1808–1812

Anasetti C, Martin PJ, Morishita Y, Badger CC, Bernstein ID, Hansen JA (1987) Human large granular lymphocytes express high affinity receptors for murine monoclonal antibodies of the IgG3 subclass. J Immunol 138:2979–2981

Anegon I, Cuturi MC, Trinchieri G, Perussia B (1988) Interaction of Fc receptor (CD16) with ligands induces transcription of interleukin 2 receptor (CD25) and lymphokine genes and expression of their products in human natural killer cells. J Exp Med 167:452–472

Aramburu J, Azzoni L, Rao A, Perussia B (1995) Activation and expression of the nuclear factors of activated T cells, NFATp and NFATc in human natural killer cells: regulation upon CD16 ligand binding. J Exp Med 182:801–810

Arase H, Arase N, Saito T (1995) Fas-mediated cytotoxicity by freshly isolated natural killer cells. J Exp Med 181:1235–1238

Azzoni L, Kamoun M, Salcedo TW, Kanakaraj P, Perussia B (1992) Stimulation of Fc-gamma RIIIA results in phospholipase C-gamma1 tyrosine phosphorylation and $p56^{lck}$ activation. J Exp Med 176:1745–1750

Azzoni L, Anegon I, Calabretta B, Perussia B (1995) Stimulation of IL-2 activated NK cells via Fc gamma RIII induces c-myc-dependent apoptosis. J Immunol 154:491–499

Balboa MA, Balsinde J, Aramburu J, Mollinedo F, Lopez-Botet M (1992) Phospholipase D activation in human natural killer cells through the Kp43 and CD16 surface antigens takes place by different mechanisms. Involvement of the phospholipase D pathway in tumor necrosis factor alpha synthesis. J Exp Med 176:9–17

Bennett IM, Zatsepina O, Zamai L, Azzoni L, Mikeeva T, Perussia B (1996) Definition of an NKR-P1A+/CD56–/CD16– functionally immature human NK cell subset that differentiates in vitro in the presence of IL-12. J Exp Med 184:1845–1856

Binstadt BA, Brumbaugh KM, Dick CJ, Scharenberg AM, Williams Bl, Colonna M, Lanier LL, Kinet J, Abraham RT, Leibson PJ (1996) Sequential involvement of Lck and SHP-1 with MHC-recognizing receptors on NK cells inhibits FcR-initiated tyrosine kinase activation. Immunity 5:629–638

Biron CA, Byron KS, Sullivan JL (1989) Severe herpesvirus infections in an adolescent without natural killer cells. N Engl J Med 89:1731–1735

Blank U, Ra C, Miller L, White K, Metzger H, Kinet J (1989) Complete structure and expression in transfected cells of high affinity IgE receptor. Nature 377:187–189

Bonnema JD, Karnitz LM, Schoon RA, Abraham RT, Leibson PJ (1994) Fc receptor stimulation of phosphatidylinositol 3-kinase in Natural Killer cells is associated with protein kinase C-independent granule release and cell-mediated cytotoxicity. J Exp Med 180:1427–1435

Bonnerot C, Amigorena S, Choquet D, Pavlovich R, Choukroun V, Friedman WH (1992) Role of associated gamma-chain in tyrosine kinase activation via murine Fc gamma RIII. EMBO J 11:2747–2757

Borrego F, Pena J, Solana R (1993) Regulation of CD69 expression on human natural killer cells: differential involvement of protein kinase C and protein tyrosine kinases. Eur J Immunol 23:1039–1043

Borrego F, Lopez-Beltran A, Pena J, Solana R (1994) Downregulation of Fc gamma receptor IIIA alpha (CD16-II) on natural killer cells induced by anti-CD16 mAb is independent of protein tyrosine kinases and protein kinase C. Cell Immunol 158:208–217

Burshtyn DN, Scharenberg AM, Wagtmann N, Rajagopalan S, Berrada K, Yi T, Kinet J, Long EO (1996) Recruitment of tyrosine phosphatase HCP by the killer inhibitory receptor. Immunity 4:77–85

Cambier JC (1995) The awesome power of the immunoreceptor tyrsine-based activation motif (ITAM). J Immunol 155:3281–3285

Campbell KS, Dessing M, Lopez-Botet M, Cella M, Colonna M (1996) Tyrosine phsphorylation of a human killer inhibitory receptor recruits protein tyrosine phosphatase 1C. J Exp Med 184:93–100

Cassatella MA, Anegon I, Cuturi MC, Griskey P, Trinchieri G, Perussia B (1989) Fc gamma R(CD16) interaction with ligand induces Ca2+ mobilization and phosphoinositide turnover in human natural killer cells. Role of Ca2+ in Fc gamma R(CD16)-induced transcription and expression of lymphokine genes. J Exp Med 169:549–567

Chan AC, Desai DM, Weiss A (1994) The role of protein tyrosine kinases and protein tyrosine phosphatases in T cell antigen receptor signal transduction. Annu Rev Immunol 12:555–592

Cone JC, Lu Y, Trevillyan JM, Bjorndahl JM, phillips CA (1993) Association of the p56 lck protein tyrosine kinase with the Fc gamma RIIIA/CD16 complex in human natural killer cells. Eur J Immunol 23:2488–2497

Cuturi MC, Anegon I, Sherman F, Loudon R, Clark SC, Perussia B, Trinchieri G (1989) Production of hematopoietic colony-stimulating factors by human natural killer cells. J Exp Med 169:569–583

D'Ambrosio D, Hippen KL, Minskoff SA, Mellman I, Pani G, Siminovitch KA, Cambier JC (1995) Recruitment and activation of PTP1C in negative regulation of antigen receptor signaling by Fc gamma RIIB1. Science 268:293–297

Darby C, Geahlen RL, Schreiber AD (1994) Stimulation of macrophage Fc gamma RIIIA activates the receptor-associated protein tyrosine kinase Syk and induces phosphorylation of multiple proteins including p95 Vav and p62/GAp-associated protein. J Immunol 152:5429–5437

Dato ME, Wierda WG, Kim YB (1992) A triggering structure recognized by G7 monoclonal antibody on porcine lymphocytes and granulocytes. Cell Immunol 140:468–477

Dehaas M, Koene HR, Kleijer M, DeVries E, Simsek S, Vantol MJD, Roos D, Vondemborne AEGK (1996) A triallelic Fc-gamma receptor type IIIA polymorphism influences the binding of human IgG by NK cell Fc-gamma-RIIIA. J Immunol 156:2948–2955

DeVries E, Koene HR, Vossen JM, Gratama JW, Vondemborne AEGK, Waaijer JLM, Haraldsson A, Dehaas M, Vantol MJD (1996) Identification of an unusual Fc-gamma-receptor IIIA (CD16) on natural killer cells in a patient with recurrent infections. Blood 88:3022–3027

Ebnet K, Hausmann M, Lehmann-Grube F, Mullbacher A, Kopf M, Lamers M, Simon MM (1995) Granzyme A-deficient mice retain potent cell-mediated cytotoxicity. EMBO J 14:4230–4239

Eischen CM, Schilling JD, Lynch DH, Krammer PH, Leibson PJ (1996) Fc receptor-induced expression of Fas ligand on activated NK cells facilitates cell-mediated cytotoxicity and subsequent autocrine NK cell apoptosis. J Immunol 156:2693–2699

Farber DL, Giorda R, Nettleton MY, Trucco M, Kochan JP, Sears DW (1993) Rat Class III Fc gamma receptor isoforms differ in IgG subclass-binding specificity and fail to associate productively with rat CD3 zeta. J Immunol 150:4364–4375

Flamand V, Shores EW, Tran T, Huang K, Lee F, Greenberg A, Kinet J, Love PE (1996) Delayed maturation of CD4(–)CD8(–) Fc-gamma-RII/III+ T and natural killer cell precursors in Fc-epsilon-RI-gamma transgenic mice. J Exp Med 184:1725–1735

Fleit HB, Wright SD, Unkeless JC (1982) Human neutrofil Fc gamma receptor distribution and structure. Proc Natl Acad Sci USA 79:3275–3279

Fleit HB, Wright SD, Durie CJ, Valinsky JE, Unkeless JC (1984) Ontogeny of Fc receptors and complement receptor (CR3) during human myeloid differentiation. J Clin Invest 73:516–525

Fleit HB, Kobasiuk CD, Peress NS, Fleit SA (1992) A common epitope is recognized by monoclonal antibodies prepared against purified human neutrophil Fc gamma RIII (CD16). Clin Immunol Immunopathol 62:16–24

Fry AM, Lanier LL, Weiss A (1996) Phosphotyrosines in the killer cell inhibitory receptor motif of NKB1 are required for negative signaling and for association with protein tyrosine phosphatase 1C. J Exp Med 184:295–300

Galandrini R, Palmieri G, Piccoli M, Frati L, Santoni A (1996) CD16-mediated p21 ras activation is associated with Shc and p36 tyrosine phosphorylation and their binding with Grb2 in human natural killer cells. J Exp Med 183:179–186

Galatiuc C, Gherman M, Metes D, Sulica A, DeLeo AB, Whiteside TL, Herberman RB (1995) natural killer (NK) activity in human responders and non responders to stimulation by anti-CD16 antibodies. Cell Immunol 163:167–177

Gessner JE, Grussenmeyer T, Dumbsky M, Schmidt RE (1996) Separate promoters from proximal and medial control regions contribute to the natural killer cell-specific transcription on the human Fc-gamma-RIII-A (CD16-A) receptor gene. J Biol Chem 271:30755–30764

Gismondi A, Mainiero F, Morrone S, Palmieri G, Piccoli M, Frati L, Santoni A (1992) Triggering through CD16 or phorbol esters enhances adhesion of NK cells to laminin via very late antigen 6. J Exp Med 176:1251–1257

Halloran PJ, Sweeney SE, Strohmeier CM, Kim YB (1994) Molecular cloning and identification of the porcine cytolytic trigger molecule G7 as a Fc gamma RIII alpha (CD16) homologue. J Immunol 153:2631–2641

Harrison D, Phillips JH, Lanier LL (1991) Involvement of a metalloprotease in spontaneous and phorbol ester-induced release of natural killer cell-associated Fc gamma RIII (CD16-II). J Immunol 147:3459–3465

Hazenbos WLW, Gessner JE, Hofhuis FMA, Kuipers H, Meyer D, Heijnen IAFM, Schmidt RE, Sandor M, Capel PJA, Daeron M, Wandewinkel JGJ, Verbeek JS (1996) Impaired IgG-dependent anaphylaxis and Arthus reaction in Fc-gamma-RIII (CD16) deficient mice. Immunity 5:181–188

Henkart PA (1985) Mechanism of lymphocyte-mediated cytotoxicity. Annu Rev Immunol 3:31–58

Hibbs ML, Tolvanen M, Carpen O (1994) Membrane-proximal Ig-like domain of Fc gamma RIII (CD16) contains residues critical for ligand binding. J Immunol 152:4466–4474

Hombach A, Jung W, Pohl C, Renner C, Sahin U, Schmits R, Wolf J, Kapp U, Diehl V, Pfreundschuh M (1993) A CD16/CD30 bispecific monoclonal antibody induces lysis of Hodgkin's cells by unstimulated natural killer cells in vitro and in vivo. Int J Cancer 55:830–836

Hou J, Dietrich J, Geisler NOC (1996) The cytoplasmic tail of Fc gamma RIII alpha is involved in signaling by the low affinity receptor for immunoglobulin G. J Biol Chem 271:22815–22822

Huizinga TWJ, Kleijer M, Roos D, Von dem Borne AEG (1997) Differences between human FcRIII of human neutrophils and human K/NK lymphocytes in relation to the NA antigen system. In: Knapp W et al (eds) Leukocyte typing pp 582–585

Hulett MD, Hogarth PM (1997) Molecular basis of Fc receptor function. Adv Immunol 57:1–127

Jawar S, Moody C, Chan M, Finberg R, Geha R, Chatila T (1996) natural killer (NK) cell deficiency associated with an epitope-deficient Fc receptor type IIIA (CD16-II). Clin Exp Immunol 103:408–413

Kagi D, Ledermann B, Burki K, Seiler P, Odermatt B, Olsen KJ, Podack ER, Zinkernagel RM, Hengartner H (1994) Cytotoxicity mediated by T cells and natural killer cells is greatly impaired in perforin-deficient mice. Nature 369:31–35

Kanakaraj P, Duckworth B, Azzoni L, Kamoun M, Cantley LC, Perussia B (1994) PI-3-kinase activation induced upon Fc gamma RIIIA-ligand interaction. J Exp Med 179:551–558

Kaufman Ds, Schoon RA, Leibson PJ (1993) MHC class I expression on tumor targets inhibits natural killer cell-mediated cytotoxicity without interfering with target recognition. J Immunol 150:1429–1436

Kindt GC, van de Winkel JGJ, Moore SA, Anderson CL (1991) Identification and structural characterization of Fc gamma receptors on pulmonary alveolar macrophages. Am J Physiol 260:403–411

Kipps TJ, Parham P, Punt J, Herzenberg LA (1985) Importance of immunoglobulin isotype in human antibody dependent, cell-mediated cytotoxicity directed by murine monoclonal antibodies. J Exp Med 161:1–17

Kurosaki T, Ravetch JV (1989) A single amino acid in the GPI attachment domain determines the membrane topology of Fc gamma RIII. Nature 342:805–807

Kurosaki T, Gander I, Wirthmueller U, Ravetch JV (1992) The beta subunit of the Fc epsilon RI is associated with the Fc gamma RIII on mast cells. J Exp Med 175:447–451

Lanier LL, Phillips JH (1995) NK cell recognition of major histocompatibility complex class I molecules (review). Semin Immunol 95:75–82

Lanier LL, Kipps TJ, Phillips JH (1985) Functional properties of a unique subset of cytotoxic CD3+ T lymphocytes that express Fc receptors for IgG (CD16/Leu-11 antigen). J Exp Med 162:2089–2106

Lanier LL, Riutenberg JJ, Phillips JH (1988) Functional and biochemical analysis of CD16 antigen on natural killer cells and granulocytes. J Immunol 141:3478–3485

Lanier LL, Cwirla S, Yu G, Testi R, Phillips JH (1989) Membrane anchoring of a human IgG Fc receptor (CD16) determined by a single amino acid. Science 246:1611–1613

Leibson PJ (1995) MHC-recognizing receptors: they're not just for T cells anymore. Immunity 3:5–8

Letourneur O, Kennedy ICS, Brini AT, Ortaldo JR, O'Shea JJ, Kinet J (1991) Characterization of the family of dimers associated with Fc receptors (Fc epsilon RI and Fc gamma RIII). J Immunol 147:2652–2656

Li M, Wirthmueller U, Ravetch JV (1996) Reconstitution of human Fc-gamma-RIII type specificity in transgenic mice. J Exp Med 183:1259–1263

Ljunggren HG, Karre K (1990) In search of the 'missing self': MHC molecules and NK cell recognition. Immunol Today 11:7–10

Manciulea M, Rabinowich H, Sulica A, Lin WC, Whiteside TL, DeLeo AB, Herberman RB, Correy SJ (1996) Divergent phosphotyrosine signaling via Fc gamma RIIIA on human NK cells. Cell Immunol 167:63–71

Mates D, Galatiuc C, Maldovan I, Morel PA, Chambers WH, DeLeo AB, Rabinowich H, Schall R, Whiteside TL, Sulica A et al (1994) Expression and function of Fc gamma RII on human natural killer cells. Nat Immunity 13:289–300

McCaffrey PG, Luo C, Kerppola TK, Jain J, Badalian TM, Ho AM, Burgeon E, Lane WS, Lambert JN, Curran T, Verdine GL, Rao A, Hogan PG (1993) Isolation of the cyclosporin-sensitive T cell transcription factor NFATp. Science 262:750–754

Mellman I, Unkeless JC (1980) Purification of a functional Fc receptor through the use of a monoclonal antibody. J Exp Med 152:1048–1069

Moingeon P, Lucich JL, Reinherz EL (1992) Characterization of Fc epsilon RI gamma in human natural killer cells. Int Immunol 4:955–958

Moingeon P, Rodewald HR, McConkey D, Mildonian A, Awad K, Reinherz EL (1993) Generation of natural killer cells from both Fc gamma RII/III+ and Fc gamma RII/III-murine fetal liver progenitors. Blood 82:1453–1462

Montel AH, Bochan MR, Hobbs JA, Lynch DH, Brahmi Z (1995) Fas involvement in cytotoxicity mediated by human NK cells. Cell Immunol 166:236–246

Moretta L, Ciccone E, Mingari MC, Biassoni R, Moretta A (1994) Human natural killer cells: origin, clonality, specificity, and receptors. Adv Immunol 55:341–380

Muta T, Kurosaki T, Misulovin Z, Sanchez M, Nussenzweig MC, Ravetch JV (1994) A 13-amino-acid motif in the cytoplasmic domain of Fc gamma RIIB modulates B-cell receptor signalling. Nature 369:340–342

Nagler A, Lanier LL, Cwirla S, Phillips JH (1989) Comparative studies of human FcRIII-positive and negative natural killer cells. J Immunol 143:3183–3191

Nakagomi H, Petersson M, Magnusson I, Juhlin C, Matsuda M, Mellstedt H, Taupin JL, Vivier E, Anderson P, Kiessling R (1993) Decreased expression of the signal-transducing zeta chains in tumor-infiltrating T-cells and NK cells of patients with colorectal carcinoma. Cancer Res 53:5610–5612

Ono M, Bolland S, Tempst P, Ravetch JV (1996) The role of the inositol phosphatase SHIP in negative regulation of the immune system by the receptor Fc gamma RIIB. Nature 383:263–266

Orloff DG, Ra C, Frank D, Klausner RD, Kinet J (1990) Family of disulfide-linked dimers containing the zeta and gamma chains of the T cell receptor and the gamma chain of Fc receptors. Nature 347:189–191

Ortaldo JR, Mason AT, O'Shea JJ (1995) Receptor-induced death in human natural killer cells: involvement of CD16. J Exp Med 181:339–344

Ortaldo JR, Winklerpickett RT, Nagata S, Ware CF (1997) Fas involvement in human NK cell apoptosis. Lack of a requirement for CD16-mediated events. J Leukoc Biol 61:209–215

O'Shea JJ, Weissman AM, Kennedy ICS, Ortaldo JR (1991) Engagement of the natural killer cell IgG Fc receptor results in tyrosine hosphorylation of the zeta chain. Proc Natl Acad Sci USA 88:350–354

O'Shea JJ, McViar DW, Kuhns DB, Ortaldo JR (1992) A role for protein tyrosine kinase activity in natural cytotoxicity as well as antibody-dependent cellular cytotoxicity. Effects of herbimycin A. J Immunol 148:2497–2502

Peltz GA, Grundy HO, Labo RV, Yssel H, Barsh GS, Moore KW (1989) Human Fc gamma RIII, cloning, expression, and identification of the chromosomal locus of two Fc receptors for IgG. Proc Natl Acad Sci USA 86:1013–1017

Perussia B, Ravetch JV (1991) Fc gamma RIII (CD16) on human macrophages is a functional product of the Fc gamma RIII-2 gene. Eur J Immunol 21:425–429

Perussia B, Trinchieri G (1981) Inactivation of natural killer cell cytotoxic activity after interaction with target cells. J Immunol 126:754–758

Perussia B, Trinchieri G (1984) Antibody 3G8, specific for the human neutrophil Fc receptor, reacts with natural killer cells. J Immunol 158:1410–1415

Perussia B, Trinchieri G (1988) Structure and functions of NK cell Fc receptor. J Immunol Immunopharmacol 8:147–150

Perussia B, Trinchieri G, Cerrottini JC (1979) Functional studies of Fc receptor-bearing human lymphocytes: effect of treatment with proteolytic enzymes. J Immunol 123:681–687

Perussia B, Acuto O, Terhorst C, Faust J, Fanning V, Lazarus R, Trinchieri G (1983a) Human natural killer cell analyzed by B73.1, a monoclonal antibody blocking FcR functions. II. Studies of B73.1 antibody-antigen interaction on the lymphocyte membrane. J Immunol 130:2142–2148

Perussia B, Starr S, Abraham S, Fanning V, Trinchieri G (1983b) Human natural killer cells analyzed by B73.1, a monoclonal antibody blocking Fc receptor functions. I. Characterization of the lymphocyte subset reactive with B73.1. J Immunol 130:2133–2141

Perussia B, Trinchieri G, Jackson A, Warner NL, Faust J, Rumpold H, Kraft D, Lanier LL (1984) The Fc receptor for IgG on human natural killer cells: phenotypic, functional, and comparative studies with monoclonal antibodies. J Immunol 133:180–189

Perussia B, Tutt MM, Qiu WQ, Kuziel WA, Tucker PW, Trinchieri G, Bennett M, Ravetch JV, Kumar V (1989) Murine natural killer cells express functional Fc gamma receptor II encoded by the Fc gamma R alpha gene. J Exp Med 170:73–86

Phillips JH, Chang CW, Lanier LL (1991) Platelet-induced expression of Fc gamma RIII (CD16) on human monocytes. Eur J Immunol 21:895–899

Pignata C, Prasad KV, Robertson MJ, Levine H, Rudd CE, Ritz J (1993) Fc gamma RIIIA-mediated signaling involves src-family lck in human natural killer cells. J Immunol 151:6794–6800

Podack ER, Young JD-E, Cohn ZA (1985) Isolation and biochemical and functional characterization of perforin 1 from cytolytic T-cell granules. Proc Natl Acad Sci USA 82:8629–8633

Pricop L, Rabinowich H, Morel PA, Sulica A, Whiteside TL, Herberman RB (1993) Characterization of the Fc mu receptor on human natural killer cells. Interaction with its physiologic ligand, human normal IgM, specificity of binding, and functional effects. J Immunol 151:3018–3029

Qiu WQ, De Bruin, Brownstein BH, Pearse R, Ravetch JV (1990) Organization of the human and mouse low-affinity Fc gamma R genes: duplication and recombination. Science 248:732–735

Ra C, Jouvin M-H, Kinet J (1989) Complete structure of the mouse mast cell receptor for IgE (Fc epsilon RI) and surface expression of chimeric receptors (rat-mouse-human) on transfected cells. J Biol Chem 264:15323–15327

Rabinowich H, Manciulea M, Mates D, Sulica A, Herberman RB, Corey SJ, Whiteside TL (1996) Physical and functional association of Fc-mu receptor on human natural killer cells with the zeta- and Fc-epsilon-RI gamma-chains and with src family protein tyrosine kinases. J Immunol 157:1485–1491

Raulet DH, Held W (1995) Natural killer cell receptors: the offs and ons of NK cell recognition. Cell 82:697–700

Ravetch JV, Kinet JP (1991) Fc receptors. Annu Rev Immunol 9:457–492

Ravetch JV, Perussia B (1989) Alternative membrane forms of Fc gamma RIII (CD16) on human natural killer cells and neutrophils. Cell type-specific expression of two genes that differ in single nucleotide substitutions. J Exp Med 170:481–497

Reth M (1989) Antigen receptor tail clue. Nature 338:383–384

Rodewald HR, Moingeon P, Lucich JL, Dosiou C, Lopez P, Reinherz EL (1992) A population of early fetal thymocytes expressing Fc gamma RII/RIII contains precursors of T lymphocytes and natural killer cells. Cell 69:139–150

Salcedo TW, Azzoni L, Wolf SF, Perussia B (1993a) Modulation of perforin and granzyme messenger RNA expression in human natural killer cells. J Immunol 151:2511–2520

Salcedo TW, Kurosaki T, Kanakaraj P, Ravetch JV, Perussia B (1993b) Physical and functional association of $p56^{lck}$ with Fc gamma RIIIA (CD16) in natural killer cells. J Exp Med 177:1475–1480

Scallon BJ, Scigliano E, Freedman VH, Miedel MC, Pan YC, Unkeless JC, Kochan JP (1989) A human immunoglobulin G receptor exists in both polypeptide-anchored and phosphatidylinositol-glycan-anchored forms. Proc Natl Acad Sci USA 86:5079–5083

Scharenberg AM, Kinet J (1996) The emerging field of receptor-mediated inhibitory signaling: SHP or SHIP? Cell 87:961–964

Selvaraj P, Carpen O, Hibbs ML, Springer TA (1989) Natural killer cell and granulocyte Fc gamma receptor III (CD16) differ in membrane anchor and signal transduction. J Immunol 143:3283–3288

Silla LM, Chen J, Zhong RK, Whiteside TL, Ball ED (1995) Potentiation of lysis of leukaemia cells by a bispecific antibody to CD33 andCD16 (Fc gamma RIII) expressed by human natural killer (NK) cells. Br J Haematol 89:712–718

Stahls A, Liwszyc GE, Couture C, Mustelin T, Andersson LC (1994) Triggering of human natural killer cells trhough CD16 induces tyrosine phosphorylation of the p72 syk kinase. Eur J Immunol 24:2491–2496

Sulica A, Gataliuc C, Manciulea M, Bancu AC, DeLeo AB, Whiteside TL, Herberman RB (1993) Regulation of human natural cytotoxicity by IgG. IV. Association between binding of monomeric IgG to the Fc receptors on large granular lymphocytes and inhibition of natural killer (NK) cell activity. Cell Immunol 147:397–410

Sweeney SE, Halloran PJ, Kim YB (1996) Identification of a unique porcine Fc-gamma-RIIIA-alpha molecular complex. Cell Immunol 172:92–99

Takai T, Li M, Sylvestre D, Clynes R, Ravetch JV (1994) FcR gamma chain deletion results in pleiotropic effector cell defects. Cell 76:519–529

Takizawa F, Adamczewski M, Kinet J (1992) Identification of the low affinity receptor for immunoglobulin E on mouse mast cells and macrophages as Fc gamma RII and Fc gamma RIII. J Exp Med 176:469–475

Tamm A, Schmidt RE (1996) The binding epitopes of human CD16 (Fc gamma RIII) monoclonal antibodies. Implications for ligand binding. J Immunol 157:1576–1581

Ting AT, Einspahr KJ, Abraham RT, Leibson PJ (1991) Fc gamma receptor signal transduction in natural killer cells: coupling to phospholipase C via a G-protein independent, but tyrosine kinase-dependent pathway. J Immunol 147:3122–3127

Ting AT, Karnitz LM, Schoon RA, Abraham RT, Leibson PJ (1992a) Fc gamma receptor activation induces the tyrosine phosphorylation of both phospholipase C (PLC)-gamma 1 and PLC-gamma 2 in natural killer cells. J Exp Med 176:1751–1755

Ting AT, Schoon RA, Abraham RT, Leibson PJ (1992b) Interaction between protein kinase C-dependent and G protein-dependent pathways in the regulation of natural killer cell granule exocytosis. J Biol Chem 267:23957–23962

Trinchieri G (1989) Biology of natural killer cells. Adv Immunol 47:187–376

Trinchieri G, O'Brien T, Shade M, Perussia B (1984) Phorbol esters enhance spontaneous cytotoxicity of human lymphocytes, abrogate Fc receptor expression and inhibit antibody-dependent lymphocyte-mediated cytotoxicity. J Immunol 133:1869–1877

Trotta R, Kanakaraj P, Perussia B (1996) Fc gamma R-dependent MAP kinase activation in leukocytes: a common signal transduction event necessary for expression of TNF-alpha and early activation genes. J Exp Med 184:1027–1035

Trounstine M, Peltz GA, Yssel H, Huizinga TW, Von dem Borne AEG, Spits H, Moore KW (1990) Reactivity of clones, expressed human Fc gamma RIII isoforms with monoclonal antibodies which distinguish cell-type-specific and allelic forms of Fc gamma RIII. Int Immunol 2:303–310

Uciechowski P, Gessner JE, Schindler R, Schmidt RE (1992) Fc gamma RIII activation is different in CD16+ cytotoxic T lymphocytes and natural killer cells. Eur J Immunol 22:1635–1638

Unkeless JC (1979) Characterization of a monoclonal antibody directed against mouse macrophage and lymphocyte Fc receptors. J Exp Med 150:580–596

Vance BA, Huizinga TW, Guyre PM (1992) Functional polymorphism of Fc gamma RIII on human LGL/NK cells. FASEB J 6:1620A

Vance BA, Huizinga TW, Wardwell K, Guyre PM (1993) Binding of monomeric human IgG defines an expression polymorphism of Fc gamma RIII on Large Granular Lymphocyte/natural killer cells. J Immunol 151:6429–6439

Vivier E, Mortin C, O'Brien C, Drucker B, Schlossman SF, Anderson P (1991) Tyrosine phosphorylation of Fc gamma RIII (CD16): zeta complex in human natural killer cells. Induction by antibody-dependent cytotoxicity but not natural killing. J Immunol 146:206–212

Vivier E, Rochet N, Ackerly M, Petrini J, Levine H, Daley JF, Anderson P (1992) Signaling function of reconstituted CD16: zeta: gamma receptor complex isoforms. International Immunology 4:1313–1323

Vivier E, da Silva A, Ackerly M, Levine H, Rudd CE, Anderson P (1993) Association of a 70-kDa tyrosine phosphoprotein with the CD16: zeta: gamma complex expressed in human natural killer cells. Eur J Immunol 23:1872–1876

Walsh CM, Matloubian M, Liu CC, Ueda R, Kurahara CG, Christensen JL, Huang MT, Young JD, Ahmed R, Clark WR (1994) Immune function in mice lacking the perforin gene. Proc Natl Acad Sci USA 91:10854–10858

Weiner LM, Clark JI, Ring DB, Alpaugh RK (1995) Clinical development of 2B1, a bispecific murine monoclonal antibody targeting c-erbB-2 and Fc gamma RIII. J Hematother 4:453–456

Weishank RL, Luster AD, Ravetch JV (1988) Function and regulation of a murine macrophage-specific IgG Fc receptor, Fc gamma R-alpha. J Exp Med 167:1909–1925

Weiss A, Littman DR (1994) Signal transduction by lymphocyte antigen receptors. Cell 76:263–274

Werner G, von dem Borne AEGK, Tromp JF, van der Plas-van Dalen CM, Visser FJ, Engelfriet CP, Tetteroo PA (1988) Localization of the human NA1 alloantigen on neutrofil Fc-gamma receptors. Leukocyte Typing 3 (3):109–121

Wing MG, Moreau T, Greenwood J, Smith RM, Hale G, Isaacs J, Waldman H, Lachmann PJ, Compston A (1996) Mechanism of first-dose cytokine-release syndrome by CAMPATH 1-H. Involvement of CD16 (Fc-gamma-RIII) and CD11/18 (LFA-1) on NK cells. J Clin Invest 98:2819–2826

Xu XL, Chong SF (1996) Vav in natural killer cells is tyrosine phosphorylted upon cross-linking of Fc-gamma-RIIIA and is constiutively associated wth a serine/threonine kinase. Biochem J 318:527–532

Yano H, Nakanishi S, Kimura K, Nanai Y, Saitoh Y, Fukui Y, Nonamura Y, Matsuda Y (1993) Inhibition of histamin secretion by wortmannin through the blockade of phosphatidylinositol-3 kinase in RBL 2H3 cells. J Biol Chem 268:25846–25856

Young JD-E, Cohn ZA (1986) Cell-mediated killing. A common mechanism. Cell 46:641–642

Zupo S, Azzoni L, Massara R, D'Amato A, Perussia B, Ferrarini M (1993) Fc-gamma receptor III-positive T lymphocytes express functional IL-2 receptor b chain. J Clin Immunol 13:228–236

Adhesion in NK Cell Function

T.S. HELANDER and T. TIMONEN

1 Introduction

NK cells express various adhesion molecules in greater abundance than do other circulating mononuclear cells. In vitro they are the most adhesive of freshly isolated lymphocytes. The adhesion molecule expression of NK cells is altered by activation. Both high-affinity conformation of β_2-integrins and upregulation of various adhesion molecules takes place, especially after the stimulation with interleukin (IL) 2.

With their adhesion receptors NK cells bind to endothelium, extracellular matrix, stromal cells, and actual target cells. Thus the adhesion receptor repertoire of NK cells provide a fundamental basis for their homing, infiltration characteristics, and target cell recognition.

2 Binding to Endothelium and Extracellular Matrix

In their endogenous state NK cells are present particularly in the blood stream and spleen. There are indications, however, that NK cells are capable of extravasation. For example, NK cells infiltrate allogeneic organ transplants before T cells (NEMLANDER et al. 1983), and parenchymal NK cells have been detected in infectious inflammatory lesions and malignant tumors (MACINTYRE and WELSH 1986; NATUK

Department of Pathology, Haartman Institute, University of Helsinki, P.O. Box 21 (Haartmaninkatu 3), Helsinki, Finland

and WELSH 1987; INVERARDI et al. 1992; FOGLER et al. 1996). A considerable amount of new data has recently accumulated on the molecular mechanisms of NK cell adhesion to endothelium and subsequent adhesion phenomena in transendothelial migration and NK cell infiltration in intercellular space.

According to the currently accepted theory, leukocyte and lymphocyte binding and transmigration takes place in various steps (SPRINGER 1994). First, inflammatory mediators cause vasodilation and upregulate endothelial adhesion molecules, including E- and P-selectins as well as the integrin ligands ICAM-1 and VCAM-1. Vasodilation causes lymphocyte pavementing which in turn enables the selectin-dependent loose rolling of lymphocytes along endothelium. The rolling is followed by the activation of integrins on the loosely attaching lymphocytes. The conformational change in the integrins is probably induced by chemokines, cytokines, and endothelial adhesion molecule ligands. The next step is the integrin-mediated firm adhesion of leukocytes to the endothelium and subsequent induction of migration, probably by β_1- and β_2-integrins.

This sequence of events, although well established for granulocytes, has not been directly confirmed in the NK system. However, NK cells express the carbohydrate SLe^x (sialyl Lewis ^{x}, the ligand of selectins) and L-selectin detecting carbohydrate ligands on endothelium, meaning that the molecular prerequisites for rolling in the NK system exist (MÄENPÄÄ et al. 1993; PINOLA et al. 1994). In the NK system also $\alpha_4\beta_7$–VCAM-1 pathway has been implicated in rolling. NK cells express abundantly the α_4/β_1 (VLA-4) integrin, and therefore their ligand VCAM-1 probably also serves as a target in the firm adhesion of NK cells to endothelium (MÄENPÄÄ et al. 1993). Indeed, anti-VCAM-1 antibodies inhibit NK cell homing into experimental melanoma metastasis in vivo (FOGLER et al. 1996). Anti-β_2-integrin and anti-ICAM-1 antibodies are known to inhibit NK cell adhesion to cultured endothelial cells (BIANCHI et al. 1993), implicating CD11/CD18 as important adhesion molecules in NK cell endothelial cell interaction. Although the amount of the other endothelial β_2-integrin ligand ICAM-2 is not increased in inflammation, NK cells are capable of detecting pathological redistribution and the resulting local increase in the concentration of ICAM-2 on target cells (HELANDER et al. 1996). Additional adhesion molecules suggested to be involved in the binding of NK cells to endothelium include CD44 (GALANDRINI et al. 1994), CD2 (ANASETTI et al. 1987), CD31 (PECAM-1) (BERMAN et al. 1996) on NK cells, and VAP-1 and L-VAP-2 (SALMI and JALKANEN 1992; AIRAS et al. 1993) on endothelium. It appears that NK cells and T cells probably use largely overlapping receptors in adhering to vessel walls.

In vitro NK cells respond to chemotactic stimuli such as the members of C-C family of chemokines (β chemokines), *N*-formyl-methionyl-leucyl-phenylalanine tripeptide (fMLP), casein, CD5a (the cleavage product of the fifth component of complement), and as IL-12 (PUNTURIERI et al. 1989; DOBOS et al. 1992; ALLAVENA et al. 1994; MAGHAZACHI et al. 1994; TAUB et al. 1995; LOETSCHER et al. 1996). The fact that NK cells are found in allografts, malignant tumors, and inflammatory lesions, strongly suggests that NK cells are indeed capable of responding to chemotactic stimuli also in vivo. We have recently shown that a peptide derived from ICAM-2 activates NK cell migration (SOMERSALO et al. 1995). As ICAM-2 is also a potential target structure in the actual cytotoxic event, the finding raises the possibility that

Table 1. Binding molecules in NK cell adhesion to endothelium and subsequent transmigration and infiltration

Phase	NK cell receptor	Ligand
Rolling	L-Selectin	sLe^x
	sLe^x	E- and P-selectin
	$\alpha 4/\beta_7$	VCAM-1, fibronectin, MadCAM-1
	CD57	P- and L-selectin
Endothelial adhesion	β_2-Integrins (LFA-1)	ICAM-1,-2
	$\alpha 4/\beta_1$ (VLA-4)	VCAM-1, fibronectin
	Unknown	VAP1, L-VAP2
	CD2	CD58 (LFA-3)
	CD31 (PECAM-1)	CD31
Transmigration and infiltration	α_1-α_2/β_1 (VLA-1,-2)	Collagen, laminin
	α_4-α_5/β_1 (VLA-4,-5)	Fibronectin
	$\alpha 6/\beta_1$ (VLA-6)	Laminin
	CD44	Hyaluronic acid (HA), fibronectin, collagen
	CD2	CD58 (LFA-3)

some molecules function as chemoattractants in soluble form and low concentration, whereas in membrane-bound form and high concentration they serve as actual target structures. In fact, it has been shown that, for example, C5a at low concentrations increases neutrophil migration whereas at high concentrations it triggers effector functions (Dobos et al. 1992).

The existence of NK cells in pathological lesions further suggests that they are capable of infiltrating three-dimensional tissue in vivo. In vitro evidence shows that NK cells infiltrate tumor spheroids (Jääskeläinen al. 1992) and apparently utilize both β_1- and β_2-integrins for the locomotion. The ligands of β_2-integrins may be cell-bound ICAM molecules, but NK cells may in some circumstances facilitate migration by producing ligands for their own β_2-integrins (Somersalo et al. 1992). The extracellular matrix (ECM) is also involved in NK cell migration. NK cells recognize fibronectin through α_4/β_1- and α_5/β_1-integrins, and fibronectin facilitates NK cell migration (Somersalo and Saksela 1991). The α_1-α_2/β_1-integrins are expressed by long-term activated NK cells. Laminin and collagen I are recognized by activated NK cells, probably through α_1/β_1-receptors (Mäenpää et al. 1993; Shibuya et al. 1996).

Altogether, the present evidence shows that NK cells are highly capable of extravasation and migration. They respond to several chemotactic stimuli and utilize both cellular and ECM ligands for their locomotion. The adhesion molecules involved in these phenomena are listed in Table 1.

It is noteworthy that NK cells, unlike resting T cells, do not recirculate. Therefore their extravasation is always associated with inflammatory antigenic changes in endothelium. Even ICAM-2, suggested to be important in recirculation of unactivated lymphocytes and present in resting endothelium, is recognized by NK cells only after a pathological redistribution of ICAM-2. It is also noteworthy that, in theory, NK cell pavementing, rolling, extravasation, and chemotactic migration towards the target, can all occur in the absence of T cell activation. Rolling occurs through the S-Le^x-selectin pathway already utilized by unactivated NK cells. Binding can be mediated by integrins, and chemotaxis would be induced by chemokines and IL-12, all produced by cells outside the T cell system. Thus it is plausible that NK cells can reach the target before the T cells. This supports the suggestion that NK cells participate in directing T cell response to Th1 phenotype by providing interferon-γ and tumor necrosis factor before and during the subsequent activation of dormant T cells (Kos and Engleman 1996).

3 Binding in Target Cell Recognition

The main consequence of target cell recognition by NK cells is cytotoxicity. However, some target cells are protected from NK cells through receptor-mediated inactivation. Furthermore, contact of NK cells with other cells may also lead to NK cell proliferation and cytokine production. These functions depend on the presence of soluble cytokines and can be supported by cells not sensitive to NK cytotoxicity. According to present practice, the term target cell recognition refers to regulation of the effector cell cytolytic machinery mediated by target cell recognizing NK cell receptors.

Target cell recognition can be divided into two phases, binding of the NK cell to the target and triggering or inactivation, i.e., receptor-mediated regulation of the cytolytic machinery. Receptors and target molecules involved in these phases have been extensively studied. It has become evident that triggering of the lytic machinery is the sum effect of positive and negative signals (Moretta et al. 1994; Chambers and Brissette-Storkus 1995; Colonna and Samaridis 1995; Gumperz and Parham 1995; Raulet and Held 1995; Lanier and Phillips 1996; Lòpez-Botet et al. 1996). Especially the identification and characterization of the negatively signaling receptors leading to the inhibition of cytotoxicity (the so called killer inhibitory receptors [KIRs] and C-type lectins) has recently developed rapidly. On the other hand, knowledge of the receptors delivering positive triggering signals is less advanced.

Candidate triggering NK receptors frequently mentioned in the recent literature include CD16, NKR-P1, NK-TR1, 2B4, and p38 (Chambers and Brissette-Storkus 1995; Raulet and Held 1995). Recently some evidence of the existence of target structures for NKG2 has also been presented, and a formation of heterodimeric receptors consisting of NKG2A and CD94 has been reported (Duchler et al. 1995; Lazetic et al. 1996). Only CD16 and NKR-P1 can be regarded as established NK cell receptors, whereas the actual NK cell receptor status of the others is still preliminary or controversial. In addition, some of the members of KIRs may trigger NK cells. These receptors are called killer activating receptors (KARs). Moreover, some forms of CD94 and Ly-49 may trigger cytolysis. Thus it seems that the triggering of lysis is a function of multiple receptors, as is the case in the protection from lysis.

There is very little information on the binding capacity of the candidate triggering receptors. Recognition of target-bound antibodies by CD16 is associated with increased binding, which is mediated by integrins and CD2 (VOLTARELLI et al. 1993). The binding affinity of the other candidate NK cell receptors is probably quite low. It is generally believed that, as in T cells, the triggering receptors themselves contribute little the adhesion. However, through lateral cross-talk they activate adhesion receptors, such as β_2-integrins, and thus create a positive feedback loop in which triggering facilitates adhesion and vice versa. It will be of interest to see whether the inactivating receptors downregulate the expression of high avidity β_2-integrins or inhibit the expression of adhesion receptors.

The actual adhesion receptors of NK cells are relatively well characterized (TIMONEN et al. 1990; ROBERTSON et al. 1990). However, it is increasingly unclear whether these receptors serve merely in binding, or whether they also participate in triggering as signal transducing receptors.

CD2 is an adhesion molecule which provides an alternative pathway in T cell activation. Coligation of CD2 and CD16 in NK cells activates cytotoxicity and cytokine production (ANASETTI et al. 1987). Blockade of CD2 by monoclonal antibodies inhibits NK activity to a modest degree (TIMONEN et al. 1990), indicating that CD2-CD58 (LFA-3) pathway may be involved in NK binding and cytotoxicity, although it apparently is not the major mechanism of binding or triggering. Probably the main function of CD2 is costimulation. Other suggested costimulatory/stimulatory NK cell receptors include CD7, CD27, CD44, CD69, and a still unknown NK counterreceptor (other than CD28 and CTL-4) of the costimulatory molecule CD80 (B7-1) (MORETTA et al. 1991; GALANDRINI et al. 1994; RABINOWICH et al. 1994; OKUBO et al. 1995; CHAMBERS et al. 1996; YANG et al. 1996). The binding capacity of these receptors in NK recognition has not been established.

It is clear that in NK cytotoxicity the prerequisite of triggering is the binding of NK cells to the target. NK cells express relatively many adhesion molecules, including three β_2-integrins (CD11a/CD18, CD11b/CD18, CD11c/CD18) (TIMONEN et al. 1990; ROBERTSON et al. 1990; MÄENPÄÄ et al. 1993), the recently described DNAM-1 (SHIBUYA et al. 1996), CD2 (TIMONEN et al. 1990; MÄENPÄÄ et al. 1993) as well as α_1, α_2 α_4, α_5/β_1-integrins (RABINOWICH et al. 1994, 1995; GISMONDI et al. 1995; PERÉZ-VILLAR et al. 1996), α_4/β_7 integrin, CD44 (GALANDRINI et al. 1994), CD56 (NAGLER et al. 1989; BENNET et al. 1996), and L-selectin (MÄENPÄÄ et al. 1993). The β_1- and β_7-integrins, CD56, and L-selectin probably participate mostly in the homing and migration of NK cells, whereas their involvement in target cell recognition is apparently of minor importance.

The β_2-integrin–ICAM pathway is instrumental in the binding of both endogenous and IL-2-activated NK cells to their targets. It was long thought that β_2-integrins function in NK cells as they do in T cells: first the triggering receptor (in T cells TcR; in NK cells NKR-P1, for example) activates the killer cell and induces an adhesive conformation in killer cell β_2-integrins (DUSTIN and SPRINGER 1989). The integrins mediate binding and further facilitate triggering by creating a closer contact between triggering receptors and their ligands. This positive feedback loop, although functional in T cells, has remained hypothetical in the NK system.

4 Are There Bifunctional Receptors That Mediate Both Binding and Triggering?

It is known that β_2-integrin activation in NK cells can also take place through cytokine stimulation (DAMLE et al. 1987; TIMONEN et al. 1990), and therefore the increase in the binding capacity through β_2-integrins does not necessarily require the engagement of target-recognizing triggering receptors. It is unclear whether the activated β_2-integrins serve straight as signal transducing receptors in the triggering of the cytolytic machinery. Ligation of CD11a/CD18 is known to induce calcium influx and phosphoinositide turn over on NK cells (PARDI et al. 1989; MELERO et al. 1993; POGGI et al. 1996), and anti-CD11a antibodies as well as integrin-binding peptide from ICAM-2 induce tyrosine phosphorylation in NK cell proteins (SOMERSALO et al. 1995). Glucans enhance NK cytotoxicity through CD11b/CD18 (DI RENZO et al. 1991). In addition, β_2-integrins have been shown to serve as promiscuous signal transduction receptors by recruiting other activating membrane molecules through lateral communication (LUB et al. 1995; PETTY and TODD 1996). All this information suggest that β_2-integrins may under some circumstances serve as signal transduction molecules, i.e., as triggering NK receptors.

What is the mechanism by which NK cell receptors distinguish altered cells from normal ones? The answer is easy in the case of antibody-detecting CD16, but the basis of target cell selectivity of other candidate receptors has remained elusive. Certainly the modulation of MHC-I renders target cells unrecognizable by the inhibitory receptors and allows the lysis to occur. However, is the subsequent triggering automatic, or are pathological triggering ligands required in conjunction with altered MHC-I, as a kind of double-check for the permission to kill?

The capacity of NK cells to destroy a variety of normal autologous cells indicates that the triggering ligands are not necessarily anything foreign, as are nonself peptides foreign when presented to T cells.

We have recently suggested that β_2-integrins distinguish their target cells through changes in the distribution of target ICAM-2 molecules (HELANDER et al. 1996). We showed in a BW5147 mouse thymoma model that the thymoma cells become sensitive to IL-2 activated human NK cells when hybridized with human chromosome 6 (HELANDER et al. 1991). The killing was dependent on CD11/CD18-ICAM-2 pathway, although sensitive and resistant target cells expressed equal amounts of ICAM-2. However, in the sensitive target cells ICAM-2 was distributed as concentrates to the tip of uropods whereas in the resistant cells it was evenly distributed on cell membrane. The results reveal a novel form of NK cell recognition: target structures are already present on normal cells and only become recognizable through abnormal planar distribution, which raises the local adhesion molecule concentration above the threshold level for triggering. This recognition pattern bears some resem-

Table 2. Adhesion molecules involved in the target cell recognition of NK cells

CD11a/CD18 (LFA-1)	ICAM-1,-2
CD11b-c/CD18 (Mac-1; p150,95)	ICAM-1,-2, β-glucans, C3bi
CD2	CD58 (LFA-3)
DNAM-1	Unknown
CD16 (FcγRIIIa)	Target bound antibodies
CD44	HA[a], fibronectin, collagen, Mad CAM-1

[a] Not shown to be involved in NK cell recognition.

blance to that used by collectins. For example, the mannose binding lectin – an important component of innate immunity – binds to bacterial cell walls with a high concentration of mannose but does not bind to eukaryotic cells which usually do not expose high amounts of mannose residues (Turner 1996).

We also showed that the distribution of ICAM-2 is controlled by the cytoskeleton-membrane linker protein ezrin. It is of interest that ezrin is known to redistribute to newly formed microvilli in herpes simplex virus infected fibroblasts (Pakkanen et al. 1988). Thus it is possible that the ezrin-directed redistribution of adhesion molecule ligands – and perhaps some other adhesion ligands in addition to ICAM-2 – also sensitizes virus-infected cells to NK cytotoxicity.

As MHC-I molecules are major protective elements of target cells, it will be of interest to study whether ezrin also redistributes MHC-I. It is tempting to speculate that the redistribution of ICAM-2 on top of cellular projections would also serve as means to diminish local inhibitory MHC-I concentration. On the other hand, it could as well be postulated that the MHC-I foreign peptide complexes are coredistributed with ICAM, thus facilitating the antigen presentation for T cells. We are currently testing these two hypotheses in our BW5147 and virus infection models.

Adhesion molecules most probably involved in the target cell recognition of NK cells are listed in Table 2.

5 Concluding Remarks

NK cells form a distinct third class of lymphocytes in addition to T and B cells. They have diverse biological functions, including resistance towards infections and neoplasms as well as regulation of lymphohematopoiesis. Resting NK cells circulate in blood. Upon activation they are capable of transmigration, extravasation and infiltration towards the target cells. Several adhesion pathways and chemotactic compounds that control these phenomena have recently been identified.

NK cells recognize their target cells by multiple different receptors. The receptors roughly fall into four different categories: (a) adhesion molecules, (b) triggering receptors, (c) inhibitory receptors, and (d) costimulatory receptors. Ambivalent receptors that are either triggering or inhibitory may possibly form a fifth category. However, there is no evidence that structurally identical receptors would be ambivalent: one member of Ly-49 is stimulatory, others inhibitory; inhibitory CD94 is structurally different from the activating one, and the intracytoplasmic and transmembrane domains of KARs differ from those of KIRs.

The prerequisite of the function of the inhibitory or activatory NK cell receptors is the binding of NK cell to its target. The major adhesion molecules of the NK system are β_2-integrins and CD2. However, several other adhesion pathways have been described, and their overall contribution to binding is not yet well established and probably depends on target cell type.

The biological function of NK inhibitory receptors apparently is to monitor MHC-I status. The receptors recognize normal MHC-I and prevent unnecessary cytotoxicity. If the amount of MHC-I is reduced, and/or the MHC-I is occupied by foreign peptide (in both cases the amount of self peptide-MHC-I complexes is reduced), the inhibitory receptors do not recognize their normal target and permit the lysis.

It is unclear whether the license to kill from the inhibitory receptors is always sufficient for the triggering, or whether additional alterations from the normal are required by the triggering activatory receptors to engage. The search for mysterious NK target antigens has so far been unsuccessful. However, two models have been described in which also the triggering is associated with pathological alterations in target cell membrane: CD16 requires target cell bound antibodies, and thus indirectly detects foreign structures, and CD11a/CD18 detects pathologically redistributed ICAM-2 on target cells. Also CD2 is known to function as a signal transducing molecules, in addition to its binding capacity. Thus NK cell binding and triggering may, at least in some instances, be mediated by same receptors.

References

Airas L, Salmi M, Jalkanen S (1993) Lymphocyte-vascular adhesion protein-2 is a novel 70-kDa molecule involved in lymphocyte adhesion to vascular endothelium. J Immunol 151:4228–4238

Allavena P, Paganin C, Zhou D, Bianchi G, Sozzani S, Mantovani A (1994) Interleukin-12 is chemotactic for natural killer cells and stimulates their interaction with vascular endothelium. Blood 84:2261–2268

Anasetti C, Martin PJ, June CH, Hellström KE, Ledbetter JA, Rabinovitch PS, Morishita Y, Hellström I, Hansen JA (1987) Induction of calcium flux and enhancement of cytolytic activity in natural killer cells by cross-linking of the sheep erythrocyte biding protein (CD2) and Fc-receptor (CD16). J Immunol 139:1772–1779

Bennett IM, Zatsepina O, Zamai L, Azzoni L, Mikheeva T, Perussia B (1996) Definition of a natural killer NKR-P1A+/CD56–/CD16– functionally immature human NK cell subset that differentiates in vitro in the presence of interleukin 12. J Exp Med 184:1845–1856

Berman ME, Die Y, Muller WA (1996) Roles of platelet/endothelial cell adhesion molecule-1 (PECAM-1, CD31) in natural killer cell transendothelial migration and beta 2 integrin activation. J Immunol 156:1515–1524

Bianchi G, Sironi M, Ghibaudi E, Selvaggini C, Elices M, Allavena P, Mantovani A (1993) Migration of natural killer cells across endothelial cell monolayers. J Immunol 151:5135–5144

Chambers BJ, Salcedo M, Ljunggren H-G (1996) Triggering of natural killer cells by the costimulatory molecule CD80 (B7-1). Immunity 5:311–317

Chambers WH, Brissette-Storkus CS (1995) Hanging in the balance: natural killer cell recognition of target cells. Chem Biol 2:429–435

Colonna M, Samaridis J (1995) Cloning of immunoglobulin-superfamiliy members associated with HLA-C and HLA-B recognition by human natural killer cells. Science 268:405–408

Damle NK, Doyle LV, Bender JR, Bradley EC (1987) Interleukin-2-activated human lymphocytes exhibit enhanced adhesion to normal vascular endothelial cells and cause their lysis. J Immunol 138:1779–1785

Di Renzo L, Yefenof E, Klein E (1991) The function of human NK cells is enhanced by beta glucan, a ligand of CR3 (CD11b/CD18). Eur J Immunol 21:1755–1758

Dobos GJ, Norgauer J, Eberle M, Schollmeyer PJ, Traynor-Kaplan, AE (1992) C5a reduces formyl peptide-induced actin polymerization and phosphatidylinositol (3,4,5)-triphosphate formation, but not phaphatidylinositol (4,5)biphosphate hydrolysis and superoxide production, in human neutrophils. J Immunol 149:609–614

Duchler M, Offterdinger M, Holzmuller H, Lipp J, Chu CT, Aschauer B, Bach FH, Hofer E (1995) NKG2-C is a receptor on human natural killer cells that recognizes structures on K562 target cells. Eur J Immunol 25:2923–2931

Dustin ML, Springer TA (1989) T-cell receptor cross-linking transiently stimulates adhesiveness through LFA-1. Nature 341:619–624

Fogler WE, Volker K, McCormick KL, Watanabe M, Ortaldo JR, Wiltrout RH (1996) NK cell infiltration into lung, liver, and subcutaneous B16 melanoma is mediated by VCAM-1/VLA-4 interaction. J Immunol 156:4707–4714

Galandrini R, De Maria R, Piccoli M, Frati L, Santoni A (1994) CD44 triggering enhances human NK cell cytotoxic functions. J Immunol 153:4399–4407

Gismondi A, Milella M, Palmieri G, Piccoli M, Frati L, Santoni A (1995) Stimulation of protein tyrosine phosphorylation by interaction of NK cells with fibronectin via alpha 4 beta 1 and alpha 5 beta 1. J Immunol 154:3128–3137

Gumperz JE, Parham P (1995) The enigma of the natural killer cell. Nature 378:245–248

Helander T, Timonen T, Kalliomäki P, Schröder J (1991) Recognition of chromosome 6-associated target structures by human lymphokine-activated killer cells. J Immunol 147:2063–2067

Helander TS, Carpén O, Turunen O, Kovanen PE, Vaheri A, Timonen T (1996) ICAM-2 redistributed by ezrin as a target for killer cells. Nature 382:265–268

Inverardi L, Samaja M, Motterlini R, Mangili F, Bender JR, Pardi R (1992) Early recognition of a discordant xenogeneic organ by human circulating lymphocytes. J Immunol 149:1416–1423

Jääskeläinen J, Mäenpää A, Patarroyo M, Gahmberg CG, Somersalo K, Tarkkanen J, Kallio M, Timonen T (1992) Migration of recombinant IL-2-activated T and natural killer cells in the intercellular space of human H-2 glioma spheroids in vitro. A study on adhesion molecules involved. J Immunol 149:260–268

Kos FJ, Engleman EG (1996) Immune regulation: a critical link between NK cells and CTLs. Immunol Today 17:174–176

Lanier LL, Phillips JH (1996) Inhibitory MHC class I receptors on NK cells and T cells. Immunol Today 17:86–91

Lazetic S, Chang C, Houchins JP, Lanier LL, Phillips JH (1996) Human natural killer cell receptors involved in MHC class I recognition are disulfide-linked heterodimers of CD94 and NKG2 subinits. J Immunol 157:4741–4745

Loetscher P, Seitz M, Clark-Lewis I, Boggiolini M, Moser B (1996) Activation of NK cells by C-C cytokines: chemotaxis, Ca2+ mobilization and enzyme release. J Immunol 156:322–327

Lpez-Botet M, Moretta L, Strominger J (1996) NK-cell receptors and recognition of MHC class I molecules. Immunol Today 17:212–214

Lub M, van Kooyk Y, Figdor CG (1995) Ins and outs of LFA-1. Immunol Today 16:479–483

MacIntyre KW, Welsh RM (1986) Accumulation of natural killer and cytotoxic T large granular lymphocytes in the liver during virus infection. J Exp Med 164:1667–1681

Mäenpää A, Jääskeläinen J, Carpén O, Patarroyo M, Timonen T (1993) Expression of integrins and the other adhesion molecules on NK cells: impact of IL-2 on short and long-term cultures. Int J Cancer 53:850–855

Maghazachi AA, Al-Aoukaty A, Schall TJ (1994) C-C chemokines induce the chemotaxis of NK and IL-2 activated NK cells. J Immunol 153:4969–4977

Melero I, Balboa MA, Alonso JL, Yague E, Pivel JP, Sanchez-Madrid R, López-Botet M (1993) Signalling through the LFA-1 leukocyte integrin actively regulates intercellular adhesion and tumor necrosis factor-alpha production in natural killer cells. Eur J Immunol 23:1859–1865

Moretta A, Poggi A, Pende D, Tripodi G, Orengo AM, Pella N, Augugliaro R, Bottino C, Ciccone E, Moretta L (1991) CD69-mediated pathway of lymphocyte activation: anti-CD69 monoclonal antibodies trigger the cytolytic activity of different lymphoid effector cells with the exception of cytolytic T lymphocytes expressing T cell receptor α/β. J Exp Med 174:1393–1398

Moretta L, Ciccone E, Mingari MC, Biassone R, Moretta A (1994) Human natural killer cells: origin, clonality, specificity and receptors. Adv Immunol 55:341–380

Nagler A, Lanier LL, Cwirla S, Phillips JH (1989) Comparative studies of human FcRIII-positive and negative natural killer cells. J Immunol 143:3183–3191

Natuk RJ, Welsh RM (1987) Accumulation and chemotaxis of natural killer/large granular lymphocytes at sites of virus replication. J Immunol 138:877–883

Nemlander A, Saksela E, Häyry P (1983) Are "natural killer" cells involved in allograft rejection? Eur J Immunol 13:348–350

Okubo Y, Teshigawara K, Wei Y, Zhao X, Uchida A (1995) Requirement of the co-receptor signals for the activation and the prevention of cell death of natural killer cells. Nat Immun 14:85

Pakkanen R, Bonsdorff C-H, Turunen O, Wahlström T, Vaheri A (1988) Redistribution of M_r 75 000 plasma membrane protein, cytovillin, into newly formed microvilli in herpes simplex and Semliki Forest virus infected human embryonal fibroblasts. Eur J Cell Biol 46:435–443

Pardi R, Bender JR, Dettori C, Giannazza E, Engleman EG (1989) Heterogenous distribution and transmembrane signalling properties of lymphocyte function-associated antigen (LFA-1) in human lymphocyte subsets. J Immunol 143:3157–3166

Peréz-Villar JJ, Melero I, Gismondi A, Santoni A, López-Botet M (1996) Functional analysis of $\alpha1/\beta1$ integrin in human natural killer cells. Eur J Immunol 26:2303–2029

Petty HR, Todd RF III (1996) Integrins as promiscuous signal transduction devices. Immunol Today 17:209–212

Pinola M, Renkonen R, Majuri M-L, Tiisala S, Saksela E (1994) Characterization of the E-selectin ligand on NK cells. J Immunol 152:3586–3594

Poggi A, Spada F, Costa P, Tomasello E, Revello V, Pella N, Zocchi MR, Moretta L (1996) Dissection of lymphocyte function-associated antigen 1-dependent adhesion and signal transduction in human natural killer cells shown by the use of cholera or pertussis toxin. Eur J Immunol 26:967–965

Punturieri A, Santoni A, Ming JW, Nobili N, Mantovani A, Bottazzi B (1989) In vitro migration of rat large granular lymphocytes. Cell Immunol 123:257–263

Rabinowich H, Lin WC, Herberman RB, Whiteside TL (1994) Signalling via CD7 molecules on human NK cells. Induction of tyrosine phosphorylation and beta 1 integrin-mediated adhesion to fibronectin. J Immunol 153:3504–3513

Rabinowich HL, Lin WC, Manciulea M, Herberman RB, Whiteside, TL (1995) Induction of protein tyrosine phosphorylation in human natural killer cells by triggering via alpha 4 beta 1 or alpha 5 beta 1 integrins. Blood 85:1858–1864

Raulet DH, Held W (1995) Natural killer cell receptors: the offs and ons of NK cell recognition. Cell 82:697–700

Robertson MJ, Caligiuri MA, Manley TJ, Levine H, Ritz J (1990) Human natural killer cell adhesion molecules. Differential expression after activation and participation in cytolysis. J Immunol 145:3194–3201

Salmi M, Jalkanen S (1992) Induction and function of vascular adhesion protein-1 at sites of inflammation. Science 257:1407–1409

Shibuya A, Campbell D, Hannum C, Yssel H, Franz-Bacon K, McClanahan T, Kitamura T, Nicholl J, Sutherland GR, Lanier LL, Phillips JH (1996) DNAM-1, a novel adhesion molecule involved in the cytolytic function of T lymphocytes. Immunity 4:573–581

Somersalo K, Saksela E (1991) Fibronectin facilitates the migration of human natural killer cells. Eur J Immunol 21:35–42

Somersalo K, Tarkkanen J, Patarroyo M, Saksela E (1992) Involvement of beta-2 integrins in the migration of human natural killer cells. J Immunol 149:590–598

Somersalo K, Carpen O, Saksela E (1994) Stimulated natural killer cells secrete factors with chemotactic activity, including NAP-1/IL-8, which supports VLA-4 and VLA-5 mediated migration of T-lymphocytes. Eur J Immunol 24:2957–2965

Somersalo K, Carpén O, Saksela E, Nortamo P, Gahmberg CG, Timonen T (1995) Activation of NK cell migration by leukocyte binding peptide from ICAM-2. J Biol Chem 270:8629–8636
Springer TA (1994) Traffic signals for lymphocyte recirculation and leukocyte migration: the multistep paradigm. Cell 76:301–314
Taub DD, Sayers TJ, Carter CR, Ortaldo JR (1995) Alpha and beta chemokines induce NK cell migration and enhance NK-mediated cytolysis. J Immunol 155:3877–3888
Timonen T, Gahmberg CG, Patarroyo M (1990) Participation of CD11a-c/CD18, CD2 and RGD-binding receptors in endogenous and interleukin-2-stimulated NK activity of CD3-negative large granular lymphocytes. Int J Cancer 46:1035–1040
Turner MW (1996) Mannose-binding lectin: the pluripotent molecule of the innate immune system. Immunol Today 17:532–540
Voltarelli JC, Gjerset G, Anasetti C (1993) Adhesion of CD16+ K cells to antibody-coated targets is mediated by CD2 and CD18 receptors. Immunology 79:509–511
Yang FC, Agematzu K, Nakazawa T, Mori T, Ito S, Morimoto C, Komiyama A (1996) CD27/CD70 interaction directly induces natural killer cell killing activity. Immunology 88:289–293

B. Activation of NK Cells and Effector Functions

Signal Transduction During NK Cell Activation: Balancing Opposing Forces

K.M. Brumbaugh, B.A. Binstadt, and P.J. Leibson

1 Introduction

Natural killer (NK) cells are lymphocytes that mediate cytotoxicity and secrete cytokines in response to certain virally infected cells, tumor targets, and some normal hematopoietic cells (Trinchieri 1989). Unlike T lymphocytes, NK cells mediate these effector functions without prior sensitization and in a non-MHC restricted fashion. Despite the efforts of many, a single activating receptor responsible for triggering natural cytotoxicity has yet to be elucidated. In fact, the emerging picture is that a combination of structurally distinct activating and inhibitory receptors influence the ability of NK cells to lyse specific target cells or to secrete regulatory cytokines.

Department of Immunology, Mayo Clinic and Foundation, Rochester, MN 55905, USA

When the receptors on the NK cells bind to their specific soluble or cell-associated ligand, this recognition must be translated into intracellular second messengers in order to initiate specific functional responses. For example, Fc receptor (FcR)-initiated activation of antibody-dependent cellular cytotoxicity (ADCC) depends on early protein tyrosine kinase (PTK) activation, followed by phospholipase C (PLC)-γ dependent phosphoinositide hydrolysis, and mobilization of intracellular calcium (Bonnema and Leibson 1996). The receptors initiating natural killing are less well defined, and therefore our understanding of the relevant signaling events is less clear. Characterizations to date suggest some overlap with FcR-initiated signaling (e.g., a requirement for rapid PTK activation and calcium signaling), yet there is also clear evidence that some signaling elements are utilized differently during ADCC vs. natural cytotoxicity (Bonnema and Leibson 1996).

However, the ultimate ability of an NK cell to undergo full activation is not determined solely by the signals generated from "triggering" receptors. Rather, there are inhibitory receptors on NK cells, which upon ligand binding can potently block cellular activation even in the presence of activating costimuli. For example, MHC-recognizing inhibitory receptors (e.g., murine Ly-49, human killer cell inhibitory receptors, human CD94) are responsible for the observation that NK cells preferentially kill targets lacking MHC class I expression (Ljunggren and Kärre 1990; Trinchieri 1994; Leibson 1995a; Yokoyama 1995; Ciccone et al. 1996; Colonna 1996; Gumperz and Parham 1996; Lanier and Phillips 1996; Moretta et al. 1996; Raulet 1996). In fact, a tumor target cell that would be normally killed by NK cells (and therefore most effectively bind to triggering receptors on NK cells) can become fully resistant to lysis if the cell is genetically manipulated to increase its MHC class I expression. Thus the balance between potentially activating and inhibitory receptors determines the outcome of the cellular response. This chapter focuses on defining these alternative receptor-initiating signaling events.

2 Activation Signals

NK cells are unique among lymphocytes in that they do not rearrange their T cell receptor (TCR) or immunoglobulin (Ig) genes and are phenotypically defined as $CD3^-$, $CD16^+$, $CD56^+$ (Reynolds and Ortaldo 1987). The alternative modes of cellular cytotoxicity mediated by these cells are initiated by different sets of receptors. ADCC is triggered by engagement of FcγRIIIA (CD16) on NK cells with the Fc portion of antibodies bound to cell-associated antigens. In contrast, the receptors initiating natural killing against tumor cells, virus-infected cells, and some normal hematopoietic targets are less well defined, although investigators have implicated roles for certain C-type lectins, CD69, CD2, Lag-3, and several other receptors. Because the receptor/ligand interactions required to initiate natural cytotoxicity are heterogeneous and not precisely defined, we begin the review by describing the more completely characterized FcγR-initiated signal events. Comparisons are then made with known signaling elements involved with natural killing.

2.1 ADCC

FcγRIIIA is a multichain receptor complex that consists of a low-affinity ligand-binding α chain (CD16) as well as two subunits required for receptor expression and signal transduction (TRINCHIERI and VALIANTE 1993; LEIBSON 1995b). These associated chains are disulfide-linked homo- or heterodimers of TCRζ and FcεRIγ (WEISSMAN et al. 1988; ANDERSON et al. 1989, 1990; LANIER et al. 1989, 1991; ORLOFF et al. 1990; VIVIER et al. 1993). The ζ and γ chains do not possess intrinsic enzymatic activity, but they contain tyrosine-based motifs known as immunoreceptor tyrosine-based activation motifs (ITAMs) in their cytoplasmic tails (RETH 1989; CAMBIER 1995). It is through ITAMs that multisubunit immune recognition receptors (TCR, B cell antigen receptors, FcR) couple to downstream signaling events. In addition to participating in signal transduction, the γ chain has also been shown to increase the FcγRIIIA affinity for ligand (MILLER et al. 1996); a similar role has not been proposed for ζ.

2.1.1 Protein Tyrosine Kinases

One of the earliest detectable signaling events following receptor cross-linking is increased tyrosine kinase activity (OSHEA et al. 1991; VIVIER et al. 1991; EINSPAHR et al. 1991; WIRTHMUELLER et al. 1992). In fact, pharmacological inhibition of FcR-initiated PTK activation (e.g., using herbimycin A or genistein) blocks ADCC (EINSPAHR et al. 1991; OSHEA et al. 1992). Two specific families of PTK have been implicated in FcγRIII-initiated signaling: the src family (which in NK cells includes Lck, Fyn, Yes, and Lyn) and the syk family (which in NK cells includes Syk and ZAP-70). The src family kinase Lck physically associates with the FcγRIII complex (CONE et al. 1993; PIGNATA et al. 1993; SALCEDO et al. 1993) and may play a critical role in the phosphorylation of the ζ/γ ITAMs (WEISS and LITTMAN 1994). The phosphorylation of ζ/γ provides a potential docking site for the SH2 domain-containing syk family members (VAN OERS and WEISS 1995). This is clearly the case for ZAP-70 (VIVIER et al. 1993) but has been more difficult to detect for Syk (TING et al. 1995). Once ZAP-70/Syk assembles into the signaling complex, their tyrosine phosphorylation (possibly involving Lck) leads to their activation (CHAN et al. 1995; WANGE et al. 1995).

This sequential tyrosine kinase activation (see Fig. 1) parallels models of TCR, B cell receptor, and FcεRI signaling in which src family kinases are activated prior to syk family PTK (WEISS and LITTMAN 1994; RAVETCH 1994). The specific kinases involved in each model vary depending on the structural elements of specific receptor subunits (e.g., their ITAMs) and on the cell-specific expression of certain PTK. Although there may be certain levels of redundancy between members of each PTK family, distinct roles have also been identified. For example, in vitro analysis of overexpressed Lck in NK cells suggest that it can couple to the FcR, whereas other src family members (e.g., Fyn or c-Src) cannot (TING et al. 1995). However, Lck-deficient as well as dominant-negative Lck transgenic mice have normal ADCC NK cell function (in spite of profound T cell developmental abnormalities) (MOLINA et

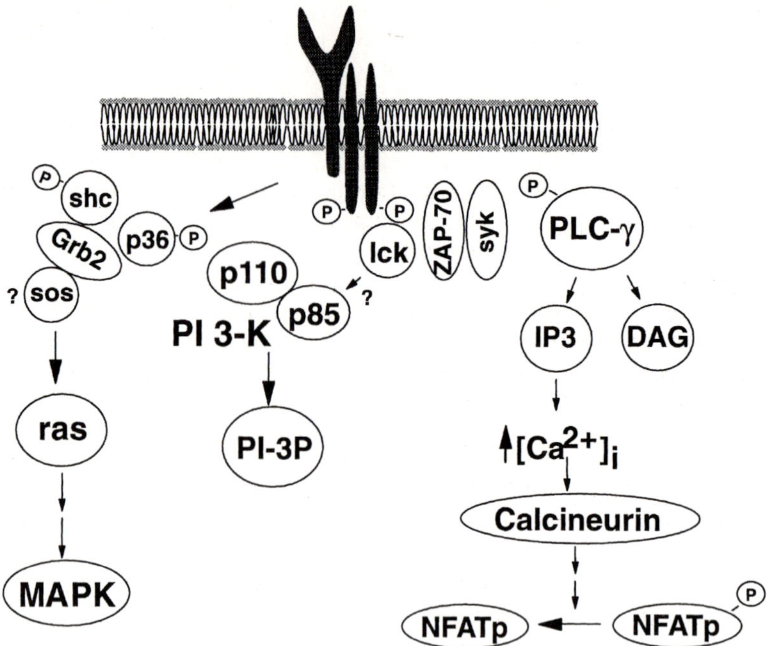

Fig. 1. FcR ligation induces the activation of proximal PTKs. This PTK activation initiates a number of different downstream signaling cascades leading to cytokine secretion, ADCC, and/or activation-induced cell death

al. 1992; LEVIN et al. 1993; WEN et al. 1995). This implies potential redundancy with an as yet unidentified src family member or the possibility of an FcR-initiated src family-independent, syk family-dependent signaling pathway.

In the case of syk family PTK there also appear to be both distinct and redundant elements to their function. Comparisons of chimeric receptors composed of extracellular CD16 and either intracellular Syk or ZAP-70 show that Syk activation is sufficient for generating a cytotoxic response whereas ZAP-70 requires costimulation with a src family PTK (KOLANUS et al. 1993). However, the normal NK cell mediated ADCC and natural cytotoxicity in ZAP-70-deficient conditions (e.g., ZAP-70 knockout mice and ZAP-70 deficient patients) (ARPAIA et al. 1994; CHAN et al. 1994; ELDER et al. 1994; NEGISHI et al. 1995) implies that either Syk can subserve ZAP-70s normal FcR-related function, or that an alternative Syk-independent pathway can be employed.

The ability of ADCC to function in the absence of Lck or ZAP-70 is consistent with observations using CD45-deficient mice. CD45 is a membrane-spanning protein tyrosine phosphatase (PTP) required for TCR and B cell receptor initiated signaling (TROWBRIDGE and THOMAS 1994). During T cell activation CD45 dephosphorylates the negative regulatory site on Lck, thus allowing its activation. However, CD45-deficient mice exhibit normal ADCC and natural cytotoxicity (YAMADA et al. 1996).

Because of the putative essential role for CD45 in Lck activation, these results are, again, consistent with the lack of requirement for Lck in NK cell mediated killing.

2.1.2 Phospholipase C-γ

Once the FcγRIII complex assembles its activated kinases, a number of downstream effectors can be activated. One of the downstream effectors in FcR-initiated signal transduction is PLC-γ. PLC-γ cleaves membrane phosphoinositides to generate inositol-1,4,5-trisphosphate and *sn*-1,2-diacylglycerol, resulting in increased intracellular free calcium concentrations ($[Ca^{2+}]_i$) and protein kinase C (PKC) activation, respectively. Both PLC-γ_1 and PLC-γ_2 are tyrosine phosphorylated and activated following FcγRIII cross-linking (Azzoni et al. 1992; Ting et al. 1992), leading to the subsequent increase in inositol phosphates and $[Ca^{2+}]_i$ (Windebank et al. 1988; Cassatella et al. 1989). Lck overexpression in NK cells augments PLC-γ tyrosine phosphorylation (Ting et al. 1995), suggesting that a src family member is part of the signaling mechanism coupling the FcγR to PLC-γ. In addition, experiments using the CD16-PTK chimeric receptors show that either ZAP-70 or Syk lead to calcium mobilization (Kolanus et al. 1993). These observations are consistent with a model in which FcγR-initiated, src family-dependent activation of syk family PTKs result in PLC-γ activation and the subsequent increase in $[Ca^{2+}]_i$.

2.1.3 Phosphatidylinositol 3-Kinase

Another downstream effector of the FcγR-induced tyrosine kinase cascade is phosphatidylinositol 3 kinase (PI3-K). PI3-K is a lipid kinase consisting of a p85 regulatory subunit and a p110 catalytic subunit (Kapeller and Cantley 1994). Following FcγR ligation PI3-Ks ability to phosphorylate inositol phospholipids at the D-3 position of the inositide ring is enhanced (Kanakaraj et al. 1994; Bonnema et al. 1994a). The critical role for PI3-K in FcR-initiated NK cell function is supported by the observation that wortmannin, a fungal metabolite that inhibits PI3-K by binding irreversibly to its p110 catalytic subunit, blocks ADCC (Bonnema et al. 1994a). PI3-K in other cell types is known to influence cytoskeletal structure, and therefore its downstream targets in NK cells may include proteins controlling cytoskeletal functions leading to granule release.

2.1.4 G Proteins

In addition to tyrosine kinases activating downstream enzymes such as PLC-γ and PI3-K, certain families of low molecular weight, guanine nucleotide binding (G) proteins are activated after FcγR cross-linking. Ras, a G protein involved in many mitogenic signaling cascades (McCormick 1994), is activated following FcγR ligation (Galandrini et al. 1996). As in T cells, the adaptor proteins p36 and p52^{shc} (Pastor et al. 1995) are tyrosine phosphorylated after receptor stimulation, which allows the adaptor Grb2 to bind via its SH2 domains to Shc and p36. Ras is subsequently activated by its guanine nucleotide exchange factor-mediated binding to GTP. One of the downstream molecules activated by Ras is the serine/threonine kinase MAPK. Pharmacological studies suggest that the Ras/MAPK signaling pathway is important in NK cells for FcR-initiated transcriptional control of tumor necrosis factor (TNF) and c-fos (TROTTA et al. 1996).

Other G proteins have been implicated in NK cell effector functions. The low molecular weight rho family G proteins are expressed in NK cells and their inactivation with the toxin C3 exoenzyme inhibits cell-mediated killing (LANG et al. 1992). In addition, pertussis toxin sensitive G proteins have been implicated in NK cell chemotaxis, killing (WHALEN et al. 1992), and FcR-induced apoptosis (CARRACEDO et al. 1995). Pertussis toxin treated NK cells can form normal conjugates with target cells and undergo normal phosphoinositide hydrolysis (WHALEN et al. 1992), suggesting a role for these G proteins in separate regulatory functions.

2.1.5 Transcriptional Regulation

Although many second messengers are known to be activated upon FcγR cross-linking, less is known regarding the nuclear factors acting downstream of these second messengers. Nuclear factor of activated T cells (NFATp) is a cyclosporin A (CsA) sensitive transcription factor known to regulate transcription of several cytokines (FLANAGAN et al. 1991; JAIN et al. 1992; MCCAFFREY et al. 1993; NORTHROP et al. 1994). Since FcR-induced signals can stimulate TNF-α, granulocyte-macrophage colony-stimulating factor (GM-CSF), and interferon (IFN)-γ cytokine production in a CsA-sensitive manner, one candidate transcription factor that binds to the promoters of cytokine genes is NFATp (COCKERILL et al. 1993; GOLDFELD et al. 1993; MASUDA et al. 1993). NFATp is constitutively expressed in the cytosol of unstimulated cells in a phosphorylated state. Upon receptor activation the phosphatase calcineurin dephosphorylates NFATp allowing it to traverse to the nucleus. Calcineurin is the target of the CsA/cyclophilin drug complex, and therefore the inactivation of calcineurins phosphatase activity prevents NFATp from migrating to the nucleus. NFATc is a related protein that is not constitutively expressed in most cells but is inducible by agents that activate PKC and/or increase $[Ca^{2+}]_i$. FcR stimulation of NK cells produces NFAT-like binding activity that was identified as NFATp by supershifting antibodies; this NFAT activity can activate transcription of GM-CSF and TNF-α (ARAMBURU et al. 1995). However, FcR stimulation also induces transcription of NFATc. Thus the NFATp binding activity in GM-CSF and TNF-α promoters does not contain the NFATc component although its message induction after FcR cross-linking indicates other genes may be regulated by NFATc. Despite its CsA sensitivity there are no NFAT binding sites in the IFN-γ promoter, and a CsA-sensitive factor other than NFAT must therefore be involved in IFN-γ gene induction.

2.2 Natural Cytotoxicity

Direct antitumor and antiviral NK cell mediated killing is initiated by the interaction of NK cell receptors with triggering epitopes on susceptible targets. However, except for a handful of putative receptors (discussed below) little is known about the molecular identity of the relevant activating NK cell receptors. This has seriously hindered studies on signal transduction since studies using cellular targets as stimulating ligands results in the binding of multiple different NK cell surface receptors. In spite of this limitation information has emerged suggesting the participation of certain key signaling pathways. Both natural cytotoxicity and ADCC are dependent on rapid PTK activation, PLC-catalyzed release of phosphoinositides, and elevations in $[Ca^{2+}]_i$ (GERRARD et al. 1987; SEAMAN et al. 1987; CHOW et al. 1988; STEELE and BRAHMI 1988; WINDEBANK et al. 1988; STAHLS and CARPEN 1989; TING et al. 1991). In contrast, recent experiments suggest that some signaling elements are used differentially during natural cytotoxicity vs. ADCC. For example, whereas natural cytotoxicity against prototypic NK-sensitive targets, such as K562, can be controlled by PKC-dependent, PI3-K independent pathways, FcR-initiated granule release and killing can be regulated by PI3-K dependent, PKC-independent mechanisms (BONNEMA et al. 1994a). Given the number of potential receptors involved in natural cytotoxicity, natural killing of different targets is likely to be regulated by different second messengers. For example, certain virus-infected and "lymphokine-activated killer cell"-sensitive targets appear to trigger NK-mediated killing in the absence of detectable PLC-dependent calcium signaling (ZANOVELLO et al. 1989; PAYA et al. 1990). This heterogeneity must always be kept in mind when trying to formulate generalizable conclusions.

2.2.1 Adhesion Molecules

Clearly a variety of adhesion molecules on NK cells can modulate the development of natural cytotoxicity, but their precise role in triggering versus costimulation is often difficult to establish. Among the adhesion molecules expressed on NK cells, most of the analyses to date have focused on the β_1 and β_2 integrins. The β_1 integrins are expressed on NK cells with the α_4 or α_5 subunits to mediate adherence to fibronectin. Cross-linking these β_1 integrins with monoclonal antibodies or fibronectin induces tyrosine kinase activity (GISMONDI et al. 1995; RABINOWICH et al. 1995); one of the phosphorylated substrates is paxillin (RABINOWICH et al. 1995), which is a cytoskeletal protein. In addition, cross-linking other NK cell receptors, such as CD7, increases β_1 integrin adherence to fibronectin (RABINOWICH et al. 1994). The relevance of these β_1 integrins to NK cell cytotoxic activity was recently shown in that NK cells in the presence of immobilized fibronectin have enhanced cytotoxicity against ADCC and NK-sensitive but not NK-resistant targets (PALMIERI et al. 1995). The enhancement of cytotoxicity required $[Ca^{2+}]_i$ increase. Thus β_1 integrins appear to serve as coactivators which enhance NK cytotoxicity.

The β_2 integrin LFA-1, expressed as CD11a/CD18 on NK cells, acts to mediate hetero- and homotypic adhesion, induce phosphatidylinositol turnover, $[Ca^{2+}]_i$ increase, granule release, and cytokine secretion (Kohl et al. 1984; Schmidt et al. 1985; Timonen et al. 1988; Melero et al. 1993). Most evidence supports a role for LFA-1 as a coreceptor rather than a triggering receptor. However, one mechanism proposed for LFA-1 as a receptor able to mediate natural cytotoxicity involves the redistribution of its ligand ICAM-2 on diseased versus normal cells (Helander et al. 1996).

2.2.2 Activating Forms of MHC-Recognizing Receptors

Although NK cells are not MHC-restricted in their killing, there is abundant in vitro and in vivo data suggesting that MHC recognition potently modulates their activation. Although the major focus has been on inhibitory MHC-recognizing receptors, separate MHC-recognizing receptors have been identified that trigger NK cell activation after their ligation (Mason et al. 1994, 1996; Rolstad et al. 1994; Moretta et al. 1995; Murphy et al. 1995; Perez-Villar et al. 1995; Brumbaugh et al. 1996). The most compelling evidence of NK cell mediated killing of specific allo-MHC target cells has been in the rat system (Rolstad et al. 1994). Extensive immunogenetic studies in this model suggest positive recognition of allogeneic class I molecules, notably nonclassical class I. Analysis using G protein-specific antibodies and permeabilized rat NK cells suggests roles for the G proteins G_o and G_z in allo-triggered killing (Maghazachi et al. 1996). In humans MHC-recognizing p50 molecules have been identified which share the extracellular ligand binding domains of p58 killer cell inhibitory receptors (KIR), but whose truncated cytoplasmic tail lack the inhibitory motif (Colonna and Samaridis 1995; Wagtmann et al. 1995a; Biassoni et al. 1996). p50-specific antibodies activate NK cells to kill FcR-bearing targets in a redirected lysis assay (Moretta et al. 1995). Presumably the charged residue in the transmembrane domain of p50 facilitates its interaction with a separate subunit (or subunits) transducing the activating signal. Similar receptors with truncated cytoplasmic tails and charged transmembrane residues are present in the human CD94/NKG2 family (Chang et al. 1995; Houchins et al. 1991). This family has been used to evaluate the intracellular activating signals generated after receptor ligation. CD94 ligation results in rapid PTK activation, PLC-γ tyrosine phosphorylation, inositol phosphate release, calcium signaling, and PI3-k activation (Brumbaugh et al. 1996). Despite these striking similarities with FcR-initiated signaling, the ζ and γ subunits are not tyrosine phosphorylated following CD94 ligation, suggesting the utilization of separate transducing subunits.

2.2.3 Other Activating Receptors

A series of other receptors have been identified which, upon antibody-mediated receptor ligation (in a redirected lysis assay) induce a cytotoxic response. However, in each case additional information is needed to implicate them as having major roles in initiating natural cytotoxicity. NKR-P1 is a receptor family with C-type lectin homology (Giorda et al. 1990). Homologous family members have been described on rat, mouse, and human NK cells (Giorda et al. 1990; Giorda and Trucco 1991;

LANIER et al. 1994). Ligation of NKR-P1 on the rat NK leukemic line RNK-16 induces inositol release and increases in $[Ca^{2+}]_i$ (RYAN et al. 1991). A recently generated NKR-P1 deficient mutant of RNK-16 was selectively deficient in killing certain tumor cell lines (RYAN et al. 1995). Genetically restored expression of a single NKR-P1 family member (NKR-P1A) restored signaling (inositol phosphate release) and a cytotoxic response to certain tumor lines. These data are consistent with a role for NKR-P1 in certain modes of natural cytotoxicity mediated by rat NK cells.

Additional receptors include NK-TR1 and LAG3. NK-TR1 is a type II transmembrane receptor with a cyclophilinlike domain (BINO et al. 1992; ANDERSON et al. 1993). NK cell transfection with NK-TR1 antisense cDNA reduces non-MHC restricted killing (GIARDINA et al. 1995), and antibody reactive with NK-TR1 induces granule exocytosis, IFN-γ secretion and reverse ADCC (FREY et al. 1991). The cellular localization and the associated signaling pathways are yet to be defined. LAG3 is a transmembrane protein of the Ig superfamily with restricted CD4 homology. NK cells from mice with a Lag-3 null mutation exhibit defects in natural cytotoxicity against a restricted subset of NK-sensitive targets (MIYAZAKI et al. 1996). The role of LAG3 in "triggering" versus "conjugate formation" and its potential signaling mechanisms remain unclear.

2.3 Cytokine Receptors

NK cells express cytokine receptors that respond to a variety of differentiation factors and alter NK cell effector functions (PERUSSIA 1991). Recent investigations have focused heavily on interleukin (IL)-2, IL-12 and IFN-α because of their shared abilities to enhance NK cell mediated cytotoxicity (HENNEY et al. 1981; ORTALDO et al. 1984; TRINCHIERI et al. 1984; WELSH 1984; LANIER et al. 1985; LONDON et al. 1986; KOBAYASHI et al. 1989; STERN et al. 1990; ROBERTSON et al. 1992; BONNEMA et al. 1994b). The interaction of these cytokines with their receptors on NK cells leads to the activation of multiple signaling molecules, including proximally the Janus family of tyrosine kinases (e.g., IL-2 activation of Jak-1 and Jak-3; MIYAZAKI et al. 1994; RUSSELL et al. 1994) and IL-12 activation of Jak-2 and Tyk-2 (BACON et al. 1995a) and the family of "signal transducers and activators of transcription" (STAT) proteins. The potentially unique roles of individual STAT proteins was recently highlighted by experiments evaluating STAT4. Although STAT4 is widely expressed, evaluations to date suggest that it is only tyrosine phosphorylated after stimulation of lymphocytes with IL-12 (BACON et al. 1995b). Mice with targeted disruption of the STAT4 gene are viable, fertile, and have no detectable defect in hematopoiesis, yet all IL-12 functions are disrupted, including IFN-γ induction, mitogenesis, T_H1 differentiation, and enhancement of NK cytolytic function (KAPLAN et al. 1996; THIERFELDER et al. 1996). These results suggest that although certain cytokine receptors overlap in their activation of common JAKs and STATs, others are uniquely coupled to family members that are essential for their downstream biological functions. Multiple cytokines positively regulate NK cell activation (e.g., IL-2, IL-12, IL-15, IFN-α, c-kit) and therefore a description of signal transduction by their receptors on NK cells goes beyond the scope of this chapter. The reader is referred to several recent reviews on specific cytokine receptor signaling mechanisms (Karnitz and Abraham 1995; Taniguchi 1995; Lamont and Adorini 1996; Tagaya et al. 1996; Theze et al. 1996).

3 Inhibitory Signals

Potent NK cellular functions (e.g., cell-mediated killing and the secretion of pleiotropic cytokines) must be tightly regulated in order to avoid the development of pathological conditions. As discussed in the initial part of this chapter, some of this regulation occurs by the limited expression of activating ligands and their receptors. In addition, NK cells have generated a series of inhibitory mechanisms that can block cellular activation. For example, MHC class I recognition by specific subpopulations of NK cells can completely block the generation of cellular cytotoxicity. The recent cloning of families of MHC-recognizing receptors has provided a molecular basis upon which to analyze the mechanism of this inhibition (Yokoyama et al. 1989; Smith et al. 1994; Colonna and Samaridis 1995; DAndrea et al. 1995; Wagtmann et al. 1995a; Mason et al. 1995; Stoneman et al. 1995). Additional inhibitory processes are engaged after NK cell activation in order to downregulate the immune response. These range from the development of an unresponsive state (i.e., anergy) to receptor-induced NK cell apoptosis.

3.1 Inhibitory MHC-Recognizing Receptors

There has been broad interest in recent data showing that receptor-mediated recognition of MHC class I complexes on target cells can block NK cell and T cell cytotoxic function in vitro and in vivo (Ljunggren and Kärre 1990; Trinchieri 1994; Leibson 1995a; Yokoyama 1995; Ciccone et al. 1996; Colonna 1996; Gumperz and Parham 1996; Lanier and Phillips 1996; Moretta et al. 1996; Raulet 1996). Among the novel MHC-recognizing receptors defined to date are human KIR (two or three Ig superfamily domains in their extracellular regions) (Colonna and Samaridis 1995; DAndrea et al. 1995; Wagtmann et al. 1995a; Dohring et al. 1996; Pende et al. 1996), human CD94/NKG2 (both subunits are members of the C-type lectin superfamily) (Houchins et al. 1991; Moretta et al. 1994; Chang et al. 1995; Lazetic et al. 1996; Perez-Villar et al. 1996; Phillips et al. 1996), and murine Ly-49 (type II disulfide-linked dimeric integral membrane proteins with homology to the C-type lectin superfamily) (Yokoyama et al. 1989; Smith et al. 1994; Mason et al. 1995; Stoneman et al. 1995). Different MHC-recognizing receptors have differing specificities for distinct MHC class I molecules, and clonal subpopulations of NK cells differ in their expression of specific MHC-recognizing receptors. Despite the structural heterogeneity emerging evidence suggests that a common inhibitory mechanism is utilized by the diverse MHC-recognizing receptors. This mechanism is best defined for the KIR family of receptors and includes three steps: (a) tyrosine

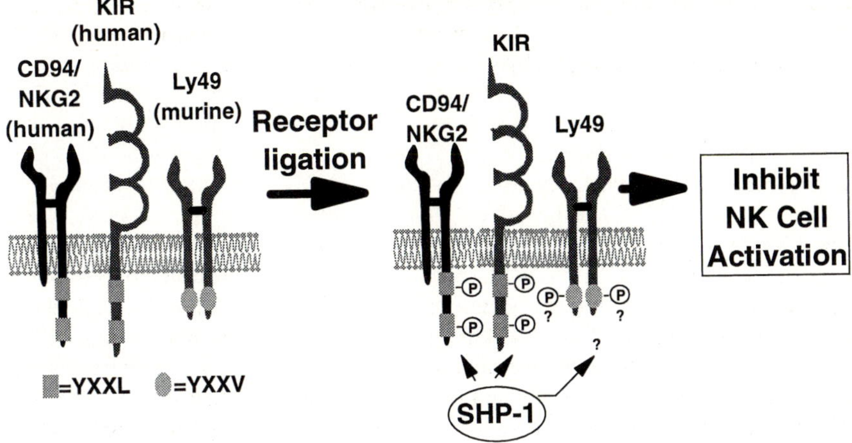

Fig. 2. MHC-recognizing receptors mediate inhibition of NK cell activation by recruiting SHP-1 to tyrosine phosphorylated ITAMs. Following receptor ligation, cytoplasmic ITAMs become tyrosine phosphorylated, allowing the association with the SH2-domain containing tyrosine phosphatase SHP-1. SHP-1 recruitment is necessary for the inhibition of NK cell activation

phosphorylation of the cytoplasmic tail of the receptor, (b) association of the receptor with the SH2-domain containing tyrosine phosphatase SHP-1, and (c) SHP-1 dependent inhibition of proximal protein tyrosine kinases (see Fig. 2).

3.1.1 Tyrosine Phosphorylation of MHC-Recognizing Receptors

Transfer and expression of p58 or p70 KIR is sufficient to confer inhibitory function to an NK cell upon class I recognition (WAGTMANN et al. 1995b). This suggests that monomeric KIR contain all the structural motifs required for the generation of the inhibitory signaling pathway. Detailed analysis of the cytoplasmic tails of the human KIR has provided some initial insights into the mechanisms by which these receptors can inhibit NK cell activation. The cytoplasmic tails of the p58 and p70 varieties of KIR contain the amino acid sequence D/E $(X)_2$ YXXL $(X)_{26}$ YXXL (COLONNA and SAMARIDIS 1995; WAGTMANN et al. 1995a; DANDREA et al. 1995). The similarity of this motif to ITAMs suggests that the phosphorylation of tyrosine residues by src$^-$ family tyrosine kinases may lead to association with SH2 domain containing proteins. In fact, KIR cross-linking does result in the tyrosine phosphorylation of this modified ITAM (BURSHTYN et al. 1996; BINSTADT et al. 1996; CAMPBELL et al. 1996; FRY et al. 1996; OLCESE et al. 1996), and genetic analysis suggests that the src family PTK Lck plays a central role in this process (BINSTADT et al. 1996). The cytoplasmic tails of the Ly-49A and NKG2 receptors also contain residues similar to those surrounding the first tyrosine of the KIR modified ITAM (BURSHTYN et al. 1996), suggesting that a common intracellular mechanism is employed by diverse MHC-recognizing receptor families.

3.1.2 Tyrosine Phosphatase Recruitment

Once the modified ITAM tyrosines are phosphorylated, there is a binding site for SH2 domain-containing proteins. In fact, the tyrosine phosphorylation of KIR by pharmacological stimulation, antibody-mediated cross-linking, or incubation with specific MHC class I bearing targets results in the phosphotyrosine-dependent association of KIR with the tyrosine phosphatase SHP-1 (BURSHTYN et al. 1996; BINSTADT et al. 1996; CAMPBELL et al. 1996; FRY et al. 1996; OLCESE et al. 1996). SHP-1 binding to the tyrosine phosphorylated residues increases its catalytic activity (BURSHTYN et al. 1996; CAMPBELL et al. 1996), and experiments in which the catalytically inactive (dominant negative) form of SHP-1 is expressed suggest that its catalytic activity is required for KIR-mediated inhibition (BURSHTYN et al. 1996; BINSTADT et al. 1996). Recently we have also defined a role for SHP-1 in the inhibition mediated by CD94/NKG2 (Brumbaugh et al., unpublished observations). The tyrosine phosphorylated subunit recruits SHP-1, and experiments with dominant negative SHP-1 again suggest an essential role for its catalytic activity in the NK cell inhibition.

3.1.3 Interruption of NK Cell Activation

Information is just beginning to emerge as to how KIR-associated SHP-1 can inhibit NK cell activation. Studies evaluating KIR effects on natural cytotoxicity have been limited by our incomplete understanding of activating signals during this process and the heterogeneous activating receptors engaged. In spite of these limitations KIR engagement can block the inositol phosphate release and calcium signaling induced by binding to NK-sensitive targets (KAUFMAN et al. 1995). More detailed analyses of the effects of KIR ligation on FcR-initiated signaling demonstrated inhibition of the tyrosine phosphorylation of ζ, ZAP-70, and PLC-γ, as well as subsequent increases in inositol phosphate release and $[Ca^{2+}]_i$ (BINSTADT et al. 1996). Inhibitory CD94/NKG2 also blocks the generation of these same second messengers (BRUMBAUGH et al. 1996). In each case the expression of a dominant negative SHP-1 restores the normal proximal activation signals, supporting its central role in these regulatory events (BINSTADT et al. 1996; Brumbaugh et al., unpublished observations). Additional studies are required to determine the specific targets of the KIR-associated SHP-1.

3.2 Target Cell-Induced Inactivation

When NK cells are coincubated with unlabeled NK-sensitive targets, there is a time-dependent and temperature-dependent decrease in their capacity subsequently to mediate killing of additional tumor targets (PERUSSIA and TRINCHIERI 1980; BRAHMI et al. 1985; ABRAMS and BRAHMI 1986, 1988a,b; XIAO and BRAHMI 1989). These inactivated NK cells have a reduced ability to kill a broad range of different NK-sensitive and antibody-coated targets. Although depletion of critical effector molecules can limit the effectiveness of cell-mediated killing, studies also suggest modified intracellular signaling (Bajpai and Brahmi 1994). NK cell restimulation with IL-2 increases cellular responsiveness and recovery of cytotoxic function (Abrams and Brahmi 1986, 1988a; Xiao and Brahmi 1989; Bajpai and Brahmi 1994).

3.1.3 Activation-Induced Cell Death

After an NK cell delivers its lethal hit to susceptible targets, it may either recycle (to kill again), become inactivated (see above section), or undergo activation-induced cell death (AICD). The autocrine induction of NK cell death has best been described for IL-2 and/or IL-12 activated NK cells receiving chronic FcR stimulation (Azzoni et al. 1995; Ortaldo et al. 1995). In this case FcR-initiated NK cell death is dependent on tyrosine kinase activation and calcium signaling. Recent data suggest that the FcR-initiated induction of Fas ligand (FasL) expression on the activated NK cells is central to this process (Eischen et al. 1996). In fact the observation that antibodies blocking FasL/Fas interactions inhibit FcR-initiated AICD is consistent with a model in which autocrine FasL/Fas interaction leads to the NK cells demise (Eischen et al. 1996). Additional studies are needed to determine whether similar processes are initiated after NK cells mediate natural cytotoxicity.

4 Summary

Significant progress has been made in our understanding of the basic signaling mechanisms regulating NK cell activation. Advances have been fueled in part by the molecular characterization of specific activating receptors (e.g., the FcγRIII multi-subunit complex) and inhibitory receptors (e.g., novel MHC-recognizing inhibitory receptors). However, certain aspects of these analyses are complicated by the heterogeneous nature of the receptor-ligand interactions utilized during the development of a cytotoxic response. Future advances will depend in part on the further molecular characterization of the involved receptors and second messengers and on the development of experimental models for genetically manipulating the signaling elements. It will remain important to understand both activating and inhibitory signaling pathways as the emerging theme is that the balance of these two opposing forces determines the functional outcome of an NK cells interaction with its target.

Acknowledgements. The data discussed from the authors laboratory were supported by the Mayo Foundation and by the National Institutes of Health grant CA47752. We thank Theresa Lee for her skillful assistance with the preparation of the manuscript

References

Abrams SI, Brahmi Z (1986) The functional loss of human natural killer cell activity induced by K562 is reversible via an interleukin-2-dependent mechanism. Cell Immunol 101:558–570

Abrams SI, Brahmi Z (1988a) Target cell directed NK inactivation. Concomitant loss of NK and antibody-dependent cellular cytotoxicity activities. J Immunol 140:2090–2095

Abrams SI, Brahmi Z (1988b) Mechanism of K562-induced human natural killer cell inactivation using highly enriched effector cells isolated via a new single-step sheep erythrocyte rosette assay. Ann Inst Pasteur/Immunol 139:361–381

Anderson P, Caligiuri M, Ritz J, Schlossman SF (1989) CD3-negative natural killer cells express ζ TCR as part of a novel molecular complex. Nature 341:159–162

Anderson P, Caligiuri M, O'Brien C, Manley T, Ritz J, Schlossman SF (1990) Fcγ receptor type III (CD16) is included in the ζ NK receptor complex expressed by human natural killer cells. Proc Natl Acad Sci USA 87:2274–2278

Anderson SK, Callinger S, Roder, J, Frey J, Young HA, Ortaldo JR (1993) A cyclophilin-related protein involved in the function of natural killer cells. Proc Natl Acad Sci USA 90:542–546

Aramburu J, Azzoni L, Rao A, Perussia B (1995) Activation and expression of the nuclear factors of activated T cells, NFATp and NFATc, in human natural killer cells: Regulation upon CD16 ligand binding. J Exp Med 182:801–810

Arpaia E, Shahar M, Dadi H, Cohen A, Rolfman CM (1994) Defective T cell receptor signaling and $CD8^+$ thymic selection in humans lacking Zap-70 kinase. Cell 76:947–958

Azzoni L, Kamoun M, Salcedo TW, Kanakaraj P, Perussia B (1992) Stimulation of FcγRIIIA results in phospholipase C-γ1 tyrosine phosphorylation and $p56^{lck}$ activation. J Exp Med 176:1745–1750

Azzoni L, Anegon I, Calabretta B, Perussia B (1995) Ligand binding to FcγR induces c-myc-dependent apoptosis in IL-2-stimulated NK cells. J Immunol 154:491–499

Bacon CM, McVical DW, Ortaldo JR, Rees RC, O'Shea JJ, Johnston JA (1995a) Interleukin 12 (IL-12) induces tyrosine phosphorylation of JAK2 and TYK2: differential use of janus family tyrosine kinases by IL-2 and IL-12. J Exp Med 181:399–404

Bacon CM, Petricoin EF III, Ortaldo JR, Rees RC, Larner AC, Johnston JA, O'Shea JJ (1995b) Interleukin 12 induces tyrosine phosphorylation and activation of STAT4 in human lymphocytes. Proc Natl Acad Sci USA 92:7307–7311

Bajpai A, Brahmi Z (1994) Target cell-induced inactivation of cytolytic lymphocytes. J Biol Chem 269:18864–18869

Biassoni R, Cantoni C, Falco M, Verdiani S, Bottino C, Vitale M, Conte R, Poggi A, Moretta A, Moretta L (1996) The human leukocyte antigen (HLA)-C-specific "activatory" or "inhibitory" natural killer cell receptors display highly homologous extracellular domains but differ in their transmembrane and intracytoplasmic portions. J Exp Med 183:645–650

Bino T, Frey JL, Ortaldo JR (1992) Mechanism of target cell recognition by $CD3^-$ LGL. I. Development of a monoclonal antibody to a K562-associated target cell antigen. Cell Immunol 142:28–39

Binstadt BA, Brumbaugh KM, Dick CJ, Scharenberg AM, Williams BL, Colonna M, Lanier LL, Kinet J-P, Abraham RT, Leibson PJ (1996) Sequential involvement of Lck and SHP-1 with MHC-recognizing receptors on NK cells inhibits FcR-initiated tyrosine kinase activation. Immunity 5:629–638

Bonnema JD, Leibson PJ (1996) Signal transduction during NK cell activation. In: Moretta L (ed) Molecular basis of NK cell recognition and function. Karger, Basel, pp 28–43

Bonnema JD, Karnitz LM, Schoon RA, Abraham RT, Leibson PJ (1994a) Fc receptor stimulation of phosphatidylinositol 3-kinase in natural killer cells is associated with protein kinase C-independent granule release and cell-mediated cytotoxicity. J Exp Med 180:1427–1435

Bonnema JD, Rivlin KA, Ting AT, Schoon RA, Abraham RT, Leibson PJ (1994b) Cytokine-enhanced NK cell-mediated cytotoxicity. Positive modulatory effects of IL-2 and IL-12 on stimulus-dependent granule exocytosis. J Immunol 152:2098–2104

Brahmi Z, Bray RA, Abrams SI (1985) Evidence for an early calcium-independent event in the activation of the human natural killer cell cytolytic mechanism. J Immunol 135:4108–4113

Brumbaugh KM, Perez-Villar JJ, Dick CJ, Schoon RA, Lopez-Botet M, Leibson PJ (1996) Clonotypic differences in signaling from CD94 (kp43) on NK cells lead to divergent cellular responses. J Immunol 157:2804–2812

Burshtyn DN, Scharenberg AM, Wagtmann N, Rajagopalan S, Berrada K, Yi, T, Kinet, J-P, Long EO (1996) Recruitment of tyrosine phosphatase HCP by the killer cell inhibitory receptor. Immunity 4:77–85

Cambier JC (1995) Antigen and Fc receptor signaling. The awesome power of the immunoreceptor tyrosine-based activation motif (ITAM). J Immunol 155:3281–3285

Campbell KS, Dessing M, Lopez-Botet M, Cella M, Colonna M (1996) Tyrosine phosphorylation of a human killer inhibitory receptor recruits protein tyrosine phosphatase 1C. J Exp Med 184:93–100

Carracedo J, Ramirez R, Marchetti P, Pintado OC, Baixeras E, Martinez-A C, Kroemer G (1995) Pertussis toxin-sensitive GTP-binding proteins regulate activation-induced apoptotic cell death of human natural killer cells. Eur J Immunol 25:3094–3099

Cassatella MA, Anegon I, Guturi MC, Griskey P, Trinchieri G, Perussia B (1989) FcγR(CD16) interaction with ligand induces Ca^{2+} mobilization and phosphoinositide turnover in human natural killer cells. Role of Ca^{2+} in FcγR(CD16)-induced transcription and expression of lymphokine genes. J Exp Med 169:549–567

Chan AC, Kadlecek TA, Elder ME, Filipovich AH, Kuo W-L, Iwashima M, Parslow TG, Weiss A (1994) ZAP-70 deficiency in an autosomal recessive form of severe combined immunodeficiency. Science 264:1599–1601

Chan AC, Dalton M, Johnson R, Kong G-H Wang T, Thoma R, Kurosaki T (1995) Activation of ZAP-70 kinase activity by phosphorylation of tyrosine 493 is required for lymphocyte antigen receptor function. EMBO 14:2499–2508

Chang C, Rodriguez A, Carretero M, Lopez-Botet M, Phillips JH, Lanier LL (1995) Molecular characterization of human CD94: a type II membrane glycoprotein related to the C-type lectin superfamily. Eur J Immunol 25:2433–2437

Chow SC, NGJ, Nordstedt C, Fredholm BB, Jondal M (1988) Phosphoinositide breakdown and evidence for protein kinase C involvement during human NK killing. Cell Immunol 114:96–103

Ciccone E, Grossi CE, Velardi A (1996) Opposing functions of activatory T-cell receptors and inhibitory NK-cell receptors on cytotoxic T cells. Immunol Today 17:450–453

Cockerill PN, Shannon MF, Bert AG, Ryan GR, Vadas MA (1993) The granulocyte-macrophage colony-stimulating factor/interleukin 3 locus is regulated by an inducible cyclosporin A-sensitive enhancer. Proc Natl Acad Sci USA 90:2466–2470

Colonna M (1996) Natural killer cell receptors specific for MHC class I molecules. Curr Opin Immunol 8:101–107

Colonna M, Samaridis J (1995) Cloning of immunoglobulin-superfamily members associated with HLA-C and HLA-B recognition by human natural killer cells. Science 268:405–408

Cone JC, Lu Y, Trevillyan JM, Bjorndahl JM, Phillips CA (1993) Association of the $p56^{lck}$ protein tyrosine kinase with the FcγRIIIA/CD16 complex in human natural killer cells. Eur J Immunol 23:2488–2497

D'Andrea A, Chang C, Franz-Bacon K, McClanahan T, Phillips JH, Lanier LL (1995) Molecular cloning of NKB1. A natural killer cell receptor for HLA-B allotypes. J Immunol 155:2306–2310

Dohring C, Scheidegger D, Samaridis J, Cella M, Colonna M (1996) A human killer inhibitory receptor specific for HLA-A. J Immunol 156:3098–3101

Einspahr KJ, Abraham RT, Binstadt BA, Uehara Y, Leibson PJ (1991) Tyrosine phosphorylation provides an early and requisite signal for the activation of natural killer cell cytotoxic function. Proc Natl Acad Sci USA 88:6279–6283

Eischen CM, Schilling JD, Lynch DH, Krammer PH, Leibson PJ (1996) Fc receptor-induced expression of Fas ligand on activated NK cells facilitates cell-mediated cytotoxicity and subsequent autocrine NK cell apoptosis. J Immunol 156:2693–2699

Elder ME, Lin D, Clever J, Chan AC, Hope TJ, Weiss A, Parslow TG (1994) Human severe combined immunodeficiency due to a defect in ZAP-70, a T cell tyrosine kinase. Science 264:1596–1599

Flanagan JM, Corthesy B, Bram RJ, Crabtree GR (1991) Nuclear association of a T-cell transcription factor blocked by FK-506 and cyclosporin A. Nature 352:803–807

Frey JL, Bino T, Kantor RRS, Segal DM, Giardina SL, Roder J, Anderson S, Ortaldo JR (1991) Mechanism of target cell recognition by natural killer cells: characterization of a novel triggering molecule restricted to $CD3^-$ large granular lymphocytes. J Exp Med 174:1527–1536

Fry AM, Lanier LL, Weiss A (1996) Phosphotyrosines in the killer cell inhibitory receptor motif of NKB1 are required for negative signaling and for association with protein tyrosine phosphatase 1C. J Exp Med 184:295–300

Galandrini R, Palmieri G, Piccoli M, Frati L, Santoni A (1996) CD16-mediated p21^{ras} activation is associated with Shc and p36 tyrosine phosphorylation and their binding with Grb2 in human natural killer cells. J Exp Med 183:179–186

Gerrard JM, Hildes E, Atkinson EA, Greenberg AR (1987) Activation of inositol cycle in large granular lymphocyte leukemia RNK following contact with an NK-sensitive tumor. In: Samuelsson B, Paoletti R, Ramwell PW (eds) Advances in prostaglandin, thromboxane, and leukotriene research, vol 17. Raven, New York, pp 573–576

Giardina SL, Anderson SK, Sayers TJ, Chambers WH, Palumbo GA, Young HA, Ortaldo JR (1995) Selective loss of NK cytotoxicity in antisense NK-TR1 rat LGL cell lines. Abrogation of antibody-independent tumor and virus-infected target cell killing. J Immunol 154:80–87

Giorda R, Trucco M (1991) Mouse NKR-P1. A family of genes selectively coexpressed in adherent lymphokine-activated killer cells. J Immunol 147:1701–1708

Giorda R, Rudert WA, Vavassori C, Chambers WH, Hiserodt JC, Trucco M (1990) NKR-P1, a signal transduction molecule on natural killer cells. Science 249:1298–1300

Gismondi A, Milella M, Palmieri G, Piccoli M, Frati L, Santoni A (1995) Stimulation of protein tyrosine phosphorylation by interaction of NK cells with fibronectin via α4β1 and α5β1. J Immunol 154:3128–3137

Goldfeld AE, McCaffrey PG, Strominger JL, Rao A (1993) Identification of a novel cyclosporin-sensitive element in the human tumor necrosis factor α gene promoter. J Exp Med 178:1365–1379

Gumperz JE, Parham P (1995) The enigma of the natural killer cell. Nature 378:245–248

Helander TS, Carpen O, Turunen O, Kovanen PE, Vaheri A, Timonen T (1996) ICAM-2 redistributed by ezrin as a target for killer cells. Nature 382:265–268

Henney CS, Kuribayashi K, Kern DE, Gillis S (1981) Interleukin-2 augments natural killer cell activity. Nature 291:335–338

Houchins JP, Yabe T, McSherry C, Bach FH (1991) DNA sequence analysis of NKG2, a family of related cDNA clones encoding type II integral membrane proteins on human natural killer cells. J Exp Med 173:1017–1020

Jain J, McCaffrey PG, Valge-Archer VE, Rao A (1992) Nuclear factor of activated T cells contains Fos and Jun. Nature 356:801–804

Kanakaraj P, Duckworth B, Azzoni L, Kamoun M, Cantley LC, Perussia B (1994) Phosphatidylinositol-3 kinase activation induced upon FcγRIIIA-ligand interaction. J Exp Med 179:551–558

Kapeller R, Cantley LC (1994) Phosphatidylinositol 3-kinase. Bioessays 16:565–576

Kaplan MH, Sun Y-L, Hoey T, Grusby MJ (1996) Impaired IL-12 responses and enhanced development of Th2 cells in Stat4-deficient mice. Nature 382:174–177

Karnitz LM, Abraham RT (1995) Cytokine receptor signaling mechanisms. Curr Opin Immunol 7:320–326

Kaufman DS, Schoon RA, Robertson MJ, Leibson PJ (1995) Inhibition of selective signaling events in natural killer cells recognizing major histocompatibility complex class I. Proc Natl Acad Sci USA 92:6484–6488

Kobayashi M, Fitz L, Ryan M, Hewick RM, Clark SC, Chan S, Loudon R, Sherman F, Perussia B, Trinchieri G (1989) Identification and purification of natural killer cell stimulatory factor (NKSF), a cytokine with multiple biologic effects on human lymphocytes. J Exp Med 170:827–845

Kohl S, Springer TA, Schmalstieg FC, Loo LS, Anderson DC (1984) Defective natural killer cytotoxicity and polymorphonuclear leukocyte antibody-dependent cellular cytotoxicity in patients with LFA-1/OKM-1 deficiency. J Immunol 133:2972–2978

Kolanus W, Romeo C, Seed B (1993) T cell activation by clustered tyrosine kinases. Cell 74:171–183

Lamont AG, Adorini L (1996) IL-12: a key cytokine in immune regulation. Immunol Today 17:214–217

Lang P, Guizani L, Vitte-Mony I, Stancou R, Dorseuil O, Gacon G, Bertoglio (1992) ADP-ribosylation of the ras-related, GTP-binding protein RhoA inhibits lymphocyte-mediated cytotoxicity. J Biol Chem 267:11677–11680

Lanier LL, Phillips JH (1996) Inhibitory MHC class I receptors on NK cells and T cells. Immunol Today 17:86–91

Lanier LL, Benike CJ, Phillips JH, Engleman EG (1985) Recombinant interleukin 2 enhanced natural killer cell-mediated cytotoxicity in human lymphocyte subpopulations expressing the Leu7 and Leu11 antigens. J Immunol 134:794–801

Lanier LL, Yu G, Phillips JH (1989) Co-association of CD3ζ with a receptor (CD16) for IgG Fc on human natural killer cells. Nature 342:803–805

Lanier LL, Yu G, Phillips JH (1991) Analysis of FcγRIII (CD16) membrane expression and association with CD3ζ and FcεRI-γ by site-directed mutation. J Immunol 146:1571–1576

Lanier LL, Chang C, Phillips JH (1994) Human NKR-P1A. A disulfide-linked homodimer of the C-type lectin superfamily expressed by a subset of NK and T lymphocytes. J Immunol 153:2417–2428

Lazetic S, Chang C, Houchins JP, Lanier LL, Phillips JH (1996) Human natural killer cell receptors involved in MHC class I recognition are disulfide-linked heterodimers of CD94 and NKG2 subunits. J Immunol 157:4741–4745

Leibson PJ (1995a) MHC-recognizing receptors: they're not just for T cells anymore. Immunity 3:5–8

Leibson PJ (1995b) Viewpoint: signal transduction during natural killer cell activation. Nat Immun 14:117–122

Levin SD, Anderson SJ, Forbush KA, Perlmutter RM (1993) A dominant-negative transgene defines a role for $p56^{lck}$ in thymopoiesis. EMBO 12:1671–1680

Ljunggren H-G, Kärre K (1990) In search of the 'missing self': MHC molecules and NK cell recognition. Immunol Today 11:237–244

London L, Perussia B, Trinchieri G (1986) Induction of proliferation in vitro of resting human natural killer cells: IL2 induces into cell cycle most peripheral blood NK cells, but only a minor subset of low density T cells. J Immunol 137:3845–3854

Maghazachi AA, Al-Aoukaty A, Naper C, Torgersen KM, Rolstad B (1996) Preferential involvement of G_o and G_z proteins in mediating rat natural killer cell lysis of allogeneic and tumor target cells. J Immunol 157:5308–5314

Mason LH, Yagita H, Ortaldo JR (1994) LGL-1: a potential triggering molecule on murine NK cells. J Leukoc Biol 55:362–370

Mason LH, Ortaldo JR, Yound HA, Kumar V, Bennett M, Anderson SK (1995) Cloning and functional characteristics of murine large granular lymphocyte-1: a member of the Ly-49 gene family (Ly-49G2). J Exp Med 182:293–303

Mason LH, Anderson SK, Yokoyama WM, Smith HRC, Winkler-Pickett R, Ortaldo JR (1996) The Ly-49D receptor activates murine natural killer cells. J Exp Med 184:2119–2128

Masuda ES, Tokumitsu H, Tsuboi A, Shlomai J, Hung P, Arai K-I, Arai N (1993) The granulocyte-macrophage colony-stimulating factor promoter cis-acting element CLE0 mediates induction signals in T cells and is recognized by factors related to AP1 and NFAT. Mol Cell Biol 13:7399–7407

McCaffrey PG, Perrino BA, Soderling TR, Rao A (1993) NF-AT_p, a T lymphocyte DNA-binding protein that is a target for clacineurin and immunosuppressive drugs. J Biol Chem 268:3747–3752

McCormick F (1994) Activators and effectors of ras p21 proteins. Curr Opin Genet Dev 4:71–76

Melero I, Balboa MA, Alonso JL, Yague E, Pivel JP, Sanchez-Madrid F, Lopez-Botet M (1993) Signaling through the LFA-1 leucocyte integrin actively regulates intercellular adhesion and tumor necrosis factor-α production in natural killer cells. Eur J Immunol 23:1859–1865

Miller KL, Duchemin A-M, Anderson CL (1996) A novel role for the Fc receptor γ subunit: enhancement of FcγR ligand affinity. J Exp Med 183:2227–2233

Miyazaki T, Kawaharea A, Fujii H, Nakagawa Y, Minami Y, Liu Z-J, Oishi I, Silvennoinen O, Witthuhn BA, Ihle JN, Taniguchi T (1994) Functional activation of Jak1 and Jak3 by selective association with IL-2 receptor subunits. Science 266:1045–1047

Miyazaki T, Dierich A, Benoist C, Mathis D (1996) Independent modes of natural killing distinguished in mice lacking Lag3. Science 272:405–408

Molina TJ, Kishihara K, Siderovski DP, van Ewijk W, Narendran A, Timms E, Wakeham A, Paige CJ Hartmann K-U, Veillette A, Davidson D, Mak TW (1992) Profound block in thymocyte development in micc lacking $p56^{lck}$. Nature 357:161–164

Moretta A, Vitale M, Sivori S, Bottino C, Morelli L, Auguliaro R, Barbaresi M, Pende D, Ciccone E, Lopez-Botet M, Moretta L (1994) Human natural killer cell receptors for HLA-Class I molecules. Evidence that the Kp43 (CD94) molecule functions as receptor for HLA-B alleles. J Exp Med 180:545–555

Moretta A, Sivori S, Vitale M, Pende D, Morelli L, Augugliaro R, Bottino C, Moretta L (1995) Existence of both inhibitory (p58) and activatory (p50) receptors for HLA-C molecules in human natural killer cells. J Exp Med 182:875–884

Moretta A, Bottino C, Vitale M, Pende D, Biassoni R, Mingari MC, Moretta L (1996) Receptors for HLA class-I molecules in human natural killer cells. Annu Rev Immunol 14:619–648

Murphy WJ, Raziuddin A, Mason L, Kumar V, Bennett M, Longo DL (1995) NK cell subsets in the regulation of murine hematopoiesis. I. $5E6^+$ NK cells promote hematopoietic growth in $H\text{-}2^d$ strain mice. J Immunol 155:2911–2917

Negishi I, Motoyama N, Nakayama K-I, Nakayama K, Senju S, Hatakeyama S, Zhang Q, Chan AC, Loh DY (1995) Essential role for ZAP-70 in both positive and negative selection of thymocytes. Nature 376:435–438

Northrop JP, Ho SN, Chen L, Thomas DJ, Timmerman LA, Nolan GP, Admon A, Crabtree GR (1994) NF-AT components define a family of transcription factors targeted in T-cell activation. Nature 369:497–502

Olcese L, Long P, Vely F, Cambiaggi A, Marguet D, Blery M, Hippen KL, Biassoni R, Moretta A, Moretta L, Cambier JC, Vivier E (1996) Human and mouse killer-cell inhibitory receptors recruit PTP1C and PTP1D protein tyrosine phosphatases. J Immunol 156:4531–4534

Orloff DG, Ra C, Frank SJ, Klausner RD, Kinet J-P (1990) Family of disulphide-linked dimers containing the ζ and η chains of the T-cell receptor and the γ chain of Fc receptors. Nature 347:189–191

Ortaldo JR, Mason AT, Gerard JP, Henderson LE, Farrar W, Hopkins RF III, Herberman RB, Rabin H (1984) Effects of natural and recombinant IL 2 on regulation of IFNγ production and natural killer activity: lack of involvement of the TAC antigen for these immunoregulatory effects. J Immunol 133:779–783

Ortaldo JR, Mason AT, O'Shea JJ (1995) Receptor-induced death in human natural killer cells: involvement of CD16. J Exp Med 181:339–344

O'Shea JJ, Weissman AM, Kennedy ICS, Ortaldo JR (1991) Engagement of the natural killer cell IgG Fc receptor results in tyrosine phosphorylation of the ζ chain. Proc Natl Acad Sci USA 88:350–354

O'Shea JJ, McVicar DW, Kuhns DB, Ortaldo JR (1992) A role for protein tyrosine kinase activity in natural cytotoxicity as well as antibody-dependent cellular cytotoxicity. J Immunol 148:2497–2502

Palmieri G, Serra A, DeMaria R, Gismondi A, Milella M, Piccoli M, Frati L, Santoni A (1995) Cross-linking of $\alpha 5\beta 1$ fibronectin receptors enhances natural killer cell cytotoxic activity. J Immunol 155:5314–5322

Pastor MI, Reib K, Cantrell D (1995) The regulation and function of $p21^{ras}$ during T-cell activation and growth. Immunol Today 163:159–164

Paya CV, Schoon RA, Leibson PJ (1990) Alternative mechanisms of natural killer cell activation during herpes simplex virus infection. J Immunol 144:4370–4375

Pende D, Biassoni R, Cantoni C, Verdiani S, Falco M, Di Donato C, Accame L, Bottino C, Moretta A, Moretta L (1996) The natural killer cell receptor specific for HLA-A allotypes: a novel member of the p58/p70 family of inhibitory receptors that is characterized by three immunoglobulin-like domains and is expressed as a 140-kD disulphide-linked dimer. J Exp Med 184:505–518

Perez-Villar JJ, Melero I, Rodriguez A, Carretero M, Aramburu J, Sivori S, Orengo AM, Moretta A, Lopez-Botet M (1995) Functional ambivalence of the Kp43 (CD94) NK cell-associated surface antigen. J Immunol 154:5779–5788

Perez-Villar JJ, Carretero M, Navarro F, Melero I, Rodriguez A, Bottino C, Moretta A, Lopez-Botet M (1996) Biochemical and serologic evidence for the existence of functionally distinct forms of the CD94 NK cell receptor. J Immunol 157:5367–5374

Perussia B (1991) Lymphokine-activated killer cells, natural killer cells and cytokines. Curr Opin Immunol 3:49–55

Perussia B, Trinchieri G (1980) Inactivation of natural killer cell cytotoxic activity after interaction with target cells. J Immunol 126:754–758

Phillips JH, Chang C, Mattson J, Gumperz JE, Parham P, Lanier LL (1996) CD94 and a novel associated protein (94AP) form a NK cell receptor involved in the recognition of HLA-A, HLA-B, and HLA-C allotypes. Immunity 5:163–172

Pignata C, Prasad KVS, Robertson MJ, Levine H, Rudd CE, Ritz J (1993) FcγRIIIA-mediated signaling involves src-family lck in human natural killer cells. J Immunol 151:6794–6800

Rabinowich H, Lin W-C, Herberman RB, Whiteside TL (1994) Signaling via CD7 molecules on human NK cells. Induction of tyrosine phosphorylation and β1 integrin-mediated adhesion to fibronectin. J Immunol 153:3504–3513

Rabinowich H, Lin W-C, Manciulea M, Herberman RB, Whiteside TL (1995) Induction of protein tyrosine phosphorylation in human natural killer cells by triggering via $\alpha_4\beta_1$ or $\alpha_5\beta_1$ integrins. Blood 85:1858–1864

Raulet DH (1996) Recognition events that inhibit and activate natural killer cells. Curr Opin Immunol 8:372–377

Ravetch JV (1994) Fc receptors: rubor redux. Cell 78:553–560
Reth M (1989) Antigen receptor tail clue. Nature 338:383–384
Reynolds CW, Ortaldo JR (1987) Natural killer activity: the definition of a function rather than a cell type. Immunol Today 8:172–174
Robertson MJ, Soiffer RJ, Wolf SF, Manley TJ, Donahue C, Young D, Herrmann SH, Ritz J (1992) Response of human natural killer (NK) cells to NK cell stimulatory factor (NKSF): cytolytic activity and proliferation of NK cells are differentially regulated by NKSF. J Exp Med 175:779–788
Rolstad B, Wonigeit K, Vaage JT (1994) Alloreactive rat natural killer (NK) cells in vivo and in vitro: the role of the major histocompatibility complex (MHC). In: Rolstad B (ed) Natural immunity to normal hemopoietic cells. CRC, Ann Arbor, pp 99–149
Russell SM, Johnston JA, Noguchi M, Kawamura M, Bacon CM, Friedmann M, Berg M, McVicar DWM Witthuhn BA, Silvennoinen O, Goldman AS, Schmalstieg FC, Ihle JN, O'Shea JJ, Leonard WJ (1994) Interaction of IL-2Rβ and γ_c chains with Jak1 and Jak3: implications for XSCID and XCID. Science 266:1042–1045
Ryan JC et al (1991) NKR-P1, an activating molecular on rat natural killer cells, stimulates phosphoinositide turnover and a rise in intracellular calxium. J Immunol 147:3244–3250
Ryan JC, Niemi EC, Nakamura MC, Seaman WE (1995) NKR-P1A is a target-specific receptor that activates natural killer cell cytotoxicity. J Exp Med 181:1911–1915
Salcedo TW, Kurosaki T, Kanakaraj P, Ravetch JV, Perussia B (1993) Physical and functional association of $p56^{lck}$ with FcγRIIIA (CD16) in natural killer cells. J Exp Med 177:1475–1480
Schmidt et al (1985) Functional characterization of LFA-1 antigens in the interaction of human NK clones and target cells. J Immunol 135:1020–1025
Seaman WE, Eriksson E, Dobrow R, Imboden JB (1987) Inositol trisphosphate is generated by a rat natural killer cell tumor in response to target cells or to crosslinked monoclonal antibody OX-34: possible signaling role for the OX-34 determinant during activation by target cells. Proc Natl Acad Sci USA 84:4239–4243
Smith HR, Karlhofer FM, Yokoyama WM (1994) Ly-49 multigene family expressed by IL-2-activated NK cells. J Immunol 153:1068
Stahls AK, Carpen O (1989) Generation of inositol phosphates during triggering of cytotoxicity in human natural killer and lymphokine-activated killer cells. Scand J Immunol 29:211–216
Steele TA, Brahmi Z (1988) Phosphatidylinositol metabolism accompanies early activation events in tumor target cell-stimulated human natural killer cells. Cell Immunol 112:402–413
Stern AS, Podlaski FJ, Hulmes JD, Pan Y-C E, Quinn PM, Wolitzky AG, Familletti PC, Stremlo DL, Truitt T, Chizzonite R, Gately MK (1990) Purification to homogeneity and partial characterization of cytotoxic lymphocyte maturation factor from human B-lymphoblastoid cells. Proc Natl Acad Sci USA 87:6808–6812
Stoneman ER, Bennett M, An J, Chesnut KA, Wakeland EK, Scheerer JB, Siciliano MJ, Kumar V, Mathew PA (1995) Cloning and characterization of 5E6(Ly-49C), a receptor molecule expressed on a subset of murine natural killer cells. J Exp Med 182:305–313
Tagaya Y, Bamford RN, DeFilippis AP, Waldmann TA (1996) IL-15: a pleiotropic cytokine with diverse receptor/signaling pathways whose expression is controlled at multiple levels. Immunity 4:329–336
Taniguchi T (1995) Cytokine signaling through nonreceptor protein tyrosine kinases. Science 268:251–255
Theze J, Alzari PM, Bertoglio J (1996) Interleukin 2 and its receptors: recent advances and new immunological functions. Immunol Today 17:481–486
Thierfelder WE, van Deursen JM, Yamamoto K, Tripp RA, Sarawar SR, Carson RT, Sangster MY, Vignali DAA, Doherty PC, Grosveld GC, Ihle JN (1996) Requirement for Stat4 in interleukin-12-mediated responses of natural killer and T cells. Nature 382:171–174
Timonen T, Patarroyo M, Gahmberg CG (1988) CD11a-c/CD18 and GP84 (LB-2) adhesion molecules on human large granular lymphocytes and their participation in natural killing. J Immunol 141:1041–1046
Ting AT, Einspahr KJ, Abraham RT, Leibson PJ (1991) Fcγ receptor signal transduction in natural killer cells. Coupling to phospholipase C via a G protein-independent, but tyrosine kinase-dependent pathway. J Immunol 147:3122–3127
Ting AT, Karnitz LM, Schoon RA, Abraham RT, Leibson PJ (1992) Fcγ receptor activation induces the tyrosine phosphorylation of both phospholipase C (PLC)-γ1 and PLC-γ2 in natural killer cells. J Exp Med 176:1751–1755

Ting AT, Dick CJ, Schoon RA, Karnitz LM, Abraham RT, Leibson PJ (1995) Interaction between lck and syk family tyrosine kinases in Fcγ receptor-initiated activation of natural killer cells. J Biol Chem 270:1–7

Trinchieri G (1989) Biology of natural killer cells. Adv Immunol 47:187–376

Trinchieri G (1994) Recognition of major histocompatibility complex class I antigens by natural killer cells. J Exp Med 180:417–421

Trinchieri G, Valiante N (1993) Receptors for the Fc fragment of IgG on natural killer cells. Nat Immun 12:218–234

Trinchieri G, Matsumoto-Kobayashi M, Clark SC, Seehra J, London L, Perussia B (1984) Response of resting human peripheral blood natural killer cells to interleukin 2. J Exp Med 160:1147–1169

Trotta R, Kanakaraj P Perussia B (1996) FcγR-dependent mitogen-activated protein kinase activation in leukocytes: a common signal transduction event necessary for expression of TNF-α and early activation genes. J Exp Med 184:1027–1035

Trowbridge IS, Thomas ML (1994) CD45: an emerging role as a protein tyrosine phosphatase required for lymphocyte activation and development. Annu Rev Immunol 12:85–116

van Oers NSC, Weiss A (1995) The syk/ZAP-70 protein tyrosine kinase connection to antigen receptor signalling processes. Semin Immunol 7:227–236

Vivier E, Morin P, O'Brien C, Druker B, Schlossman SF, Anderson P (1991) Tyrosine phosphorylation of the FcγRIII(CD16): ζ complex in human natural killer cells. Induction by antibody-dependent cytotoxicity by not by natural killing. J Immunol 146:206–210

Vivier E, da Silva AJ, Ackerly M, Levine H, Rudd CE, Anderson P (1993) Association of a 70-kDa tyrosine phosphoprotein with the CD16:ζ:γ complex expressed in human natural killer cells. Eur J Immunol 23:1872–1876

Wagtmann N, Biassoni R, Cantoni C, Verdiani S, Malnati MS, Vitale M, Bottino C, Moretta L, Moretta A, Long EO (1995a) Molecular clones of the p58 NK cell receptor reveal immunoglobulin-related molecules with diversity in both the extra- and intracellular domains. Immunity 2:439–449

Wagtmann N, Rajagopalan S, Winter CC, Peruzzi M, Long EO (1995b) Killer cell inhibitory receptors specific for HLA-C and HLA-B identified by direct binding and by functional transfer. Immunity 3:801–809

Wange RL, Guitar R, Isakov N, Watts JD, Aebersold R, Samelson LE (1995) Activating and inhibitory mutations in adjacent tyrosines in the kinase domain of ZAP-70. J Biol Chem 270:18730–18733

Weiss A, Littman DR (1994) Signal transduction by lymphocyte antigen receptors. Cell 76:263–274

Weissman AM, Hou, D, Orloff DG, Modi WS, Seuanez H, O'Brien SJ, Klausner RD (1988) Molecular cloning and chromosomal localization of the human T-cell receptor ζ chain: distinction from the molecular CD3 complex. Proc Natl Acad Sci USA 85:9709–9713

Welsh RM (1984) Natural killer cells and interferon. Crit Rev Immunol 5:55–93

Wen T, Zhang L, Kung SKP, Mollina TJ, Miller RG, Mak TW (1995) Allo-skin graft rejection, tumor rejection and natural killer activity in mice lacking $p56^{lck}$. Eur J Immunol 25:3155–3159

Whalen MM, Doshi RN, Bankhurst AD (1992) Effects of pertussis toxin treatment on human natural killer cell function. Immunology 75:402–407

Windebank KP, Abraham RT, Powis G, Olsen RA, Barna TJ, Leibson PJ (1988) Signal transduction during human natural killer cell activation: inositol phosphate generation and regulation by cyclic AMP. J Immunol 141:3951–3957

Wirthmueller U, Kurosaki T, Murakami M S, Ravetch JV (1992) Signal transduction by FcγRIII (CD16) is mediated through the γ chain. J Exp Med 175:1381–1390

Xiao J, Brahmi Z (1989) Target cell-directed inactivation and IL-2-dependent reactivation of LAK cells. Cell Immunol 122:295–306

Yamada H, Kishihara K, Kong Y-Y, Nomoto K (1996) Enhanced generation of NK cells with intact cytotoxic function in CD45 exon 6-deficient mice. J Immunol 157:1523–1528

Yokoyama WM (1995) Natural killer cell receptors specific for major histocompatibility complex class I molecules. Proc Natl Acad Sci USA 92:3081–3085

Yokoyama WM, Jacobs LB, Kanagawa O, Shevach EM, Cohen DI (1989) A murine T lymphocyte antigen belongs to a supergene family of type II integral membrane proteins. J Immunol 143:1379–1386

Zanovello P, Rosato A, Bronte V, Gerundolo V, Treves S, Di Virgilio F, Pozzan T, Biasi G, Collavo D (1989) Interaction of lymphokine-activated killer cells with susceptible targets does not induce second messenger generation and cytolytic granule exocytosis. J Exp Med 170:665–677

Effector Pathways of Natural Killer Cells

M.F. VAN DEN BROEK[1], D. KÄGI[2], and H. HENGARTNER[1]

1 Introduction

Cell-mediated cytotoxicity is an important mechanism of tumor control (MELIEF 1992) and virus elimination (ZINKEMAGEL and ROSENTHAL 1981) in vivo. Depending on the tumor target, the host has two complementary cytotoxic mechanisms at its disposal: cytotoxic T lymphocytes (CTL) and natural killer (NK) cells. NK cells are not antigen specific in the classical sense and can be activated within hours without specific priming. In contrast, CTLs are induced by specific peptides presented by major histocompatibility complex (MHC) class I molecules, are antigen-specific, and act efficiently as effector cells only after an induction and proliferation phase of 5–8 days. A tumor or an infected cell can prime acquired immunity if it presents tumor-specific peptides in the context of MHC class I and/or class II molecules to $CD8^+$ or $CD4^+$ T cells, respectively (MELIEF 1992; VAN PEL et al. 1995). Under selective pressure, however, tumors may escape immune surveillance by variants that lack MHC class I and/or II molecules (SCHRIER et al. 1983; SMITH et al. 1989; UYTTENHOVE et al. 1983), and some of these tumors have been shown to be controlled efficiently by NK cells in vivo (KÄRRE et al. 1986, 1995). In addition, some viruses have been shown to use similar strategies to avoid immunological control: herpes simplex virus types 1 and 2 (HILL et al. 1994) and murine cytomegalovirus (DEL VAL et al. 1992) downregulate MHC class I molecules upon infection, leaving only NK cells as effectors of cell-mediated cytotoxicity.

[1]Institute of Experimental Immunology, University of Zurich, Schmelzbergstr. 12, CH-8091 Zurich, Switzerland

[2]Ontario Cancer Institute, Department of Medical Biophysics and Immunology, University of Toronto, Toronto, Canada

The cytotoxic activity of NK cells is regulated both by triggering and by inhibitory signals (GUMPERZ and PARHAM 1995; RAULET 1996; MORETTA et al. 1996). It has been shown that MHC class I molecules on target cells can bind to specific receptors on NK cells and thereby prevent NK cells from lysing the target (LJUNGGREN and KÄRRE 1990; YOKOYAMA and SEAMAN 1993; KÄRRE 1995). Recently these MHC class I binding receptors have been identified as members of the Ly-49 family in mice (COLONNA and SAMARIDIS 1995) and of the killer cell inhibitor gene family in humans (WAGTMAN et al. 1995; LANIER and PHILIPS 1996). Triggering molecules on human NK cells are less well characterized than inhibiting molecules, but it has been described recently that NK cells from a small number of human donors possess triggering molecules that differ from inhibiting molecules by their transmembrane and cytoplasmic part (BIASSONI et al. 1996). In addition, a recent report has shown that the costimulatory molecule CD80 (B7-1) is able to trigger NK cells to such an extent that the negative signal provided by MHC class I molecules is overruled (CHAMBERS et al. 1996).

2 Cytotoxic Activity of NK Cells In Vitro

T cell mediated cytotoxicity is mediated by two major pathways: perforin and Fas-FasLigand (FasL) interactions (HENKART 1985; PODACK et al. 1991; ROUVIER et al. 1993; KÄGI et al. 1994b, 1996; KOJIMA et al. 1994; LOWIN et al. 1994). The use of perforin-deficient mice (KÄGI et al. 1994a; LOWIN et al. 1994; KOJIMA et al. 1994; WALSH et al. 1994), Fas-deficient mice *(lpr/lpr* mice, WATANABE-FUKUNAGA et al. 1992), and FasL-deficient mice *(gld/gld* mice, TAKAHASHI et al. 1994) contributed substantially to our current knowledge about cytolytic effector mechanisms used by CTL and by NK cells.

Using perforin-deficient (PKO) mice, we and others have demonstrated that NK cells use predominantly perforin as the lytic pathway in vitro (WALSH et al. 1994; KÄGI et al. 1994a, 1995; VAN DEN BROEK et al. 1995). NK cells were induced in C57BL/6, C57BL/6-*gld/gld*, or PKO mice by injection of poly-IC or of 10^6 plaque forming units (pfu) lymphocytic choriomeningitis virus and were subsequently tested for lytic activity on RMA cells (MHC class I^+, Fas^{low}), RMA-S cells (MHC class I^-, Fas^{low}) and on YAC-1 cells (MHC class I^-, Fas^+). We found that NK cells, independently of their inducing stimulus, derived from C57BL/6$^-$ *gld/gld* mice or from C57BL/6 mice were capable of lysing prototype murine NK target cells – MHC class I^- RMA-S and YAC-1 cells – to a similar extent, whereas MHC class I^+ RMA cells were not lysed as expected. In contrast, PKO-derived NK cells could not lyse any of the targets used (VAN DEN BROEK et al. 1995, 1996b; Table 1).

Experiments with alloreactive T cells from PKO mice show that YAC-1 cells are very sensitive to T cell dependent Fas-mediated cytolysis (KÄGI et al. 1995). In addition, susceptibility of targets to FasL-mediated cytotoxicity was tested using FasL-expressing MC57G-fibroblasts as effectors. $FasL^+$ MC57G cells were generated by infection with recombinant vaccinia virus expressing FasL (VAN DEN BROEK

Table 1. Expression of Fas and MHC class I molecules and susceptibility to NK-mediated lysis of different target cell lines

Target cell	MHC class I[a]	Fas[a]	FasL-mediated lysis[b]	Lysis by NK cells of[c]		
				C57BU6 C57BL/6	*gld/gld*	PKO
RMA	1300	30	6	0	0	0
RMA-S	20	30	6	40	33	0
MBL-2.Fas	1200	350	54	0	0	0
YAC-1	20	150	35	37	29	0

[a] Surface expression was measured by FACS analysis using biotinylated monoclonal antibodies against H-2D^b or Fas (Jo-l, PharMingen) followed by streptavidin-phycoerythrin. The values represent arbitrary units with the fluorescence of the second antibody alone set at 3 on a logarithmic scale.
[b] The percentage of FasL-mediated lytic activity was determined in a 5-h ^{51}Cr-release assay using vaccinia virus FasL (EHL et al. 1996) infected (3 h, moi=5) MC57G fibroblasts as effectors at an effector to target ratio of 10.
[c] NK cells were generated in vivo by i.v. injection of 10^6 pfu lymphocytic choriomeningitis virus WE 48 h before isolation of splenocytes. Lytic activity was determined in a 5-h ^{51}Cr-release assay, and values represent the percentage specific lysis at an effector to target ratio of 30. Spontaneous release of target cells was always %. PKO mice are perforin-deficient C57BL/6 mice (KÄGI et al. 1994a); *gld/gld* mice are FasL-deficient C57BL/6 mice (TAKAHASHI et al. 1994).

et al. 1996a; EHL et al. 1996). We observed a clear correlation between the expression of Fas on the target cell and the relative susceptibility to FasL-mediated killing (Table 1): Fas$^+$ YAC-1 cells and Fas transfected MBL-2 lymphoma cells (positive control) were lysed by FasL$^+$ effectors, whereas Fas$^-$/Fas^{low} targets (RMA, RMA-S) were not.

As shown in Table 1, NK cells obtained from PKO mice were not able to lyse MHC class I$^-$ target cells RMA-S and YAC-I, even when the latter expressed Fas and displayed susceptibility to FasL-mediated lysis. Moreover, FasL-deficient NK cells (obtained from C57BL/6-*gld/gld* mice) were shown to lyse all target cells tested to a similar extent as wild-type NK cells. Together these data demonstrate that NK cells lacking perforin as an effector molecule do not use an alternative pathway of cell-mediated cytolysis such as Fas/FasL interactions.

Recently several groups have found that murine and human NK cells may express FasL and kill via the Fas-dependent pathway. At first sight our data seem to contrast with some data published earlier which suggested a contribution of the Fas-FasL pathway to NK-mediated cytotoxicity (ARASE et al. 1995; LIU et al. 1995; EISCHEN et al. 1996). The differences may be explained by the different effector populations used in these studies: LIU et al. (1995) demonstrated that lymphokine-activated killer (LAK) cells from perforin-deficient mice are able to lyse Fas$^+$ targets in vitro, and that these effectors express mRNA for FasL. The LAK cells used, however, were probably derived from a mixture of CTL and NK cells, which makes it difficult to draw any conclusions regarding which effector cell type actually was responsible for the measured cytotoxicity in this study. In addition, the target cells used (P815, L1210) are known to express considerable amounts of MHC class I molecules, which makes them unsuitable as targets for NK cells (Kärre 1995). A recent paper (Eischen et al. 1996) has reported that human $CD3^{-}$ $CD16^{+}$ clones transcribe FasL mRNA after FcγRIII cross-linking and are able to lyse Fas^{+} target cells (Fas-transfected P815 cells). Moreover, they were shown to display FasL-dependent self-killing. Whether this observation with clones from long-term in vitro cultures can be extrapolated to freshly isolated NK cells or to murine NK cells is disputable.

The approach of using freshly isolated murine NK cells (by isolation of NKI. 1^{+} $CD3^{-}$ splenocytes) was followed by Arase et al. (Arase et al. 1995). They demonstrated that these cells – without any further activation – are able to lyse $MRL^{+/+}$ but not MRL^{-} *lpr/lpr* (Fas-deficient) thymocytes in a 12-h assay, suggesting an exclusive role for Fas-FasL interactions. Strangely enough, perforin that was presumably present in the NK effectors apparently did not suffice to kill Fas^{-} target cells. Another phenomenon which is hard to explain in the context of NK cells using solely Fas/FasL interactions (as suggested by Arase et al. 1995) is that NKI. I^{+} $CD3^{-}$ effectors from *gld/gld* (FasL-deficient) mice are as effective in lysing Fas^{+} targets. In addition, lysis of Fas-transfected tumor cells by NKI. I^{+} $CD3^{-}$ effectors has been shown. The fact that the tumor cells used also expressed MHC class I molecules makes it unlikely that NK cells as they are classically defined (Ljunggren and Kärre 1985; Kärre et al.1986) were delivering the effector function.

Finally, a recent publication (Oshimi et al. 1996) claims that freshly isolated human peripheral blood cells purified to contain 95% $CD16^{+}$ CD3 cells use Fas-FasL interactions to lyse a variety of target cells. This type of cell-mediated cytotoxicity, however, does not correspond to the classical NK-mediated cytotoxicity but rather to antibody-dependent cell-mediated cytotoxicity (ADCC) using the CD16 molecule to bind antibody. It may well be with respect to which effector pathways are used, that signaling over CD16 triggers a signaling cascade other than the one triggered via the NK receptor with respect to which effector pathways are used. In addition, the read-out system for cytotoxicity was not a ^{51}Cr-release assay as used in most other publications, but determination of apoptosis and necrosis was measured by morphological criteria.

In conclusion, none of these studies showed conclusively that the observed cytotoxic activity corresponds to the characteristic NK cell-mediated cytotoxicity, or that it is not caused by some other, non-NK cell-mediated effector cell type.

3 Cytotoxic Activity of NK Cells In Vivo

In vivo NK cells are thought to provide a first line of defense in eliminating MHC class $I^{-/low}$ aberrant cells, such as some tumor cells and virus-infected cells (Kärre et al. 1986; Schrier et al. 1983; Smith et al. 1989; Uyttenhove et al. 1983). Most in vivo data on the elucidation of cytotoxic mechanisms involved in immune

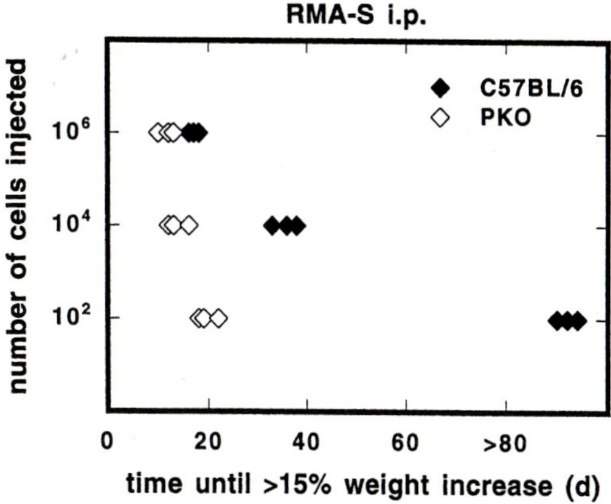

Fig. 1. Control of an intraperitoneally administered syngeneic, MHC class I lymphoma cell line, RMA-S. Male C57BL/6 (*closed symbols*) and perforin-deficient C57BL/6 (*PKO, open symbols*) were injected i.p. with 10^2, 10^4, or 10^6 live tumor cells in 0.25 ml PBS. Mice were observed daily for tumor growth by monitoring the weight of the mice, and were killed when the weight had increased by 15% compared to noninjected, age-matched controls. Each value represents an individual mouse. C57BL/6 mice injected with 10^2 RMA-S cells showed no sign of tumor growth by the end of the experiments (day 80). Similar data have been published previously (VAN DEN BROEK et al. 1995)

surveillance of allogeneic or syngeneic tumors have been generated with $CD8^+$ CTL, however. In these studies it became increasingly clear that absence of perforin has dramatic effects on the control of most syngeneic (KÄGI et al. 1994a; VAN DEN BROEK et al. 1996) and allogeneic (WALSH et al. 1996; BRAUN et al. 1996) tumors. In allogeneic systems a clear role for Fas/FasL interactions and for tumor necrosis factor has been demonstrated (WALSH et al. 1996; BRAUN et al. 1996). On the other hand, functional in vivo data on NK-mediated cytotoxicity are scarce.

We have demonstrated that a classical NK target, the MHC class I^- lymphoma cell line RMA-S, is controlled at least 100 times better by syngeneic C57BL/6 mice than by perforin-deficient C57BL/6 mice after intravenous or subcutaneous injection (VAN DEN BROEK et al. 1995; Fig. 1). This suggests a major role for perforin-dependent cytotoxicity in NK-mediated tumor control. Because RMA-S cells are not sensitive to FasL-mediated cytolysis (Table 1), this model tumor does not allow any conclusions to be drawn on the contribution of Fas/FasL interactions. In vivo experiments with Fas-transfected RMA-S or with Fas^+ YAC-1 cells are in progress in our laboratory at the moment.

A model for chemical carcinogenesis – methylcholanthrene-induced sarcomas in mice – has provided some indirect evidence for perforin playing a role as the major effector mechanism of NK cells in vivo (VAN DEN BROEK et al. 1996): We observed that perforin-deficient mice are more susceptible (faster kinetics, lower dose of carcinogen required) than wild-type C57BL/6 or CD8-deficient (FUNG-LEUNG et al. 1992) mice. Because CD8-deficient mice are known to lack functional MHC class I restricted CTL, NK cells seem to be responsible for the control of sarcomas in perforin-competent mice. In addition, ex vivo isolation of six sarcomas from six

Table 2. Expression of MHC class I molecules and Fas and susceptibility to NK-mediated lysis of methylcholanthrene-induced sarcomas

				Lysis by NK cells of[c]	
Cell line[a]	Origin[a]	MHC class I[b]	Fas[b]	C57BL/6 C57BU6	PKO
RMA-S	C57BL/6	20	30	61-45-19	0
MC57G	C57BL/6	420	10	0-0-0	0
beo	C57BL/6	35	17	72-48-27	0
kiwi	C57BL/6	40	15	49-37-18	0
ara	CD8–/–	40	16	33-25-11	0
kea	CD8–/–	30	21	68-42-30	0
ibis	PKO	25	12	52-33-16	0
mees	PKO	50	20	29-19-7	0

Beo, kiwi, ara, kea, ibis, and mees are methylcholanthrene (MCA)-induced sarcomas and were isolated from tumor-bearing mice (90–150 days after induction), trypsinized, and kept in culture. Sarcomas yielded well-growing and stable cell lines over a period of at least 3 months.

[a] RMA-S is a TAP-deficient variant of the Rauscher leukemia virus induced lymphoma RMA (LJUNGGREN et al. 1985); MC57G is an MCA-induced fibrosarcoma that was selected on high MHC class I expression and was established 20 years ago; beo and kiwi are MCA-induced sarcomas from wild-type C57BL/6 mice; ara and kea are MCA-induced sarcomas from CD8-deficient C57BL/6 mice (FUNG-LEUNG et al. 1992); ibis and mees are MCA-induced sarcomas from perforin-deficient mice (PKO, KÄGI et al. 1994a).

[b] Surface expression was measured by FACS analysis using biotinylated antibodies against H-2D^b or Fas (PharMingen) followed by streptavidin-phycoerythrin. The values represent arbitrary units with the fluorescence of the second antibody alone set at 3 on a logarithmic scale.

[c] NK cells were activated in vivo by i.p. injection of 0.1 mg poly-IC 24 h before isolation of splenocytes. Lytic activity was determined in a 5-h ^{51}Cr-release assay, and the values shown represent percentage specific lysis at an effector to target ratio of 90-30-10 (C57BL/6) or of 90 (PKO). Spontaneous release of target cells was %.

individual mice followed by surface staining for MHC class I molecules and Fas and by testing their sensitivity in vitro to NK-mediated lysis (Table 2) confirmed our assumption that methylcholanthrene-induced sarcomas, independently of their origin, are sensitive to NK cells and are probably controlled in vivo by NK cells in a perforin-dependent fashion.

4 Concluding Remarks

Together, most data generated in vitro suggest a crucial role for perforin in the lytic effector phase of NK cells, which is supported by a limited number of in vivo data. We have shown that cell lines which are clearly susceptible to FasL-mediated lysis, and which are known to be excellent NK target cells at the same time (YAC-1 cells) cannot be lysed by murine NK cells in vitro. Whether the NK cells used in our studies expressed sufficiently high levels of FasL upon in vivo activation by a physiological stimulus (virus), is not known at present. Evidence that NK cell mediated perforin-dependent cytolysis is involved in control of tumor growth in vivo is derived from experiments with MHC class I⁻ lymphoma cells (RMA-S) showing a 100-fold higher take rate in perforin-deficient mice (VAN DEN BROEK et al. 1995). A direct lytic role for NK cells in elimination of viruses is suggested by experiments carried out in *beige* mice that have normal numbers of NK cells but lack the NK lytic activity: these mice were shown to be more susceptible to infection with murine cytomegalovirus (SHELLAM et al. 1981), a virus known to downregulate MHC class I expression, thereby avoiding control by CTL.

In addition to cell-mediated cytotoxicity, NK cells have been shown to use cytokines such as interferon-γ or tumor necrosis factor-α to control some viral infections, such as vaccinia virus in mice (KARUPIAH et al. 1990) and vesicular stomatitis virus in cultured human cells (PAYA et al. 1988). There is still some room for additional effector mechanisms, such as Fas/FasL interactions, however, and future experiments using target cell lines covering the whole spectrum of MHC class I and Fas expression will shed more light on this issue.

Acknowledgements. The authors thank Daniel Binder for helpful discussions and reading of the manuscript, Stephan Ehl for providing the recombinant vaccinia virus expressing FasL, and Pierre Golstein (Marseille, France) for providing the Fas-expression vector that enabled us to generate Fas-transfected cell lines.

References

Arase H, Arase N, Saito T (1995) Fas-mediated cytotoxicity by freshly isolated natural killer cells. J Exp Med 181:1235–1238

Biassoni R, Cantoni C, Falco M, Verdiani S, Bottino C, Vitale M, Conte R, Poggi A, Moretta A, Moretta L (1996) The HLA-C-specific "activatory" or "inhibitory" natural killer cells receptors display highly homologous extracellular domains but differ in their transmembrane and intracytoplasmic portions. Eur J Immunol 25:2433–2437

Chambers BJ, Salcedo M, Ljunggren HG (1996) Triggering of natural killer cells by the costimulatory molecule CD80 (B7-1). Immunity 5:311–317

Colonna M, Samaridis J (1995) Cloning of immunoglobulin superfamily members assocoated with HLA-C and HLA-B recognition by human NK cells. Science 268:405408

Del Val M, Hengel H, Hacker H, Hartlaub U, Ruppert T, Lucin P, Koszinowski UH (1992) Cytomegalovirus prevents antigen presentaion by blocking the transport of peptide-loaded major histocompatibility complex class I molecules to the medial golgi compartment. J Exp Med 176:729–737

Doherty PC, Biddison WE, Bennink JR, Knowles BB (1978) Cytotoxic T cell response in mice infected with influenza and vaccinia virus vay in magnitude with the H-2 genotype. J Exp Med 148:534–543

Ehl S, Hoffmann-Rohrer U, Nagata S, Hengartner H, Zinkemagel RM (1996) Different susceptibility of cytotoxic T cells to CD95 (Fas/Apo-1) ligand-mediated cell death after activation in vitro versus in vivo. J Immunol 156:2357–2360

Eischen CM, Schlling JD, Lynch DH, Krammer PH, Leibson PJ (1996) Fc receptorinduced expression on activated NK cells facilitates cell-mediated cytotoxicity and subsequent autocrine NK cell apoptosis. J Immunol 156:2693–2699

Fung-Leung WP, Schilham MW, Rahemtulla A, Kiindig TM, Vollenweider M, Potter J, van Ewijk W, Mak TW (1992) CD8 is needed for development of cytotoxic T cells but not for helper T cells. Cell 65:443–45 1

Gumperz JE, Parham P (1995) The enigma of natural killer cells. Nature 378:245–248

Hahne M, Rimoldi D, Schroter M, Romero P, Schreier M, French LE, Schneider P, Bornand T, Fontana A, Lienard D, Cerottini JC, Tschopp F (1996) Melanoma cell expression of Fas (Apo-I/CD95) ligand: implications for tumor escape. Science 274:1363–1366

Henkart PA (1985) Mechanisms of lymphocyte-mediated cytotoxicity. Annu Rev Immunol 3:31–58

Hill A, Bamett BC, McMichael AJ, McGeoch DJ (1994) HLA class I molecules are not transported to the cell surface in cells infected with herpes simplex virus type 1 and 2. J Immunol 152:22736–22741

Itoh N, Yonehara S, Ishii A, Yonehara M, Mizushima SI, Saineshima M, Hase A, Seto Y, Nagata S (1991) The polypeptide encoded by the CDNA for human cell surface antigen Fas can mediate apoptosis. Cell 66:233–242

Kägi D, Ledermann B, Bürki K, Seiler P, Odermatt B, Olsen KJ, Podack E, Zinkemagel RM, Hengartner H (1994a) Cytotoxicity mediated by cytotoxic T cells and natural killer cells is greatly impaired in perforin-deficient mice. Nature 369:31–37

Kägi D, Vignaux F, Leermann B, Bürki K, Depraetere V, Nagata S, Hengartner H, Golstein P (1994b) Fas and perforin pathways as major mechanisms of T cell mediated cytotoxicity. Science 265:528–530

Kägi D, Ledermann B, Bürki K, Zinkemagel RM, Hengartner H (1995) Lymphocyte mediated cytotoxicity in vitro and in vivo: mechanisms and significance. Immunol Rev 146:95–116

Kägi D, Ledermann B, Bürki K, Zinkernagel RM, Hengartner H (1996) Molecular mechanisms of lymphocyte-mediated cytotoxicity and their role in immunological protection and pathogenesis in vivo. Annu Rev Immunol 14:207–232

Kärre K (1995) Express yourself or die: peptides, MHC molecules and NK cells. Science 267:978–979

Kärre K, Ljunggren HG, Piontek G, Kiessling R (1986) Selective rejection of H-2 deficient lymphoma variants suggests alternative immune defence strategy. Nature 319:675–678

Karupiah G, Blanden RV, Ramshaw IA (1990) Interferon gamma is involved in the recovery of athymic nude mice from recombinant vaccinial interleukin-2 infection. J Exp Med 172:1495–1500

Kojima H, Shinohara N, Hanaoka S, Someya-Shirota Y, Takagaki Y, Ohno H, Saito T, Katayama H, Yagira H, Okumura K, Shinkai Y, Alt F, Matsuzama A, Yonehawa Y, Takayama H (1994) Two distinct pathways of specific killing revealed by perforin mutant cytotoxic T lymphocytes. Immunity 1:357–364

Lanier LL, Philips JH (1996) Inhibitory MHC class I receptors on NK cells and T cells. Immunol Today 17:86–9 1

Liu CC, Walsh CM, Eto N, Clark WR, Young JDE (1995) Morphologic and functional characterization of perforin-deficient lymphokine-activated killer cells. J Immunol 155:602–608

Ljunggren HG, Kärre K (1985) Host resistance directed selectively against H-2 deficient lymphoma variants: analysis of the mechanisms. J Exp Med 162:1745–1759

Lowin B, Hahne M, MatzmannC, Tschop J (1994) Cytolytic T cell cytotoxicity is mediated through perforin and Fas lytic pathways. Nature 370:650–652

Moretta A, Bottino C, Vitale M, pende D, Biassoni R, Mingari MC, Moretta L (1996) Receptors for HLA class I molecules in human natural killer cells. Annu Rev Immunol 14:619–648

Melief CJM (1992) Tumour eradication by adoptive transfer of cytotoxic T lymphocytes. Adv Cancer Res 58:143–175

Oshimi Y, Oda S, Honda Y, Nagata S, Miyazaki S (1996) Involvement of Fas Ligand and Fas-mediated pathway in the cytotoxicity of human natural killer cells. J Immunol 157:2909–2915

Paya CV, Kenmotsu N, Schoon RA, Leibson PJ (1988) Tumor necrosis factor and lymphotoxin secretion by human natural killer cells leads to antiviral cytotoxicity. J Immunol 141:1989–2003

Podack ER, Hengartner H, Lichtenheld MG (1991) A central role of perforin in cytolysis? Annu Rev Immunol 9:129–15 1

Raulet DH (1996) Recognition events that inhibit and activate natural killer cells. Curr Opin Immunol 8:372–377

Schrier PJ, Bernards R, Vaessen TMJ, Houweling A, van der Eb AJ (1983) Expression of class I major histocompatibility antigens switched off by highly oncogenic adenovirus 12 in transformed cells. Nature 305:776–779

Shellam GR, Allan JE, Papadimitriou JM, Bancroft GJ (1991) Increased susceptibility to cytomegalovirus infection in beige mutant mice. Proc Natl Acad Sci USA 78:5104–5108

Smith MEF, Marsh SCE, Bodmer JG, Gelsthorpe K, Bodmer WF (1989) Loss of HLAA, B, C allele products and lymphocyte function associated antigen 3 in colorectal neoplasia. Proc Natl Acad Sci USA 86:5557–5561

Takahashi T, Tanaka M, Brannan Cl, Jenkins NA, Copeland NG, Suda T, Nagata S (1994) Generalized lymphoproliferative disease in mice, caused by a point mutation in the Fas ligand. Cell 76:969–976

Uyttenhove C, Maryanski J, Boon T (1983) Escape of mouse mastocytoma P815 after nearly complete rejection is due to to antigen-loss variants rather than to immunosuppression. J Exp Med 157:1040–1052

van den Broek MF, Kiigi D, Zinkemagel RM, Hengartner H (1995) Perforin dependence of natural killer cell-mediated tumor control in vivo. Eur J Immunol 25:3514–3516

van den Broek MF, Kägi D, Ossendorp F, Toes R, Vamvakas S, Lutz WK, Melief CJM, Zinkernagel RM, Hengartner H (1996a) Decreased tumor surveillance in perforindeficient mice. J Exp Med 184:1–10

van den Broek MF, Kägi D, Zinkemagel, RM, Hengartner H (1996b) Murine NK cells use perforin and not Fas-FasLigand interactions as their lytic effector mechanism. Submittedforpublication

van Pel A, van der Bruggen P, Coulie PC, Brichard VG, Lethé B, van den Eynde B, Uyttenhove C, Renauld JC, Boon T (1995) Genes coding for tumour antigens recognized by cytotoxic T lymphocytes. Immunol Rev 145:229–250

Wagtman N, Biassoni R, Cantoni C, Verdiani S, Malnati M, Vitale M, Bottino C, Moretta L, Moretta A, Long E (1995) Molecular clones of the p5 8 NK cell receptor reveal immunoglobulin-related molecules with diversity in both the extra- and intracellular domains. Immunity 2:439–449

Walsh CM, Matloubian M, Lui CC, Ueda R, Kurahara CG, Christensen JL, Huang MTF, Young JDE, Young R, Ahmed R, Clark WR (1994) Immune function in mice lacking the perforin gene. Proc Natl Acad Sci USA 91:10854–10858

Watanabe-Fukunaga R, Brannan Cl, Copeland, NG, Jenkins NG, Nagata S (1992) Lymphoproliferation disorder in mice explained by defects in Fas antigen that mediates apoptosis. Nature 356:314–317

Yokoyama WM, Seaman WE (1993) The Ly-49 and NKR-PI gene families encoding lectin-like receptors on natural killer cells. Annu Rev Immunol 11:613–635

Zinkernagel RM, Rosenthal KL (1981) Experiments and speculation on antiviral specificity of T and B cells. Immunol Rev 58:131–155

C. Development of NK Cells

Toward a Quantitative Analysis of the Repertoire of Class I MHC-Specific Inhibitory Receptors on Natural Killer Cells

R.E. VANCE and D.H. RAULET

Department of Molecular and Cell Biology, Division of Immunology, and Cancer Research Laboratory, 489 Life Sciences Addition, University of California at Berkeley, Berkeley, CA 94720, USA

1 Introduction

Recent research establishes that natural killer (NK) cells recognize class I MHC molecules on potential target cells. Unlike T cells, however, recognition of target cell class I molecules by NK cells inhibits their activation and prevents destruction of the target cell. The pattern of recognition exhibited by NK cells suggests that one of their key functions is to destroy self cells that have extinguished or reduced expression of some or all class I molecules.

Deficiency in the expression of all class I molecules, due to mutation of β_2-microglobulin or genes that regulate class I biosynthesis, typically renders cells sensitive to lysis by NK cells (KARRE et al. 1986; LIAO et al. 1991). However, deficiency in the expression of a subset of the cell's MHC class I molecules, rather than all of them, can also render a cell sensitive to NK cells. For example, NK cells from an F_1 ($MHC^{a/b}$) mouse can often destroy parental ($MHC^{a/a}$) cells (BENNETT 1987; CHADWICK and MILLER 1992; CUDKOWICZ and STIMPFLING 1964). A comparable situation has been generated experimentally by creating H-2^b mice transgenic for the D^d class I gene (OHLEN et al. 1989). NK cells from these mice destroy nontransgenic H-2^b target cells. NK cells also often lyse fully allogeneic cells (BENNETT 1987). In all three of these situations the target cell is missing some or all of the class I molecules expressed by the host. These patterns of lysis have led to the "missing-self" hypothesis, which postulates that NK cells destroy target cells that lack some or all class I molecules of the host (LJUNGGREN and KARRE 1990). There are exceptions to this model, in its simplest form, but these exceptions do not negate the model although they do suggest additional complexities to the system.

What is the molecular basis of the missing-self model? Recent work suggests that NK cell recognition is controlled by integrating signals from both activating and inhibitory receptors. With the exception of the NK cell's Fc receptor the activating receptors are poorly characterized and may include members of the NKR-P1 receptor family (RYAN and SEAMAN 1997). In contrast the inhibitory receptors are increasingly well understood and provide an explanation for missing-self recognition. In mice the Ly-49 family of receptors bind class I MHC molecules and thereby inhibit NK cell activity (BROWN et al. 1997; GEORGE et al. 1997; TAKEI et al. 1997). These receptors are dimeric type II membrane proteins that contain a C-terminal carbohydrate recognition domain and comprise a family of approximately ten receptors designated Ly-49A to Ly-49I, encoded by closely linked genes on chromosome 6 in the mouse. The specificities of only a few of the receptors have been investigated. The data suggest that Ly-49A reacts with D^d and D^k, Ly-49C with K^b and D^d, and Ly-49G2 with D^d and L^d. The available evidence suggests that the engagement of Ly-49 receptors inhibits activation mediated by several types of stimulating receptors, including putative NK receptors for tumor cell specific ligands, the NK cell's Fc receptor, and the T cell antigen receptor (CORREA et al. 1994; HELD et al. 1996a; KARLHOFER et al. 1992).

2 The Ly-49 Receptor Repertoire

Monoclonal antibodies reactive with at least four Ly-49 receptors have been generated (BROWN et al. 1997; GEORGE et al. 1997; MASON et al. 1995; ROLAND and CAZENAVE 1992; TAKEI et al. 1997). The JR9-318 and A1 antibodies, among others, bind Ly-49A; the SW-5E6 mAb binds Ly-49C and Ly-49I; and the 4D11 mAb reacts with Ly-49G2. With some of these antibodies the distribution of the corresponding receptors on different NK cells has been investigated and reveals a complex expression pattern. As depicted in Table 1, from 15%–60% of NK cells can react with a given anti-Ly-49 monoclonal antibody (RAULET et al. 1997). These and other analyses have permitted three important conclusions to be made: (a) NK cells commonly express Ly-49 receptors that are apparently irrelevant for the animal in the sense that they fail to react detectably with the host's class I MHC molecules; (b) NK cells commonly coexpress two or more Ly-49 receptors; and (c) unlike the T and B cell receptors, the distribution of Ly-49 receptors to different cells may not involve somatic gene recombination since normal Ly-49 expression occurs in mice harboring mutations in the recombination machinery, and no Ly-49 gene rearrangements have been detected in mature NK cell populations.

The distribution of Ly-49 receptors to different NK cell subsets underlies the capacity of NK cells to discriminate class I *different* target cells, as opposed to the

Table 1. Expression of Ly-49 receptors in MHC-different mice: the "product rule"

	Percentage of NK cells in MHC background					
	B10.D2 (H-2^d)		B6 (H-2^b)		B6-$\beta_2m^{-/-}$	
NK cell subset[a]	Observed[b]	Expected by product rule[c]	Observed[b]	Expected by product rule[c]	Observed[b]	Expected by product rule[c]
Ly-49A$^+$	15.7	–	17.9	–	25.3	–
SW-5E6$^+$	47.9	–	44.5	–	63.5	–
4D11$^+$	43.6	–	48.9	–	56.4	–
Ly-49A$^+$ SW-5E6$^+$	5.0	7.5	5.9	8.0	14.6	16.1
Ly-49A$^+$ 4D11$^+$	5.1	6.8	9.9	8.8	18.7	14.3
SW5E6$^+$ 4D11$^+$	21.1	20.9	21.6	21.8	40.0	35.8
Ly-49A$^+$ SW-5E6$^+$ 4D11$^+$	1.7	3.3	4.7	3.9	13.3	9.1

[a] Refers to cells that express the indicated receptor regardless of whether they express other receptors. 4D11 reacts at least with Ly-49G2; SW-5E6 reacts at least with Ly-49C and Ly-49I.
[b] Values are averages of percentages from at least four determinations. Data derived from HELD et al. 1996b.
[c] Calculated by multiplying the observed component frequencies, e.g., %Ly-49A+ SW5E6+= (0.157×0.479)×100.

simpler task of detecting class I *deficient* target cells. Consider the destruction of H-$2^{a/a}$ target cells by H-$2^{a/b}$ NK cells. H-$2^{a/b}$ mice can harbor various NK cell subsets, including those with inhibitory Ly-49 receptors for H-2^a and not H-2^b, a separate set with inhibitory receptors for both H-2^a and H-2^b, and a third with receptors for H-2^b and not H-2^a. It is the latter set that reject H-$2^{a/a}$ target cells (GEORGE et al. 1997). The importance of subset-specific expression of Ly-49 receptors was demonstrated by experiments in which a transgene encoding the D^d-specific Ly-49A receptor was expressed in all NK cells, as opposed to a subset as observed in normal mice. This manipulation abolished the capacity of NK cells from H-2^b mice to destroy H-2^d cells while not diminishing the capacity to destroy class I deficient target cells (HELD et al. 1996a).

2.1 The Product Rule

Coexpression of Ly-49 receptors is common and results in a complex combinatorial repertoire. Functional studies suggest that NK cells that coexpress a particular pair of Ly-49 receptors can be inhibited independently through either receptor (MASON et al. 1995; YU et al. 1996). Interestingly, the distribution pattern suggests that the expression of one receptor is to some extent independent of the expression of other receptors. Thus the fraction of NK cells reacting with any two anti-Ly-49 antibodies is roughly equal to the product of the fractions of cells reacting with each of the antibodies alone (Table 1). We have called this the "product rule," and it appears to be obeyed, to a first approximation, regardless of the MHC background of the mouse (RAULET et al. 1997). The product rule is consistent with the possibility that a stochastic process underlies the Ly-49 receptor distribution mechanism. However, as discussed at length below, there is evidence that the receptor distribution pattern is not entirely stochastic. In fact it is clear that the representation of different subsets is influenced by host MHC molecules (HELD et al. 1996b). While the distribution pattern may be created by mechanisms that incorporate stochastic components, evidence suggests that it is influenced by an MHC-dependent "education" process.

2.2 Monoallelic Expression of Ly-49 Receptors

Interestingly, Ly-49 receptors, similar to T cell receptors, B cell receptors, and odorant receptors, are expressed in a predominantly monoallelic fashion (HELD et al. 1995). This has been most clearly demonstrated in the case of the Ly-49A locus. The limited Ly-49A sequence differences in the BALB versus B6 strains (three amino acid differences in the extracellular domain) results in discrimination of these two proteins by one of the Ly-49A specific monoclonal antibodies. It was demonstrated that Ly-$49A^+$ NK cells in the (B6×BALB.B)F_1 Ly-49A heterozygote consist of an approximately equal number of cells expressing Ly-$49A^{B6}$ and cells expressing Ly-$49A^{BALB}$. Monoallelic Ly-49A expression is imposed at the level of mRNA abundance, probably at the level of transcription. Evidence was also presented that the SW-5E6 antigen is expressed in a monoallelic fashion (HELD et al. 1995). Based on recent studies that have subdivided the SW-5E6$^+$ subset into Ly-49C$^+$ and Ly-49I$^+$ cells (BRENNAN et al. 1996), the earlier results can now be interpreted to suggest that either Ly-49I or Ly-49C is expressed in a monoallelic fashion; the available data do not distinguish between these possibilities (RAULET et al. 1997). It appears likely that all members of the family are expressed in a predominantly monoallelic fashion.

Monoallelic Ly-49 gene expression may arise as a consequence of the mechanism that distributes expression of different Ly-49 genes to overlapping NK cell subsets. This mechanism may treat different alleles at the same locus independently just as it treats different loci independently. Consistent with this possibility, the data suggest that the choice of active allele occurs independently at different Ly-49 loci. A cell can express Ly-49A from one chromosome, and Ly-49I from the other (HELD et al. 1995). Another relevant observation, from analyses of short-term clones of NK cells from Ly-49A heterozygous mice, is that monoallelic expression of Ly-49A genes is incomplete. Approximately 90% of the Ly-49A$^+$ clones expressed only one or the other Ly-49A allele at nearly equal frequency. However, approximately 10% of the Ly-49A$^+$ clones expressed both Ly-49A alleles. Thus approximately 10% of all NK cells expressed one Ly-49A allele, 10% expressed the other, and 1%–2% expressed both Ly-49A alleles (Held et al. 1997b; RAULET et al. 1997). These percentages are in keeping with the product rule and suggest that the two Ly-49A alleles are activated independently. Therefore just as there is predictable overlap in the expression of different Ly-49 family members, there is predictable overlap in the expression of different Ly-49A alleles. Hence both the subset distribution and monoallelic expression of Ly-49 genes could be the result of the same stochastic mechanism in which each allele at each Ly-49 locus is conferred with a fixed probability of expression in each progenitor NK cell. As expected by this model, transgenic expression of Ly-49A on all NK cells does not fully suppress endogenous Ly-49A expression (HELD and RAULET 1997a).

2.3 NK Cells Acquire Self Specificity Somatically

Although a stochastic mechanism may underlie the distribution of Ly-49 receptors to different cells, such a system by itself would inevitably lead to the generation of autoaggressive NK cells. This is because Ly-49 genes are not linked to the MHC, and therefore are not coordinately inherited with class I alleles (BROWN et al. 1997). Furthermore, some of the receptors are expected to be non-self-specific in mice of most if not all MHC types. If the receptors were distributed to different NK cells by a purely stochastic process, some of the resulting clones would fail to express self class I specific receptors. Such clones would be expected to be autoaggressive. However, it has been observed that NK cells, at least those that have not been cultured extensively in IL-2, are generally self tolerant, meaning that they are generally inhibited better by self class I MHC molecules than foreign class I molecules (CHADWICK and MILLER 1992; DORFMAN and RAULET 1996; GEORGE et al. 1997). Experiments demonstrating that NK cell functional specificity can adapt to the presence of a class I transgene (OHLEN et al. 1989) as well as to mutations that confer class I deficiency (BIX et al. 1991) strongly suggest that the self specificity of NK cells is acquired somatically. This conclusion is further supported by the results of bone marrow chimera experiments (HOGLUND et al. 1991; WU and RAULET 1997), which demonstrate that class I$^+$ NK cells differentiating in the presence of class I deficient cells are rendered tolerant of the latter cells (WU and RAULET 1997).

Two general theories have been proposed to explain the acquisition of NK cell self specificity. One emphasizes mechanisms that ensure that each functional NK cell expresses at least one self class I specific Ly-49 receptor. This theory is discussed further below. The other theory emphasizes the quantitative effects of expressing different cell surface levels of the Ly-49 receptors. The latter model overlaps to some extent with the first model and is based on the observation that the cell surface levels of Ly-49 receptors vary with the MHC type of the host (KARLHOFER et al. 1994; OLSSON et al. 1995). In H-2^d mice, which express a Ly-49A ligand, Ly-49A$^+$ NK cells exhibit lower levels of Ly-49A per NK cell than is observed in H-2^b mice or class I deficient mice, which express no known ligand. The magnitude of this effect varies in different studies, from at least twofold to more than tenfold. This phenomenon led to the proposal that the levels of Ly-49 receptors are "calibrated" against the expressed class I molecules, increasing Ly-49 cell surface levels in order to increase sensitivity of the NK cell to weak class I ligands, and vice versa (OLSSON et al. 1995). Depending on the cross-reactivity of different Ly-49 receptors with different class I molecules and their distribution pattern this mechanism could result in each NK cell having at least one productive inhibitory interaction with any set of self class I molecules that the animal happens to express.

2.4 Critique of the Calibration Model

The notion that "calibration" of cell surface Ly-49 levels is in fact responsible for determining the self tolerance of NK cells is not easily reconciled with some recent observations. In fact, these findings appear most consistent with the hypothesis that receptor downregulation is an incidental consequence of ligand-induced receptor internalization or shedding (HELD and RAULET 1997). First, Ly-49A downregulation in normal mice is not accompanied by a decrease in the levels of Ly-49A mRNA per Ly-49A+ cell, indicating that receptor downregulation occurs posttranscriptionally perhaps at the protein level. Accordingly, ligand-induced Ly-49A downregulation occurs even with a transgenic Ly-49A receptor that is driven by heterologous regulatory elements. Moreover, in a Ly-49A transgenic line where the cell surface levels of Ly-49A are low to begin with, the presence of the ligand results in further downmodulation of the receptor. In light of these results it is difficult to argue that the levels are adjusted to a specific level to optimize the sensitivity of the cells to specific class I ligands. Rather it appears that ligand engagement results in receptor downregulation compared to whatever level pertains in the absence of the ligand. These reductions in receptor levels may alter the functional specificity of NK cells for class I molecules, but it does not appear likely that NK cells calibrate receptor levels to a *specific* level dependent on the available class I molecules. To our way of thinking, mechanisms that determine the distribution of Ly-49 receptors to functional NK cell subsets can better account for NK cell self specificity and are thus a focus of this review.

2.5 Education Processes Determine NK Cell Specificity

Our favored hypothesis to explain the acquisition of NK cell self specificity emphasizes which receptors are expressed rather than the levels of each receptor and invokes an education process that ensures that each NK cell expresses at least one type of self class I specific receptor (RAULET et al. 1997). This conclusion seems to be the simplest explanation for the results of experiments that investigated the specificity of Ly-49A^{+} NK cells from H-2^{d} mice, which express a class I ligand for Ly-49A, compared to those from H-2^{b} mice, which do not express a known ligand (DORFMAN and RAULET 1996; OLSSON et al. 1995). Neither population lysed H-2^{d} target cells. However, compared to the H-2^{d}-derived Ly-49A^{+} NK cells, the H-2^{b} derived Ly-49A^{+} NK cells were also diminished in their capacity to lyse H-2^{b} target cells. The poor lysis of H-2^{b} target cells was due to inhibition of the effector cells by H-2^{b} encoded class I molecules because these effector cells lysed class I deficient lymphoblasts efficiently. Thus these Ly-49A^{+} NK cells apparently expressed inhibitory receptor(s) for self H-2^{b} class I molecules. However, although the effector cells expressed Ly-49A, the H-2^{b} induced inhibition was apparently mediated through distinct receptors, because anti-Ly-49A F(ab')$_2$ fragments failed to block inhibition (DORFMAN and RAULET 1996). As it is well established that individual NK cells can express multiple Ly-49 receptors, it was proposed that the Ly-49A^{+} NK cells expressed other, H-2^{b} specific receptors. At least some of the comparable effector cells from H-2^{d} mice did not express H-2^{b} specific receptors. It was proposed that acquisition of self class I specificity involves a requirement that each functional cell expresses at least one self-specific receptor, while tolerating expression of irrelevant receptors.

This principle has been difficult to establish by direct analysis of the Ly-49 repertoire because the specificities of at least half of the receptors are unknown, and reagents to detect cells expressing several of the receptors do not exist. Nevertheless, the frequencies of NK cells that express different Ly-49 receptors do vary depending on the MHC class I molecules expressed by the host. The remainder of this review addresses the patterns of MHC-induced changes observed in the Ly-49 repertoire, and whether these trends are consistent with specific education processes that have been proposed.

2.6 The Effect of MHC on the Sizes of Ly-49 Defined Subsets

Considering the hypothesis that NK cells should express self-specific Ly-49 receptors, we predicted that the frequency of cells expressing Ly-49A or Ly-49G2 should be higher in H-2^{d} mice than in H-2^{b} mice (Ly-49A and Ly-49G2 react with H-2^{d} class I molecules and do not react detectably with H-2^{b} class I molecules). In fact, to our surprise the opposite was true, although the effect was only marginal (HELD et al. 1996b). More substantial effects were observed when receptor overlap was examined: NK cells that express both Ly-49A and Ly-49G2, two H-2^{d}-specific receptors, were substantially less frequent in H-2^{d} mice than in H-2^{b} mice or in class I deficient mice (HELD et al. 1996b). Thus it seems that, on one hand, NK cells are required to express self-specific receptors, and on the other, that expression of at least some particular self-specific receptors is disfavored. This represents a paradox that any model of Ly-49 repertoire formation must explain.

In terms of NK cell education, the data summarized above could result from a small bias against cells that express either Ly-49A or Ly-49G2, with the more substantial reduction in double-positive Ly-49A$^+$G2$^+$ cells a consequence of the product rule. Alternatively, there may be a stronger though incomplete bias against cells expressing multiple self-specific receptors, for example, Ly-49A$^+$G2$^+$ cells in H-2^d mice, with consequent smaller reductions in the frequencies of cells expressing Ly-49A or Ly-49G2. In the latter case one might expect that the observed frequency of Ly-49A$^+$G2$^+$ cells would be less than that predicted by the product rule. However, because the effects appear to be incomplete, it is difficult to discern whether the existing data are more consistent with one or the other of these schemes (Raulet et al. 1997) (Table 1). As an alternative approach to this question we examined the effects on the repertoire of an Ly-49A transgene that is expressed in all NK cells (Held and Raulet 1997a). In H-2^d transgenic mice it was observed that the frequency of Ly-49G2$^+$ NK cells (which also express transgenic Ly-49A) was substantially and specifically reduced in the transgenic mice compared to nontransgenic, MHC-matched littermates. The magnitude of the effect was similar to the magnitude of the reduction in Ly-49A$^+$G2$^+$ cells observed in nontransgenic H-2^d mice. The transgene had no effect in class I deficient mice and had little effect in H-2^b mice. Minimally, these results suggest that the education process disfavors NK cells expressing two self-specific receptors more than it disfavors cells expressing only one or the other.

The available data suggest that a central role of the education process is to ensure that each functional NK cell expresses at least one self-specific receptor. A straightforward means to accomplish this would be a "one-step" selection process for cells with self-specific receptors from a "random" preselection repertoire. It should be noted that an identical outcome is to be expected if selection acts *against* cells that do *not* express self-specific receptors. The latter possibility could account for the results of recent bone marrow chimera experiments (Wu and Raulet 1997). As these two mechanisms result in the same outcome in normal mice, they are discussed interchangeably with respect to the predicted changes in the repertoire. The important point is that these simple one-step selection models cannot easily account for the available data. Such models invariably predict that cells expressing a given receptor should be more prevalent in ligand-bearing mice, not less so, as was observed for Ly-49A and Ly-49G2.

2.7 Two Models to Account for the Establishment of the Ly-49 Repertoire

Since a single "one-step" selection model is inadequate, we have proposed two other models that can explain the disparate observations that NK cells generally are best inhibited by self class I molecules, while at the same time there is a reduction in the frequencies of cells expressing certain self-specific receptors and especially pairs of these receptors (Held et al. 1996b; Held and Raulet 1997; Held et al. 1995; Raulet et al. 1997). The "selection model" invokes a two-step selection process acting on a preformed randomly generated repertoire, wherein there is selection for cells expressing at least one self-specific receptor, and an additional (or coordinate) selection step against cells that express "too many" self-specific receptors. It is perhaps unlikely that either selection step is based on actually "counting" the number of self-specific receptors. More likely they would be based on overall Ly-49 dependent signaling, corresponding to some amalgam of the number of different self-specific receptors, their affinity for self class I molecules, and their expression levels.

The second model, the "sequential model," involves a marriage of the mechanisms that activate Ly-49 receptor genes and the education process. It proposes that Ly-49 gene expression occurs in a sequential, cumulative manner, though perhaps in a random order, with ongoing testing of the cells for reactivity against self class I molecules. When the cell achieves the expression of a "sufficient" number and quality of self-specific receptors, Ly-49 mediated signaling would act to prevent expression of any new receptor genes and perhaps induce functional maturation of the cell (though it is not necessary to postulate the latter step). This mechanism would demand that NK cells express some self-specific receptors but would prevent the development of cells with an excess of self-specific receptors. In its purest form such a mechanism is not a selective one as all the cells eventually achieve the desired properties. However, alternate versions involving selection are possible. For example, each cell may be allowed only a limited time period to activate Ly-49 receptors, such that some cells fail to achieve the expression of self-specific receptors. Such cells would be lost, deleted, or silenced in a subsequent or coordinate step.

2.8 Mathematical Modeling

Both models discussed above incorporate mechanisms that ensure self class I specificity and yet also limit the number of cells expressing multiple self-specific Ly-49 receptors. In order to provide more specific predictive information, we have worked out mathematical treatments of each model. These treatments provide more direct evidence that each model can account for the MHC and Ly-49 transgene dependent changes in the repertoire that have been observed. The mathematical modeling has been particularly important because the calculations have demonstrated that our intuitions about the behavior of our models were not always reliable. Equally important, the mathematical treatments reveal that the models can account for the data only under specific conditions, in terms of the composition of the Ly-49 repertoire and other variables that we define. Readers not interested in the detailed calculations (Sects. 3.1, 3.2, 4.1 and 4.2) can still obtain insights from the predictions of the models that follow. At present many basic features of the composition and specificity of the Ly-49 repertoire remain unknown. As knowledge of the system grows, however, the predictions of the mathematical models can be tested against observation. It is apparent that the models differ in various predictions, such as the effects of Ly-49 transgenes and knockouts. This information provides a basis for future tests of the models against each other and also against other possible models that can be envisaged. For the sake of clarity we contrast two "extreme" models of repertoire formation. However, it must be emphasized that the models are not in all respects mutually exclusive, that evidence for one model does not rule out the other, and that there is every reason to suppose that in reality NK cells employ a combination of mechanisms.

To ease the mathematical modeling we have made several simplifying assumptions, some or all of which may turn out to be exaggerations or even incorrect, but which nevertheless allow trends to be predicted: (a) We assume that each receptor gene has an equal initial probability of being activated in an NK cell (the fact that there may be substantially fewer Ly-49A$^+$ than, for example, Ly-49G2$^+$ cells in all strains tested already suggests that this assumption may not be correct). (b) We assume that a given receptor, in a binary fashion, either binds or does not bind to self MHC class I molecules. Receptors are therefore divided cleanly into self and non-self-specific receptors, and we treat all non-self-specific receptors equivalently to each other; similarly, we treat all self-specific receptors equivalently. (c) For reasons stated in Sect. 2.4 we ignore the effect that variations in the *levels* of Ly-49 surface expression may have; here a given receptor is assumed to be either fully expressed or fully repressed. (d) We assume that the underlying mechanisms actually "count" the number of self-specific receptors; in actuality, it is likely that the mechanisms depend on overall Ly-49 dependent signaling, corresponding to some amalgam of the number of different self-specific receptors, their affinity for self class I molecules, and their expression levels. (e) We tentatively ignore the potential role of activating receptors in Ly-49 repertoire development by holding such signals as constant between the two models. (f) For simplicity, when comparing two strains we ignore receptors that cross-react with class I molecules of both strains; this makes little difference for most of the calculations, and cross-reactive receptors can be easily incorporated into the models if desired. (g) We assume that Ly-49 receptor specificity is not modified by somatic hypermutation mechanisms. Lastly, (h) we assume that once formed the repertoire is not biased by the preferential expansion of certain NK subsets.

With these assumptions trends can be predicted. It is more difficult to predict exact frequencies of the various subsets because of several uncertainties. It should be possible eventually to incorporate into the models additional variables such as differing probabilities of Ly-49 gene activation, receptor affinity, and levels. As the information base concerning Ly-49 receptor specificity and expression grows, such modifications will become increasingly relevant.

Initially we consider only a limited number of variables, which are defined in Table 2. Despite the fact that we focus on only very few variables, we demonstrate that both models are able to account for nearly all the existing quantitative data that bear on Ly-49 repertoire development.

3 Mathematical Treatment of the Selection Model

In the selection model as we have formulated it repertoire formation begins by randomly deciding whether each Ly-49 gene is expressed or not. For simplicity we assume that the probability, p, of being expressed is initially the same for all receptors,

Table 2. Definitions of variables

General variables	
n_g	Number of non-self-specific receptor genes
s_g	Number of self-specific receptors genes
t_g	n_g+s_g
n_e	Number of non-self-specific receptors expressed on a given cell
s_e	Number of self-specific receptors expressed on a given cell
t_e	n_e+s_e
R_{s1}, R_{n1}	Denote a given self-specific, or non-self-specific receptor, respectively
Selection model variables	
s_{min}	Minimum number of permitted self-specific receptors per cell
s_{max}	Maximum number of permitted self-specific receptors per NK cell
$f_i[x]$	Fraction of cells in the initial (pre-selection) population that express x
$f_f[x]$	Fraction of cells in the final (post-selection)population that express x
$f_i[s_e]$	Fraction of cells in the initial population that express s_e self-specific receptors
$f_{se}[x]$	Fraction of cells expressing s_e self-specific receptors that express x
p	Initial probability that a given Ly-49 gene is activated
q	1–p
Sequential model variables	
s_t	Target number of self-specific receptors
$f_{ne}[x]$	Fraction of *all* cells that express n_e non-self-specific receptors *and* express x

irrespective of whether they are self- or non-self-specific. (We can also consider the probability, q=1–p, of a receptor not being expressed). Consequently, after an initial phase of Ly-49 gene activation, the total number of receptors expressed by a given NK cell (t_e) might vary anywhere from 0 to the total number of germline receptor genes, with most NK cells distributed between the two extremes. If p is large, most NK cells express a large number of receptors; conversely, if p is small, most NK cells express only a few receptors.

We are most interested in predicting the behavior of variables that are commonly measured experimentally, such as the fraction of NK cells that express any one receptor (non-self-specific or self-specific) or pair of receptors. Our strategy is to calculate the predicted representation of self-specific and non-self-specific receptors separately, since different rules apply to each.

3.1 Frequencies of NK Cells Expressing Non-Self-specific Receptors According to the Selection Model

Calculating the frequencies of cells expressing non-self-specific receptors is quite simple in the selection model. The fraction of cells that express any given receptor in the repertoire before selection, i.e., in the initial repertoire, is equal to p. Since selection acts differentially only on cells expressing different numbers of self-specific receptors, and since the number of non-self-specific receptors on a given cell is assumed to be independent of the number of self-specific receptors, the representation of a non-self-specific receptor in the final repertoire equals its initial representation. Therefore the fraction of cells expressing a given non-self-specific receptor in the final, or selected, repertoire is predicted to equal p. The non-self-specific receptor is designated R_{n1}, and the frequency of cells expressing it in the final repertoire is designated $f_f[R_{n1}]$. Thus $f_f[R_{n1}]=p$. The fraction of cells predicted to express a specific pair of non-self-specific receptors, $f_f[R_{n1}R_{n2}]$, equals p^2.

3.2 Frequencies of Cells Expressing Self-Specific Receptors in the Selection Model

The calculations for self-specific receptors in the selection model are more involved. The selection model assumes that successful progression of the NK cell to the mature compartment occurs only if it expresses some but not too many self-specific Ly-49 genes. The lower and upper limits are not currently known, and we therefore define these as variables, with s_{min} representing the minimum number of expressed self-specific genes required, and s_{max} representing the maximum.

To calculate the frequencies of cells expressing self-specific receptors it is convenient to consider separately the populations of mature NK cells that express each allowable number of self-specific receptors. From within the initially generated stochastic repertoire we first determine the fraction of the population that expresses s_{min} receptors, the fraction that expresses $s_{min}+1$ receptors etc. until we reach s_{max} receptors. Cells that express more than s_{max} or fewer than s_{min} receptors obviously need not be considered as such cells do not contribute to the final population. For each population that expresses an allowable number of self-specific receptors, we then calculate the fraction of the initially generated population that expresses any *particular* self-specific receptor. We call the self-specific receptor R_{s1}. These subpopulations can be summed and divided by the total number of cells that survive selection. This yields the desired value, the fraction of cells in the final population that express a particular self-specific receptor, $f_f[R_{s1}]$. The denominator, the fraction of all cells that survive selection, is simply the sum of the fraction of all initial cells that express s_{min}, the fraction that expresses $s_{min}+1$, etc., until we reach s_{max}, i.e., the sum of $f_i[s_e]$ for all allowable values of s_e. Using a similar strategy the fraction of cells expressing a particular *pair* of self-specific receptors, $f_f[R_{s1}R_{s2}]$, can be calculated.

An example will help illustrate the calculations (Table 3). Consider the case in which there are a total of eight Ly-49 genes encoded in the genome, of which four are specific for self MHC class I. Assume, as well that the probability of initially activating any particular Ly-49 gene is 50%, and that the minimum number of self-specific receptors required by the selection process is 1 and the maximum is 2. In this case therefore $t_g=8$, $s_g=4$, $n_g=4$, p=0.5, q=0.5, $s_{min}=1$, and $s_{max}=2$. Consider first the population of cells expressing any two, and only two, self-specific receptors, i.e., $s_e=2$. The fraction of these cells in the initial population is equal to the fraction of all cells that express any *specific* pair, i.e., 1/16, times the number of possible pairs of receptors, 6; this corresponds to $f_i[s_e=2]=0.375$. By similar reasoning, $f_i[s_e=1]=0.25$. The remaining 0.375 of the cells fail to be selected.

Table 3. Example calculations[a] for the two-step selection model

s_e	$f_i[s_e]$	$f_{se}[R_{s1}]$	$f_i[s_e]\cdot f_{se}[R_{s1}]$	$f_{se}[R_{s1}R_{s2}]$	$f_i[s_e]\cdot f_{se}[R_{s1}R_{s2}]$
Initial repertoire					
1	0.25	0.25	0.063	0	0
2	0.38	0.50	0.18	0.167	0.063
Σ	0.63		0.25		0.063
Final repertoire					
			$f_f[R_{s1}]=0.4$		$f_f[R_{s1}R_{s2}]=0.1$

[a] For the conditions: $t_g=8$; $s_g=4$; $n_g=4$; $p=0.5$; $q=0.5$, $s_{min}=1$ and $s_{max}=2$.

The general formula to calculate the fraction of cells in the initial population expressing s_e receptors can be derived with the aid of the binomial theorem[1]:

$$f_i[s_e] = p^{se}q^{[sg-se]} \cdot \binom{s_g}{s_e} = p^{se}q^{[sg-se]} \cdot \frac{s_g!}{s_e![s_g-s_e]!}$$

To calculate the fraction of the initial repertoire that survives selection the $f_i[s_e]$ values are simply summed. In our example, the result is 0.63 (Table 3).

Now that we know $f_i[s_e]$ for each value of s_e, we wish to calculate the fraction of these cells that express a *particular* self-specific receptor, R_{s1}. This fraction is designated $f_{se}[R_{s1}]$. For each cell expressing two self-specific receptors of four in the genome, the probability that a particular one is expressed is 2/4. Among cells that express one self-specific receptor, 1/4 express R_{s1}. The general expression for the fraction of cells that express R_{s1} among cells expressing s_e receptors is:

$$f_{se}\,[R_{s1}] = \frac{s_e}{s_g}$$

We also wish to calculate the fraction of cells for each s_e value that express a specific *pair* of self-specific receptors, $f_{se}[R_{s1}R_{s2}]$. This value can be easily calculated as the product of the probabilities of expressing each of them. Considering cells that have expressed one of them, the probability that the second one is expressed equals s_e-1/s_g-1. Therefore:

$$f_{se}\,[R_{s1}R_{s2}] = f_{se}[R_{s1}] \cdot \frac{s_{e-1}}{s_{g-1}} = \frac{s_e}{s_g} \cdot \frac{s_{e-1}}{s_{g-1}}$$

[1]We make use of the mathematical ‘choose’ function, whereby the number of ways to choose *x* items from a pool of *y* items, i.e., *y* choose *x*, is denoted by $\binom{y}{x}$ and equals y!/x! (y–x)!. The exclamation mark denotes the factorial function, i.e. 4!=4×3×2×1

Multiplying $f_{se}[R_{s1}]$ by $f_i[s_e]$ yields the fraction of the initial repertoire that expresses R_{s1}, for cells expressing s_e receptors. Summing all of these values yields the fraction of cells in the initial repertoire that express R_{s1} and can be selected (see Table 3). By dividing this value by the fraction of the initial repertoire that can be successfully selected, we can derive the desired value, $f_f[R_{s1}]$: the fraction of cells expressing R_{s1} in the *final* repertoire.

Similarly, to calculate $f_f[R_{s1}R_{s2}]$, the fraction of selected cells expressing both R_{s1} and R_{s2}, we multiply $f_{se}[R_{s1}R_{s2}]$ by $f_i[s_e]$ for each value of s_e, sum these values, and divide by the fraction of the initial repertoire that can be successfully selected. In our example, $f_f[R_{s1}]=0.25\div0.63=0.4$ and $f_f[R_{s1}R_{s2}]=0.63\div0.63=0.1$.

While Table 2 serves as an aid, the following general formulas can be applied to the problem:

$$f_f[R_{s1}] = \sum_{s_e=s_{min}}^{s_{max}} \left(\frac{s_e}{s_g} \cdot f_i[s_e] \right) \div \sum_{s_e=s_{min}}^{s_{max}} f_i[s_e]$$

and:

$$f_f\,[R_{s1}R_{s2}] = \sum_{s_e=s_{min}}^{s_{max}} \left(\frac{s_e}{s_g} \cdot \frac{s_{e-1}}{s_{g-1}} \cdot f_i[s_e] \right) \div \sum_{s_e=s_{min}}^{s_{max}} f_i[s_e]$$

3.3 Predictions of the Selection Model

Table 4 depicts the predictions of the selection model for various conditions. For ease of interpretation the table employs a more familiar nomenclature for the receptors and ligands, where Ly-49X1 is a particular H-2^x specific receptor, etc. As anticipated, conditions exist under which the model predicts that cells expressing Ly-49X1 are more frequent in mice that do not express a ligand (H-2^y mice) than in mice that do (H-2^x mice). However, the decrease in the frequencies of cells expressing particular self-specific receptors is not seen for all conditions. Generally three conditions favor the paradoxical decrease: (a) the relative number of self-specific receptors encoded by the genome is large (s_g/t_g is large); (b) the selection process favors cells expressing relatively few self-specific receptors per cell (s_{min} and s_{max} are low); and (c) the probability of initially expressing any given receptor is high (p is relatively large).

As already noted above, the model predicts that the frequency of Ly-49X1$^+$ cells, or Ly-49X1$^+$X2$^+$ cells, in mice that do not express a ligand, is determined only by p. Therefore these frequencies should not be affected by selection, the number of H-2^x specific receptors or the number of H-2^y specific receptors. They should also not be altered by introducing new receptor transgenes into the genome or by interfering with the selection process. In contrast, we demonstrate below that the competing sequential model predicts that usage of non-self-specific receptors should be affected by these manipulations.

Table 4. Predictions of the two-step selection model

						Predicted frequency of cells expressing:			
			Number of germline receptors specific for:			Ly-49X1		Ly-49X1 and Ly-49X2	
p	s_{min}	s_{max}	$H\text{-}2^x$	$H\text{-}2^y$	Other	In $H\text{-}2^x$	In $H\text{-}2^y$	In $H\text{-}2^x$	In $H\text{-}2^y$
0.5	1	2	4	4	0	0.40	0.50	0.10	0.25
0.3	1	2	4	4	0	0.35	0.30	0.070	0.09
0.3	1	2	6	4	0	0.25	0.30	0.035	0.09
0.3	1	2	10	10	0	0.17	0.30	0.015	0.09
0.3	1	3	10	10	0	0.22	0.30	0.040	0.09
0.3	2	3	10	10	0	0.25	0.30	0.046	0.09

4 Mathematical Treatment of the Sequential Model

In the sequential model NK cells are proposed to express Ly-49 receptors in a random sequence until a sufficient number of self-specific receptors have been turned on to ensure self tolerance. The principal feature that distinguishes this model from the selection model is that NK cells *must* be tested frequently or continuously throughout development for the expression of an appropriate number of self-specific receptors, unlike in the selection model, where such a test need occur at one point in time. The model also assumes that all developing NK cells eventually reach a stage where they express an appropriate number of self-specific receptors. No NK cell ever needs to be deleted or anergized since any cell expressing too few self-specific receptors simply continues turning on receptors until a sufficient number is expressed. In all likelihood the extreme version of the sequential model that we present here to bring out its conceptual features will prove to be inaccurate in at least some respects. In particular, it seems probable that the sequential activation of receptors will have to occur within a defined, rather than an unlimited, window of time. After this time has expired, cells that have not achieved sufficient expression of self-specific receptors may be subject to selective forces. Hence it is plausible that NK cell education involves an amalgamation of the sequential and selection models.

The sequential model that we have proposed suggests that Ly-49 genes are turned on in a random, rather than defined sequence. This assumption may well turn out to be simplistic, but it fits with much of the available data and serves as a starting point for mathematical modeling. Hence in our modeling we assume that the first receptor to be activated is equally likely to be any of the Ly-49 genes encoded by the genome. The second receptor to be activated is equally likely to be any of the remaining receptors. Whether a particular receptor is self or non-self-specific is also not relevant to the sequence in which the receptor is activated. It should be noted that other versions of the sequential model can be considered, in which the sequence of receptor expression is less random, but we have not addressed such models here.

The mechanism of Ly-49 gene activation is not known. One possibility is that relevant "gene activation factors" are limiting such that there is a defined, relatively low probability of activation of a given gene per unit time over the relevant developmental period. An alternative possibility is that gene activation is somehow tied to a periodic event in cellular physiology, such as DNA replication, such that one Ly-49 gene is activated per period. As an aid in devising a mathematical treatment, the model below incorporates the notion of "periodic" gene activation, but the model nevertheless works for both schemes. Once a gene is initially activated, we assume that it remains activated, and thus that receptor gene activation is cumulative. This assumption is in line with data that we have recently obtained (Dorfman and Raulet, in preparation), and with the observation that NK cells often express non-self-specific Ly-49 receptors. It should be noted that there is now clear evidence for mechanisms by which developmentally regulated gene expression can be maintained permanently in a cell lineage, even after the factors that initially activated gene expression have disappeared from the cell. For instance hypermethylated genes are generally transcriptionally repressed, and the methylation status of a gene is heritable in the daughters of dividing cells (Bird 1992). As another example, the trithorax and polycomb gene products stably maintain the proper activation/inactivation status of homeotic genes in *Drosophila melanogaster*, even in mature cell lineages (Paro 1995). Thus the process of Ly-49 gene activation could be easily terminated by extinguishing relevant activating factors, while expression of the already activated genes could be maintained.

4.1 Frequencies of Cells Expressing Self-Specific Receptors According to the Sequential Model

The central notion of the sequential model is that the engagement of self-specific receptors by class I molecules terminates the activation of additional receptor genes. As there is evidence that NK cells can express more than one functioning self-specific receptor (Ly-49A$^+$G2$^+$ cells are detectable, though relatively infrequent, in H-2^d mice; Table 1), we presume that in some cases signaling through more than one receptor is necessary to terminate new receptor gene activation. In practice, variations in receptor affinities and cell surface levels might lead to a situation in which signaling through one receptor is sufficient in some cases to terminate new receptor engagement, while signaling through multiple receptors is necessary in others. In order to simplify the mathematical treatment, however, we have assumed that all self-specific receptors are equivalent.

Thus our model makes the assumption that there is a specific target number of self-specific receptors, s_t, that must be activated to terminate the receptor gene activation mechanism. All mature cells therefore express s_t self-specific receptors. If the total number of self-specific receptor genes (s_g) is known, the calculations resemble to those in Sect. 3.2. It is apparent that:

$$f\,[R_{s1}] = \frac{s_t}{s_g}$$

and:

$$f[R_{s1}R_{s2}] = f[R_{s1}] \cdot \frac{s_{t-1}}{s_{g-1}} = \frac{s_t}{s_g} \cdot \frac{s_{t-1}}{s_{g-1}}$$

Note that, unlike in the selection model, we do not distinguish an initial versus a final repertoire in the sequential model. This is because there is no discrete initial repertoire in the sequential model.

4.2 Frequencies of Cells Expressing Non-Self-specific Receptors According to the Sequential Model

The distribution of non-self-specific receptors is difficult to calculate in the sequential model. It is possible that a mature NK cell would express no non-self-specific receptors, if by chance, it happened to activate only self-specific receptors. It is also possible that a mature NK cell would express *all* of its non-self-specific receptors, as is any combination between these extremes.

To illustrate our approach to calculate the distribution of non-self-specific receptors in the sequential model, consider a more concrete example, in which there are a total of six Ly-49 receptors encoded by the genome, three of which recognize self MHC, and three of which do not. Assume that the expression of two self-specific receptors is sufficient to terminate new receptor gene activation (i.e., s_t=2). A useful way to visualize the sequential model is to use a probability tree diagram (Fig. 1). In this diagram, the cell begins its developmental process with no Ly-49 genes activated. The first receptor to be turned on can be self-specific, in which case the right branch is followed. Alternatively, the first receptor to be activated can be non-self-specific, in which case the left branch is followed. Initially, the probability of turning on a self-specific receptor is 3/6, as is the probability of turning on a non-self-specific receptor. The second receptor to be activated can also either be self-specific or non-self-specific, and, again, the cell follows the right or left branches, respectively. If the first receptor to be activated was self-specific, there are only two self-specific receptors and three non-self-specific receptors remaining that can be activated. Thus in such a case the probability that the second receptor to be activated is self-specific is 2/5; the probability that the second receptor to be activated is non-self-specific is 3/5, etc. All the probabilities are indicated on the tree diagram. The cell stops activating new receptor genes when it has turned on s_t self-specific receptors (i.e., after it has made s_t moves to the right). At this point we consider that it has reached an endpoint and has become an endpoint cell.

The tree diagram illustrates that the process can be divided into sequential *periods*. Since the cells that reach their endpoint in a given period have a number of common features, our approach is to consider each period separately. Clearly, only periods in which cells reach their endpoint are relevant. Each relevant period can be defined by the number of non-self-specific receptors expressed (n_e) by endpoint cells in the period. Thus for each relevant period we determine the fraction of all endpoint cells that reach their endpoint at this period, $f[n_e]$, and the fraction of these cells that express

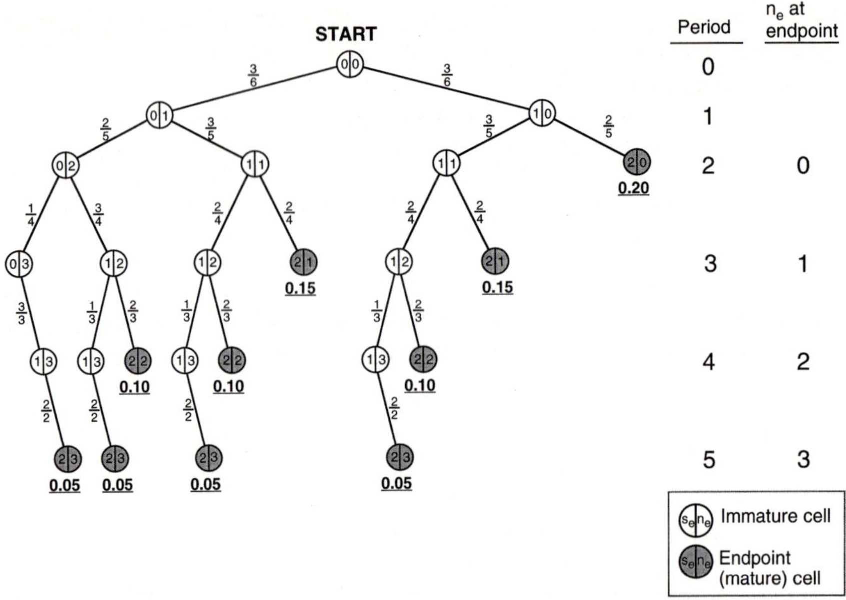

Fig. 1. Probability tree diagram of the sequential model for a system of six receptors, three of which are specific for self MHC and three of which are not. For this example, it is assumed that two self-specific receptors must be activated to terminate new receptor expression. Within each cell is indicated the number of activated self-specific receptors (*left*) and non-self-specific receptors (*right*). The immature cell begins at the top and sequentially activates receptors. Branches heading to the right arise when a cell activates a self-specific receptor; branches to the left arise when a cell activates a non-self-specific receptor. *Numbers on left and right within cells*, the numbers of expressed self and non-self-specific receptors, respectively; *fractions*, the probability of following any particular branch; *shaded circles at the end of branches*, mature enpoint cells; *underlined boldface*, the probability of reaching any particular endpoint (i.e., the endpoint probability, y, calculated by multiplying the probabilities of taking each branch along the route)

a particular non-self-specific receptor, $f_{ne}[R_{n1}]$, or pair of non-self-specific receptors, $f_{ne}[R_{n1}R_{n2}]$. Summing these values for all possible periods (i.e., for all relevant values of n_e) yields $f[R_{n1}]$, the fraction of endpoint cells that express R_{n1}, and $f[R_{n1}R_{n2}]$, the fraction of endpoint cells that express both R_{n1} and R_{n2}. The relationships are:

$$f[R_{n1}] = \sum_{n_e=0}^{n_g} f[n_e] \cdot f_{n_e}[R_{n1}]$$

$$f[R_{n1}R_{n2}] = \sum_{n_e=0}^{n_g} f[n_e] \cdot f_{n_e}[R_{n1}R_{n2}]$$

The calculation of $f[n_e]$ depends on the fact that all endpoint cells in a given period arrive at their endpoint with the same probability, regardless of the pathway taken.

Hence the fraction of cells that reach their endpoints at each period, $f[n_e]$, equals the probability of reaching an endpoint at this period (defined as y, the endpoint probability), times the number of endpoints at this period (defined as x).

The derivation of the endpoint probability, y, can be understood by considering the probability of a given pathway to an endpoint in our example (Fig. 1). At period 5 the left-most endpoint arose by expressing receptors in the order R_n, R_n, R_n, R_s, R_s. The probability of this occurring equals the product of the probabilities of each step: 3/6×2/5×1/4×3/3×2/2, or (3×2×1×3×2)/(6×5×4×3×2). The denominator is seen to equal $t_g!/(t_g\text{-}t_e)!$. The numerator can be separated into an expression that concerns non-self-specific receptors and an expression that concerns self-specific receptors: in our example (3×2×1) and (3×2). The general formulas can be seen to be $n_g!/(n_g\text{-}n_e)!$ and $s_g!/(s_g\text{-}s_t)!$, respectively. Thus the endpoint probability can be defined generally as:

$$y = \left(\frac{s_g!}{(s_g - s_t)!} \cdot \frac{n_g!}{(n_g - n_e)!}\right) \div \left(\frac{t_g!}{(t_g - t_e)!}\right)$$

The derivation of the number of endpoints, x, at each period, can also be understood by analysis of the tree diagram. Consider the fifth period. All pathways to endpoints in this or any other period must end with expression of a self-specific receptor. Therefore all the possible pathways to endpoints in this period can be described in the form: $(R_n,R_n,R_n,R_s)R_s$, where the receptors in parentheses can take all possible orders. Thus this problem reduces to determining the number of possible orders of three equivalent R_n, and one R_s, in the previous four periods. This problem can be restated in terms of only the R_n receptors: given four different periods, how many ways are there to put three R_n into them, or more generally, given t_e–1 periods, how many ways are there to put n_e receptors into them (i.e., t_e–1 choose n_e). In the example, there are four endpoints in the fifth period, where n_e=3. The general formula for the number of endpoints is:

$$x = \binom{t_e - 1}{n_e} = \frac{(t_e - 1)!}{(s_t - 1)!\, n_e!}$$

As explained above, the product of x and y equals $f[n_e]$. All the calculations for the tree in the example (s_g=3, n_g=3, s_t=2) are summarized in Table 5.

Now we need to determine the fraction of cells that express a *particular* non-self-specific receptor, R_{n1}. These values are determined for each period, defined by n_e. Consider the period where n_e=2. The question is, among cells expressing n_e different non-self-specific receptors, what is the fraction that express a particular one, R_n1? As before (Sect. 3.2), it is apparent that this value equals n_e/n_g. Similarly, the fraction of these cells that express a particular pair of receptors, R_{n1} and R_{n2}, equals $(n_e/n_g)\times(n_e-1)/(n_g-1)$. Multiplying these values by $f[n_e]$ yields $f_{ne}[R_{n1}]$, the fraction of *all* cells that express n_e receptors and express R_{n1}:

$$f_{ne}[R_{n1}] = f[n_e] \cdot \frac{n_e}{n_g}$$

Table 5. Calculations for the sequential model[a]

n_e	x	y	$f[n_e]=x\cdot y$	$f_{ne}[R_{n1}]$	$f_{ne}[R_{n1}R_{n2}]$	$n_e \times f[n_e]$
0	1	0.20	0.20	0	0	0
1	2	0.15	0.30	0.10	0	0.3
2	3	0.10	0.30	0.20	0.1	0.6
3	4	0.05	0.20	0.20	0.2	0.6
Total			1.0	$0.5=f[R_{n1}]$	$0.3=f[R_{n1}R_{n2}]$	$1.5=n_{avg}$

[a]for the conditions $s_g=3$; $n_g=3$; $s_t=2$.

Similarly:

$$f_{ne}\,[R_{n1}R_{n2}] = f[n_e]\cdot\frac{n_e}{n_g}\cdot\frac{n_e-1}{n_g-1}$$

Summing all values of $f_{ne}[R_{n1}]$ or $f_{ne}[R_{n1}R_{n2}]$ yields the desired values $f[R_{n1}]$ and $f[R_{n1}R_{n2}]$, respectively, as depicted in Table 5. Thus on average, given our initial assumptions, we can see that the sequential model predicts that 50% of mature NK cells will express a particular non-self-specific receptor, and 30% will express a particular pair of non-self-specific receptors.

Another potentially useful value that can be calculated is the average number of different non-self-specific receptors expressed on the population of cells, n_{avg}:

$$n_{avg} = \sum_{n_e=0}^{n_g} n_e \cdot f[n_e]$$

Thus in our example, the average NK cell at its endpoint expresses 1.5 non-self-specific receptors.

General expressions for $f[R_{n1}]$ and $f[R_{n1}R_{n2}]$ are:

$$f[R_{n1}] = \sum_{n_e=0}^{n_g} \left(\frac{(t_e-1)!}{(s_t-1)!n_e!}\right)\cdot\left(\frac{s_g!}{(s_g-s_t)!}\cdot\frac{n_g!}{(n_g-n_e)!}\div\frac{t_g!}{(t_g-t_e)!}\right)\cdot\left(\frac{n_e}{n_g}\right)$$

$$f[R_{n1}R_{n2}] = \sum_{n_e=0}^{n_g} \left(\frac{(t_e-1)!}{(s_t-1)!n_e!}\right)\cdot\left(\frac{s_g!}{(s_g-s_t)!}\cdot\frac{n_g!}{(n_g-n_e)!}\div\frac{t_g!}{(t_g-t_e)!}\right)\cdot\left(\frac{n_e}{n_g}\right)\cdot\frac{n_e-1}{n_g-1}$$

Table 6. Predictions of the sequential model when s_t=2

Number of germline receptors specific for:			Predicted frequency of cells expressing: Ly-49X1		Ly-49X1 and Ly-49X2	
H-2^x	H-2^y	Other	In H-2^x	In H-2^y	In H-2^x	In H-2^y
4	4	0	0.50	0.40	0.17	0.20
5	4	0	0.40	0.40	0.10	0.20
6	4	0	0.33	0.40	0.07	0.20
10	4	0	0.20	0.40	0.02	0.20
4	6	0	0.50	0.29	0.17	0.11
10	10	0	0.20	0.18	0.02	0.05
13	10	0	0.15	0.18	0.01	0.05
10	8	4	0.20	0.22	0.02	0.07

4.3 Predictions of the Sequential Model

Using these equations and the equations that govern self-specific receptor distribution (Sect. 4.1), Table 6 can be generated, which depicts the predictions of the sequential model under various conditions. For simplicity, the table addresses predictions for only a single value of s_t, 2.

We noted above that the selection model could explain one counterintuitive feature of the Ly-49 repertoire, namely, that the frequency of cells expressing a particular self-specific receptor can decrease in the presence of its ligand. We can now see that the sequential model is equally able to explain this phenomenon. As in the selection model, this behavior occurs in some but not all hypothetical repertoires and conditions. Consider a repertoire comprised of six H-2^x-specific receptors and four distinct H-2^y-specific receptors. The frequency of cells expressing a given H-2^x specific receptor, Ly-49X1, is higher in H-2^y mice (40%) than in H-2^x mice (33%). An opposite trend is observed when there are four H-2^x specific receptors and four H-2^y specific receptors. In common with the selection model, the sequential model predicts that receptor usage will decrease in ligand-expressing mice when a large proportion of all receptors are ligand-specific, and increase in ligand-expressing mice when only a small proportion of all receptors are ligand-specific. This is true over a wide range of s_t values. The frequency of cells expressing a given pair of self-specific receptors (e.g., Ly-49X1 and Ly-49X2) follows the same general trend, as illustrated in Table 6.

5 Comparisons of the Two Models

Having in hand predictions of the two models, one can ask whether either or both models are capable of accounting for the available data concerning the Ly-49 repertoire. If not, other models should be considered. Equally important is to identify the situations in which the models make different predictions, and to ask whether the available data are more consistent with one model than the other.

5.1 Do the Models Fit the Data?

It should first be noted that both models predict deviations from a strict adherence to the product rule. This is expected because both models assume that expression of different receptors is not in fact independent. This assumption is inherent in any education model because education implies a deviation from randomness. The predicted deviations, however, are not large under most conditions that we have modeled and are in line with the observed deviations from the product rule (Table 1).

The two models predict similar trends in terms of the frequencies of cells expressing a given receptor or receptor pair in strains that do or do not express an MHC ligand. Both models predict that the frequency of cells expressing Ly-49X1 is lower in H-2^x mice than in H-2^y mice only under some conditions. In general this occurs in either model only if there exists a relatively large number of H-2^x specific receptors, although other variables affect this outcome (especially p and s_{min} and s_{max} in the selection model). Is this prediction borne out by the data? The reductions in Ly-49A$^+$ and Ly-49G2$^+$ cells in H-2^d mice would fit this prediction if a relatively large number of the Ly-49 receptors are H-2^d specific. Whether this is so cannot yet be answered because of the limited data available concerning the specificity of most Ly-49 receptors. However, anecdotal evidence suggests that specificity for H-2^d may be common among Ly-49 receptors. Of four inhibitory Ly-49 receptors tested, three – Ly-49A, Ly-49G2, and Ly-49C – are reportedly reactive with D^d and/or L^d. It is also notable that H-$2^{b/d}$ mice reject H-2^d bone marrow only very inefficiently, which might suggest that expression of H-2^d-specific receptors is a common property of NK cells, at least in the case of the H-$2^{b/d}$ host (MURPHY et al. 1990). A final conclusion must await the evaluation of H-2^d reactivity of the remaining Ly-49 receptors.

5.2 The Models as Applied to Class I Deficient Mice

Any model of NK cell repertoire formation must account for the phenotype of NK cells in the class I deficient $\beta_2m^{-/-}$ mouse. These mice contain normal numbers of cells with the NK phenotype (LIAO et al. 1991), yet these cells do not attack $\beta_2m^{-/-}$ normal cells (BIX et al. 1991; HOGLUND et al. 1991; LIAO et al. 1991). The NK cells in these mice are not devoid of function, however, because they do lyse certain tumor cell lines, though with a somewhat reduced efficiency.

The phenotype of NK cells in $\beta_2m^{-/-}$ mice seems initially not to fit easily with either model or indeed with any simple model of NK cell selection by class I molecules. The sequential model in its pure form predicts that all NK cells in mice that fail to express class I molecules should express all Ly-49 receptors. The selection model would predict that such mice have no NK cells. However, it is known that $\beta_2m^{-/-}$ and $TAP^{-/-}$ mice are not completely class I deficient. They express on their cell surfaces low levels of functionally conformed class I molecules. Hence the NK cells in these mice could arise by either postulated education process, depending on interactions with low levels of class I molecules. In the sequential model the higher frequencies of NK cells expressing each tested Ly-49 receptor in $\beta_2m^{-/-}$ mice (Table 1) (HELD et al. 1996b) could result from the requirement for more receptors per cell to terminate new receptor expression when class I levels are low. In the selection model only those clones with more receptors would exhibit the appropriate reactivity with low levels of class I molecules and survive the selection process.

Alternatively, the models may well be too simplified, though some of their basic features may be correct. Perhaps the sequential process operates, but only during a limited time period in the life of a developing NK cell. After this time period, new gene activation could not occur. Cells that had not expressed self-specific receptors might then convert to an "anergized" state where they exhibit poor reactivity to all cells, or at least to normal untransformed cells, regardless of the cells' class I expression. Some or all the NK cells in class I deficient mice might be in this state. The selection model can also be adapted in a similar way. NK cells that fail selection may be induced to enter the putative anergic state. Clearly, further analysis of the NK cells in class I deficient mice is necessary to evaluate these possibilities.

5.3 Differential Predictions of the Models

What are the critical differences in the predictions of the two models? There are several, but two are most relevant in view of data that are currently being generated:

5.3.1 The Expected Effects of Ly-49 Transgenes Expressed in All NK Cells

Both models predict that a Ly-49 transgene (e.g., Ly-49A) expressed by all NK cells, in a strain that expresses a class I ligand (e.g., $H\text{-}2^d$), would result in decreased usage of other self-specific receptors (e.g., Ly-49G2). Such an effect was observed (Sect. 2.5). However, the models make different predictions concerning the effects of the transgene on non-self-specific receptors. In the selection model the transgene should have no effect on the frequencies of cells expressing non-self-specific receptors, since these frequencies are dependent only upon p. However, in the sequential model it can be seen that expression of the transgene early in all NK cells hastens the moment in which cells express s_t receptors and hence decreases the likelihood that any given non-self-specific receptor has time to be activated. A comparison of the

Table 7. Predicted effects of a Ly-49X1 transgene in the sequential versus selection models

Variables			Predicted frequencies of cells expressing			
Number of germline receptors specific for:			Ly-49X2		Ly-49Y1	
H-2^x	H-2^y	Ly-49X1 transgene?	In H-2^x	In H-2^y	In H-2^x	In H-2^y
Sequential model (s_t=2)						
4	4	-	0.50	0.40	0.40	0.50
4	4	+	0.25	0.40	0.20	0.50
6	4	-	0.33	0.40	0.29	0.50
6	4	+	0.17	0.40	0.14	0.50
13	10	-	0.15	0.18	0.14	0.20
13	10	+	0.08	0.18	0.07	0.20
Selection model (p=0.3, s_{min}=1, s_{max}=2)						
4	4	-	0.35	0.30	0.30	0.35
4	4	+	0.16	0.30	0.30	0.35
6	4	-	0.25	0.30	0.30	0.35
6	4	+	0.12	0.30	0.30	0.35
10	10	-	0.17	0.30	0.30	0.17
10	10	+	0.08	0.30	0.30	0.17

predicted effects of a Ly-49X transgene according to the two models under some specific conditions is presented in Table 7.

Does the available data bear on these predictions? It was observed that the Ly-49A transgene caused a modest decrease in the frequency of cells in H-2^d mice that stained with the Ly-49 specific SW-5E6 mAb. Unfortunately, it is so far difficult to draw a conclusion from this experiment because of the uncertainties concerning the nature and specificity of receptors detected by the SW-5E6 mAb. With these uncertainties the available data are inadequate to distinguish the sequential or selection models. However, at the present pace of research into the specificity of receptors in this family, a clean test should be forthcoming in the near future.

5.3.2 The Effects of "Irrelevant" MHC Expression on the Frequencies of Cells Expressing a Given Ly-49 Receptor

The selection model predicts that the frequency of cells expressing a Ly-49 receptor in mice that do not express a cognate class I molecule should simply equal p. This should be true equally in class I deficient mice and in mice that express noncognate class I molecules. In contrast, the sequential model predicts differences between class I deficient mice and mice that express noncognate class I molecules. In class I deficient mice new receptor gene activation continues for a longer duration in each cell than in class I$^+$ mice, although the duration may have an upper limit. Hence class I deficient mice might be predicted to harbor a higher frequency of cells expressing a given Ly-49 receptor than class I$^+$ mice expressing irrelevant class I molecules. The available data are inconclusive on this point. We have reported that there are more cells expressing Ly-49A or Ly-49G2 or both in class I deficient mice than in H-2^b mice which are thought not to express a ligand for these receptors (HELD et al. 1996b). These data might be seen to support the sequential model. We have thus far refrained from drawing this conclusion because of the possibility that one or both of these receptors reacts weakly with H-2^b encoded class I molecules (HELD and RAULET 1997).

6 Concluding Remarks

The models elaborated here make various predictions concerning the effects of specific manipulations on the NK repertoire. While available data are so far inadequate to distinguish these models or verify them, the current pace of research in this area is dramatic, and it is likely that new reagents and information will be soon forthcoming which will allow rigorous testing of the predictions of each model. We hope that the mathematical treatments described above will serve as an aid to this research.

Acknowledgements. We thank Drs. Montgomery Slatkin and George Oster for valuable advice on the mathematical modeling, and Jeffrey Dorfman for comments on the manuscript. This research was supported by National Institutes of Health grants RO1AI35021 and RO1AI39642. R.E.V. is a predoctoral fellow of the Howard Hughes Medical Institute. Those interested in obtaining a Macintosh-compatible spreadsheet designed to perform calculations for the mathematical models described in this paper should contact us by email: rvance@ocf.berkeley.edu.

References

Bennett M (1987) Biology and genetics of hybrid resistance. Adv Immunol 41:333–443

Bird A (1992) The essentials of DNA methylation. Cell 70:5–8

Bix M, Liao N-S, Zijlstra M, Loring J, Jaenisch R, Raulet D (1991) Rejection of class I MHC-deficient hemopoietic cells by irradiated MHC-matched mice. Nature 349:329–331

Brennan J, Lemieux S, Freeman J, Mager D, Takei F (1996) Heterogeneity among Ly49C NK cells: characterization of highly related receptors with differing functions and expression patterns. J Exp Med 184:2085–2090

Brown MG, Scalzo AA, Matsumoto K, Yokoyama WM (1997) The natural killer gene complex: a genetic basis for understanding natural killer cell function and innate immunity. Immunol Rev 155:53–65

Chadwick BS, Miller RG (1992) Hybrid resistance in vitro. Possible role of both class I MHC and self peptides in determining the level of target cell sensitivity. J Immunol 148:2307–2313

Correa I, Corral L, Raulet DH (1994) Multiple natural killer cell-activating signals are inhibited by major histocompatibility complex class I expression in target cells. Eur J Immunol 24:1323–1331

Cudkowicz G, Stimpfling JH (1964) Induction of immunity and of unresponsiveness to parental marrow grafts in adult F1 hybrid mice. Nature 204:450–453

Dorfman JR, Raulet DH (1996) Major histocompatibility complex genes determine natural killer cell tolerance. Eur J Immunol 26:151–155

George T, Yu YYL, Liu J, Davenport C, Lemieux S, Stoneman E, Mathew PA, Kumar V, Bennett M (1997) Allorecognition by murine natural killer cells: lysis of T-lymphoblasts and rejection of bone marrow grafts. Immunol Rev 155:29–40

Held W, Cado D, Raulet DH (1996a) Transgenic expression of the Ly49A natural killer cell receptor confers class I MHC-specific inhibition and prevents bone marrow allograft rejction. J Exp Med 184:2037–2041

Held W, Dorfman JR, Wu M-F, Raulet DH (1996b) Major histocompatibility complex class I-dependent skewing of the natural killer cell Ly49 receptor repertoire. Eur J Immunol 26:2286–2292

Held W, Raulet DH (1997a) Ly49A transgenic mice provide evidence for an MHC-dependent education process in NK cell development. Exp Med 185:2079–2088

Held W, Raulet DH (1997b) Expression of the Ly49A gene in murine natural killer cell clones is predominantly but not exclusively mono-allelic. Eur J Immunol 27:2876–2884

Held W, Roland J, Raulet DH (1995) Allelic exclusion of Ly49 family genes encoding class I-MHC-specific receptors on NK cells. Nature 376:355–358

Hoglund P, Ohlen C, Carbone E, Franksson L, Ljunggren H, Latour A, Koller B, Karre K (1991) Recognition of β2-microglobulin-negative (β2m-) T-cell blasts by natural killer cells from normal but not from $\beta 2m^-$ mice: nonresponsiveness controlled by $\beta 2m^-$ bone marrow in chimeric mice. Proc Natl Acad Sci USA 88:10332–10336

Karlhofer FM, Hunziker R, Reichlin A, Margulies DH, Yokoyama WM (1994) Host MHC class I molecules modulate in vivo expression of a NK cell receptor. J Immunol 153:2407–2416

Karlhofer FM, Ribaudo RK, Yokoyama WM (1992) MHC class I alloantigen specificity of $Ly\text{-}49^+$ IL-2 activated natural killer cells. Nature 358:66–70

Karre K, Ljunggren HG, Piontek G, Kiessling R (1986) Selective rejection of H-2-deficient lymphoma variants suggests alternative immune defense strategy. Nature 319:675–678

Liao N, Bix M, Zijlstra M, Jaenisch R, Raulet D (1991) MHC class I deficiency: susceptibility to natural killer (NK) cells and impaired NK activity. Science 253:199–202

Ljunggren HG, Karre K (1990) In search of the 'missing self': MHC molecules and NK cell recognition. Immunol Today 11:237–244

Mason LH, Ortaldo JR, Young HA, Kumar V, Bennett M, Anderson SK (1995) Cloning and functional characteristics of murine LGL-1: a member of the Ly-49 gene family (Ly-49G2). J Exp Med 182:293–303

Murphy WJ, Kumar V, Cope JC, Bennett M (1990) An absence of T cells in murine bone marrow allografts leads to an increased susceptibility to rejection by natural killer cells and T cells. J Immunol 144:3305–3311

Ohlen C, Kling G, Hšglund P, Hansson M, Scangos G, Bieberich C, Jay G, Karre K (1989) Prevention of allogeneic bone marrow graft rejection by H-2 transgene in donor mice. Science 246:666–668

Olsson MY, Karre K, Sentman CL (1995) Altered phenotype and function of natural killer cells expressing the major histocompatibility complex receptor Ly-49 in mice transgenic for its ligand. Proc Natl Acad Sci USA 92:1649–1653

Paro R (1995) Propagating memory of transcriptional states. Trends Gen 11:295–297

Raulet DH, Held W, Correa I, Dorfman J, Wu M-F, Corral L (1997) Specificity, tolerance and developmental regulation of natural killer cells defined by expression of class I-specific Ly49 receptors. Immunol Reviews 155:41–52

Roland J, Cazenave P-A (1992) Ly-49 antigen defines an αβ TCR population in i-IEL with an extrathymic maturation. Int Immunol 4:699–706

Ryan JC, Seaman WE (1997) Divergent functions of lectin-like receptors on NK cells. Immunol Rev 155:79–89

Takei F, Brennan J, Mager DL (1997) The Ly49 family: genes proteins and recognition of class I MHC. Immunol Rev 155:67–77

Wu M-F, Raulet DH (1997) Class I-deficient hematopoietic cells and nonhematopoietic cells dominantly induce unresponsiveness of NK cells to class I-deficient bone marrow grafts. J Immunol 158:1628–1633

Yu YY, George T, Dorfman J, Roland J, Kumar V, Bennett M (1996) The role of Ly49A and 5E6 (Ly49C) molecules in hybrid resistance mediated by murine natural killer cells against normal T cell blasts. Immunity 4:67–76

Ontogeny and Differentiation of Murine Natural Killer Cells and Their Receptors

P.V. SIVAKUMAR, I. PUZANOV, N.S. WILLIAMS, M. BENNETT, and V. KUMAR

1 Introduction

Cellular immunology was actively investigated during the 1960s, stimulated in large part by the development of plaque assays for antibody-forming cells (JERNE and NORDIN 1963) and the assay for cytotoxic cells (ROSENAU and MOON 1964). The discovery that the thymus and bursa of Fabricius are necessary for the development of T and B cells (MILLER and MITCHELL 1969; GLICK and WHATLEY 1967; COOPER et al. 1965) led to the concept of "central lymphoid organs." Subsequently it appeared that the effector cell responsible for rejection of bone marrow allografts following large doses of total-body irradiation is not a T or a B cell, but is eliminated by destruction of bone marrow with the bone-seeking isotope ^{89}Sr (CUDKOWICZ and

Department of Pathology and Graduate Program in Immunology, University of Texas Southwestern Medical Center, Department of Pathology, 6000 Harry Hines Blvd., Dallas, TX 75235-9072, USA

Bennett 1971; Bennett 1973). Thus these effector cells were termed "marrow-dependent" or M cells, based on the analogy with the thymus and bursa-dependent T and B cell. Later studies revealed that M cells are identical to natural killer (NK) cells.

In the early 1970s investigators studying the ability of cytolytic lymphocytes in the peripheral blood of cancer patients to kill tumor cells found that lymphocytes from healthy patients are also able to lyse the same target cells (Rosenberg et al. 1972; Takasugi et al. 1973). This killing which is spontaneous and does not require prior sensitization was termed "natural killing" and was found to be mediated by lymphocytes which had a large granular morphology. These cells were called NK cells (Kiessling et al. 1975; Heberman et al. 1975) or large granular lymphocytes (LGLs). NK activity was shown to be distinct from MHC-restricted CTL killing because both syngeneic and allogeneic targets can be lysed. It was subsequently shown that virally infected cells (Trinchieri et al. 1978) and normal cells (Nunn et al. 1977) can also be killed. It was not until a decade later, however, that NK cells were clearly characterized as a phenotypically distinct population of circulating peripheral blood mononuclear cells (Perussia et al. 1983; Lanier et al. 1986).

NK cells are now defined as lymphocytes that have a large granular morphology, have their T cell receptor (TCR) and B cell receptor (BCR) in germline configuration, do not express membrane CD3 proteins, express FCRγII/III cell surface receptor, and also express a variety of cell surface receptors that are unique to NK cells and a subset of T cells, i.e., CD56 in humans and NK1.1 and 2B4 in mice. Antigens expressed on murine NK cells can be divided into two main categories, those that are expressed on all NK cells (NK1.1 and 2B4) and receptors expressed on subsets of NK cells (Ly-49 family). Although NK killing has been considered to be nonspecific and non-MHC restricted, there is now abundant evidence that NK cells can mediate very specific lysis of untransformed cells in vitro and hematopoietic stem cells in vivo. The specificity of NK cells has been further defined by the discovery of the Ly-49 family of receptors in mice. The Ly-49 family of receptors are expressed on subsets of murine NK cells and have been shown to bind to MHC class I (reviewed in Yokoyama 1995; Raulet and Held 1995; Raulet 1996). This specific interaction leads to a negative signal that inhibits target cell lysis.

In humans the p58 family of receptors (killer inhibitory receptors) perform this same function (reviewed in Colonna 1996; Moretta et al. 1994). The specificity of target recognition by NK cells has been explained by the "missing-self" hypothesis (Ljunggren and Kärre 1990). According to this hypothesis, NK cells lyse allogeneic target cells because the NK cells lack (or are missing) receptors for allogeneic (non-self-encoded) MHC molecules. This hypothesis has been strengthened by the discovery of the Ly-49 family receptors. Although functionally NK cells have been established as a distinct population, their lineage has not been clearly defined. NK cells have been categorized as belonging to either the lymphoid or the myeloid lineage or possibly a separate lineage. It is currently unresolved how NK cells fit into the overall scheme of hematopoiesis.

This review summarizes the data and ongoing research in the field of NK ontogeny and differentiation. It focuses on the nature of the microenvironment required for NK differentiation and the possible relationship of NK cells to T cells and other lymphoid cells. We also discuss the expression of different NK receptors during ontogeny in the murine system and the possible nature of the signal(s) needed for NK receptor specificity and function.

2 Differentiation of NK Cells

NK cells have been found in a variety of tissues in both humans and rodents. The spleen is the richest source for mature functional NK cells in humans and rodents; 3%–4% of lymphocytes in the spleen are NK cells. Another compartment rich in NK cells is peripheral blood; in humans NK cells constitute around 6%–15% of blood lymphocytes. In bone marrow cytolytic activity is low and the number of NK cells represent approx. 1% of lymphocytes. Unlike recirculating T cells that are found in the white pulp of the spleen, NK cells are found in the red pulp. NK cells and LGL activity have also been demonstrated in the liver, in interstitial compartments of the lung in humans and rodents, and in the intestinal mucosa of mice and rats (TRINCHIERI 1989). There is no evidence for NK recirculation, but the levels of NK activity in various organs dramatically increases following administration of immunostimulants. A number of mechanisms could explain this alteration in activation and proliferation of preexisting NK cells in the tissues, localization of blood-borne NK cells or NK precursors, and migration of NK cells from other tissues: It is therefore essential to have a better understanding of the distribution of NK cells, the organ/tissues needed for their differentiation, and the environment needed for them to develop into mature cells capable of function during infection.

2.1 Bone Marrow Is Absolutely Essential for NK Cell Differentiation

Although the fetal liver is a good source of stem cells during the fetal and early neonatal life, hematopoiesis slowly shifts to the bone marrow in the adult animal. It is therefore only reasonable to infer that NK cells also start developing in the bone marrow from hematopoietic stem cells. Shortly after observing the existence of a circulating cytolytic population of NK cells, HALLER et al. (1977) found that progenitors of NK cells resided in the bone marrow. Bone marrow cells from mouse strains with genetically low or high NK cell activity were transplanted into recipients with low or high activity. It was found that the genotype of the transplanted bone marrow cells and not the microenvironment of the recipients dictated the level of activity of the regenerating NK cells. WIGZELL and colleagues later showed that a functional bone marrow is required for the development of cells exhibiting spontaneous cytolytic activity (HALLER and WIGZELL 1977). Treatment of mice with a bone seeking isotope, ^{89}Sr, resulted in the destruction of the cellular elements of the marrow and suppressed NK activity. In these mice the spleen takes over B and T lymphopoiesis and myelopoiesis, and the functional activity of T and B cells and macrophages remains largely intact; however, NK activity is greatly reduced (KUMAR et al. 1979).

These results demonstrate that an intact bone marrow is essential for the development of NK cells. In confirmation of this concept, mice with 17β-estradiol-induced osteopetrosis (SEAMAN et al. 1979) as well as congenitally osteopetrotic mice (mi/mi) have reduced NK activity.

More detailed analysis has revealed that the earliest stages of murine NK differentiation can occur in the absence of a fully functional bone marrow, and that an intact bone marrow is essential only for the complete maturation of these cells into cytolytic effectors (HACKETT et al. 1986a). By using antibodies to the murine NKR-P1 molecule NK1.1 it was demonstrated that a conjugate forming, noncytotoxic, immature NK1.1^{+} population was present in the spleen of marrow-ablated (^{89}Sr- or estradiol-treated) mice. These data taken together indicate that NK cells undergo a bone marrow independent stage of differentiation, maturing to the point of acquiring target binding capacity and expression of NK1.1. A marrow-dependent stage of NK development then occurs, allowing full maturation into lytic effectors. The requirement of an intact bone marrow to support the second stage can be attributed to a variety of factors. The destruction of bone marrow by estradiol or ^{89}Sr could have resulted in the elimination of stromal cells in the marrow that function to induce NK differentiation. Stromal cell induced signaling may occur through cell-cell contact or by production of soluble factors (cytokines) that are essential for NK cell maturation. It is also possible that the treatment results in the generation of abnormal cells in the spleen that inhibit NK differentiation, either by cell-cell contact or by secretion of cytokines, or it leads to the generation of cells in the spleen that are not usually found in the bone marrow. The importance of soluble factors present in the bone marrow for NK differentiation is discussed below. We are currently investigating the role of both stromal cells and cytokines in the differentiation of NK cells from 17β-estradiol treated mice to elucidate the role of marrow-dependent factors that are essential for NK development and differentiation.

2.2 Thymic Independence of NK Cell Development

In contrast to T cells, NK cell maturation can occur in the absence of a functional thymus (HEBERMAN et al. 1975). Indeed functional NK cells are present in athymic *nude* mice and rats as well as in *scid* mice that have a mutation that affects gene rearrangement and therefore lack both T and B cells (HACKETT et al. 1986b; DORSHKIND et al. 1985). In fact *nude* and *scid* mice demonstrate stronger NK activity than their normal counterparts, as if T cells normally suppress NK function. The thymus of *scid* mice also contain more cytolytic NK cells that express typical NK markers than their normal counterparts, especially after culture in IL-2 (TUTT 1988). Normal NK cell activity is also observed in patients with DiGeorge's syndrome, showing that a functional thymus is not required for either NK differentiation or function (LIPINSKI et al. 1980; PETER et al. 1982).

2.3 In Search of the NK Cell Progenitor

Hematopoietic stem cells have been defined as cells capable of differentiating into all lineages of the hematopoietic system, and possessing the capacity to self-renew and to repopulate all lymphoid and myeloid lineage cells. Pluripotent stem cells can be isolated by cell sorting using specific markers (SPANGRUDE et al. 1988; BRECHER et al. 1993; IKUTA et al. 1992). However, the question of how, where, and when pluripotent stem cells commit themselves to differentiate along a single lineage, and whether committed progenitors can be isolated from the bone marrow is currently unresolved. Early experiments using radiation-induced chromosomal markers indicated that the bone marrow contains cells restricted to the myeloid and T cell lineages (ABRAMSON et al. 1977). Various investigators have also demonstrated the existence of cells in the bone marrow and fetal liver capable of differentiating into B cells and myeloid cells when grown on stromal cell layers (OHARA et al. 1991; CUMANO et al. 1992). The physical isolation of these cells from the bone marrow has been difficult. However, recently has been isdated (AKASHI et al. 1997) a committed lymphoid stem cell in the bone marrow which has no myeloid regenerating capability.

Although a huge body of work exists on B, T, and myeloid cell differentiation, data on NK differentiation are sparse. To study transplantable progenitors of NK cells in the bone marrow an in vivo assay was developed (HACKETT et al. 1985). In this assay recipient mice are first depleted of their endogenous mature NK cells by injection of anti-ASGM1 or anti-NK1.1. They are then lethally irradiated and receive an inoculum of syngeneic bone marrow cells. Generation of lytic NK cells is determined by the ability of recipients to clear (lyse) radiolabeled YAC-1 target cells from the lung. Initial studies using this approach identified a population NK progenitors in the bone marrow that bears the phenotype Qa-2$^+$, H-2$^+$, CD24(HSA)$^+$, ASGM1$^-$, NK1.1$^-$, Thy-1$^-$, Qa-5$^-$ (HACKETT et al. 1985, 1986a). This phenotype differed from mature NK cells that are NK1.1$^+$ ASGM1$^+$. Transfer of normal bone marrow cells into osteopetrotic mice failed to generate lytic NK cells, confirming the need for an intact bone marrow environment for NK development. Transplantable NK progenitors capable of differentiating into mature NK cells are present in the spleens of osteopetrotic mice as the spleen takes over hematopoiesis after the destruction of the bone marrow.

Further phenotypic characterization of NK progenitor populations contained in murine bone marrow has been performed more recently in our laboratory (MOORE et al. 1995). Enrichment by cell sorting revealed that the NK progenitors were contained within the Ly6A/E (Sca-1)$^+$ Lin$^-$ population. These could be further divided into two populations based on the expression of c-kit. All NK progenitor activity resided in the c-kit$^+$ population. Also, all NK progenitor activity was present in the CD43^{hi} population. Four-color analysis and cell sorting identified a rare population of Ly6$^+$, Lin$^-$, c-kit$^+$, CD43^{hi}, Fall-3^{hi}, TSA-1(Sca-2)$^-$, AA4.1^{lo}, Rh123^{hi} cells that are highly enriched for NK progenitor activity when transplanted into NK depleted, lethally irradiated mice. However, while these cells lacked pluripotent stem cells, they were also enriched for other lymphoid and myeloid generating cells. A recent report documented the existence of a CD34$^+$ Lin$^-$ CD10$^+$ c-kit$^-$ Thy-1$^-$ CD38$^+$ HLA-DR$^+$ cell population in adult human bone marrow capable of giving rise to T, B, NK and dendritic cells (GALY et al. 1995). Whether this population contains multiple committed progenitors or a single multipotent progenitor is not yet clear. So far it has not been possible to identify a cell that is purely an NK progenitor. Several studies have indicated the presence of a IL-2 responsive NK precursor in the bone marrow that is phenotypically different from mature NK cells (see below, soluble factors in NK development). A variety of in vitro systems using bone marrow feeder layers have provided mixed results (see below, stromal cells in NK development). Further characterization of these cells both in vivo and in vitro using bone marrow feeder layers and cytokines is needed to gain a better understanding of hematopoiesis.

2.4 Lineage Relationship of NK Cells

While it is possible to separate mature NK cells phenotypically from mature T and B lymphocytes and myeloid cells, it has long remained a controversy whether NK cells are part of the lymphoid lineage, myeloid lineage, or an independent lineage. There is evidence to support all three possibilities although recent experimental data in both the murine and human systems provide strong support for a lymphoid rather than a myeloid lineage.

Several lines of evidence suggest a relationship between NK cells and the myeloid lineage. $F4/80^+$ macrophage precursors have been identified in bone marrow and liver, which after culture in colony-stimulating factor (CSF) and IL-2 differentiate into cells that coexpress the NK1.1 antigen (LI et al. 1989). These cells exhibit non-MHC restricted cytotoxicity and antibody-dependent cellular cytotoxicity (ADCC). When the same population is cultured in CSF, they develop into macrophages. Transfer of these precursors into irradiated allogeneic recipients restored NK activity (BACCARINI et al. 1988). Micro-ophthalmic (mi/mi) mice that are congenitally osteopetrotic have defective NK cells and myeloid cells (STECHSCHULTE et al. 1987). Scid mice which lack both T and B cells have normal NK cells and myeloid cells (DORSHKIND et al. 1985). Although these data suggest a possible relationship with the myeloid lineage, strong evidence against this comes from transplantation experiments using W/W^v or Sl/Sl^d mutant mice that are defective in c-kit and c-kit ligand (stem cell factor), respectively. Bone marrow stem cells and the bone marrow microenvironment, respectively, in W/W^v and Sl/Sl^d mice have a severe defect in supporting myeloid differentiation as assayed by colony forming units–spleen, but there is no defect in NK development (HACKETT et al. 1985).

Evidence for an independent lineage for NK cells also comes from experiments conducted using mice with the *scid* or W/W^v mutations (HACKETT et al. 1986b). Mature NK cells but not B and T cells were generated by transplanting *scid* bone marrow cells into NK-depleted, lethally irradiated mice. It was concluded that the NK progenitors were present in *scid* mice and were different from T and B cell progenitors. Similar studies performed with W/W^v marrow cells deficient in myeloid progenitor cells showed that these marrow progenitors could generate normal NK cells. Together, these two observations led to the conclusion that NK cells constitute a separate lineage.

Evidence supporting a relationship to the lymphoid lineage comes from the fact that despite the lack of thymic dependence and absence of TCR rearrangement NK cells share features with T cells regarding receptor expression and immune effector functions, including cytolytic activity and lymphokine production. Evidence that T, B, and NK cells have a common lymphoid progenitor comes from experiments performed with a zinc finger family transcription factor, *ikaros* (GEORGIOPOULOS et al. 1994). *Ikaros* was initially isolated from a screen for transcriptional factors that could bind to the CD3δ enhancer (GEORGIOPOULOS et al. 1992) and was thought to be an early mediator of T cell commitment. Surprisingly, mice homozygous for a germline mutation in the *ikaros* DNA-binding domain lacked not only mature T cells but also B and NK cells. By contrast, erythroid and myeloid cells were intact in these mutant mice. Analysis of bone marrow and thymus for early B and T progenitors using cell specific markers indicated that these mice lack pro-B, pre-B, and mature B cells as well as T cell progenitors. Therefore it was concluded that *ikaros* is required for differentiation of pluripotent stem cells into lymphoid lineages or is expressed in a common lymphoid stem cell. However, the absence of T, B, and NK cells in *ikaros* null mice does not rule out the possibility that *ikaros* is expressed independently in cells that are already committed to the three different lineages. In any case this mutant has definitely identified a factor that is needed only for the development of lymphoid but not myeloid lineage cells.

NK cells share expression of certain cell surface markers with T cells, including Thy-1, CD2, ASGM1 in mice, and CD2 and CD8 in rats and humans. Both populations can be cytolytic and can be activated to proliferate with IL-2. A small subset of T cells also expresses NK1.1 and 2B4, as do all murine NK cells. The idea that T and NK cells are related has been strengthened recently by the discovery of a distinct population of NK1.1$^+$ T cells called natural T cells (BIX and LOCKSLEY 1995). These cells express the α/β TCR and NK1.1 and are thought to be the cells that produce IL-4 that switches the immune response to a Th2 type following certain infections (MACDONALD 1995). Although there is little doubt that mature NK cells differ from mature T cells, there are some features that suggest a possible common progenitor. Initially both mouse and human NK cells were reported to lack expression of CD3ε, δ, and γ proteins or transcripts (BIRON et al. 1987). It is now clear that membrane CD3$^-$, CD7$^+$, CD56$^+$, CD45$^+$ NK cells in human fetal liver do express cytoplasmic CD3ε and δ proteins. Clones derived from human fetal liver stably express CD3εγ and CD3εδ complexes and the ζ chain but do not rearrange the TCR (PHILLIPS et al. 1992; LANIER et al. 1992). Also, in vitro activation of human NK cells results in transcription of CD3ε and expression of cytoplasmic CD3ε proteins (LANIER et al. 1992).

These observations not only demonstrate that there is a lineage relationship between T and NK cells, but also that NK cells develop before functional T cells in ontogeny. Studies by the same group with human fetal thymus have strengthened these concepts. Human immature thymocytes (CD3$^-$ CD8$^-$ CD4$^-$ CD34$^+$) that express cytoplasmic CD3ε protein were able to undergo maturation into both T and NK cells depending on the in vitro culture conditions used (SÁNCHEZ et al. 1994). When cultured with murine fetal thymic organ cultures, CD34^{bright} triple-negative (CD3$^-$, CD4$^-$, CD8$^-$) thymocytes gave rise to both T cells and CD56$^+$ CD3$^-$ NK cells while the CD34^{dim} triple-negative cells gave rise only to T cells. A clonogenic assay showed that these cells (at a single cell level) are capable of differentiating into both T and NK cells. Although this clearly established the presence of a common T/NK progenitor in the thymus, the ability of these cells to develop into either B cells or myeloid cells has not been explored rigorously. This leaves the possibility that these cells, although biased towards T/NK development, may still be multipotential. Multipotential cells that can develop into both lymphoid and myeloid lineages have been isolated from both fetal and adult thymus (ANTICA et al. 1993; WU et al. 1991a,b).

RODEWALD and colleagues (1992) described a population of 13- to 15-day mouse fetal thymocytes with the potential to differentiate into both T and NK cells, depending on the in vivo microenvironment. These cells (day 14.5 gestation), which lack expression of CD4 and CD8, express FcγRII/III several days before TCR rearrangement. When injected intrathymically, they gave rise to mature T cells but when removed from the thymic environment, either by using an intravenous method for transfer into irradiated recipients or by culturing them in vitro with IL-2, they gave rise to NK1.1^{+} CD3^{-} cells that were able to lyse YAC-1 target cells. Again, the potential of these cells to develop into B or myeloid cells was not investigated. Because these studies were carried out in bulk populations, it is also possible that the FcγRII/III^{+} cells in the fetal thymus contain two separate progenitors, one for T cells and the other for NK cells. Another group (CARLSSON et al. 1995) has shown that a population of FcγRII/III^{+} cells isolated from murine fetal liver can differentiate into B cells when cultured on S-17 stromal cells with IL-7 and can give rise to myeloid cell colonies when cultured on methyl cellulose, suggesting that FcγRII/III can actually define a population of multipotential cells. Indeed FcγRII/III is expressed on the surface of c-kit^{+} Lin^{-} cells isolated from murine bone marrow (LANTZ and HUFF 1995), and these cells are multipotential.

Development of certain genetically manipulated mouse strains has recently provided some interesting if confusing data on the T/NK relationship. Transgenic mice that expressed the human CD3ε gene under the control of the human CD3 promoter and enhancer (WANG et al. 1994) showed a peculiar immunodeficiency. Transgenic lines expressing more than 30 copies of the transgene exhibited a block in development of both T cells and NK cells but not in B cells. Mice with lesser copy numbers of the CD3 transgene had a block only in T cell development. These workers suggested that expression of the transgene induced an aberrant signal that induced cell death in either T or NK progenitors or in a common progenitor. The low copy number mice exhibited a T cell developmental arrest at a later stage (Thy-1^{+} CD44^{-}) than in the high copy number mice (Thy-1^{+} CD44^{+}), suggesting that the common NK/T progenitor probably precedes this stage. In contrast, however, CD3ε knockout mice demonstrated an arrest in T cell development (Thy-1^{+} CD44^{-}) but had normal numbers of functional NK cells (RENARD et al. 1995). This clearly indicates that even if CD3ε is expressed in a common NK/T progenitor, its function is not required for NK development but is needed for T cell development. Together these studies do not provide definite proof for a common T/NK progenitor but certainly support the possibility.

In looking for NK progenitors in the murine fetal thymus, Brooks et al. were able to obtain long-term clonal cell populations by culturing fetal thymocytes (day 14 gestation) in high doses of IL-2 (BROOKS et al. 1993). These cells not only proliferated well in response to IL-2 but were phenotypically indistinguishable from mature NK cells except for the expression of Ly-49 family members. We have been able to reproduce these experiments and have shown that these cells express the pan NK markers NK1.1(NKR-P1C), 2B4, the subset marker 10A7 (an antibody that recognizes NKR-P1A and B), and FcγRII/III but do not express surface sCD3ε or any member of the Ly-49 family for which antibodies are available (Ly-49A, C, I, D, and G2). These cells are lytic against YAC-1 targets and secrete interferon (IFN) γ and IL-3.

In collaboration with BROOKS and colleagues we have established cell lines from murine fetal liver that show similar characteristics (MANOUSSAKA et al. 1997). These cells are morphologically similar to adult NK cells and express NK1.1 and 2B4 but do not express surface CD3 nor any known member of the Ly-49 family. As with fetal thymus derived NK1.1$^+$ cells, they are lytic towards YAC-1 targets. The analysis for CD3 transcripts in both fetal liver (FL-NK) and fetal thymus (FT-NK) derived NK1.1$^+$ cells showed that expression of these transcripts is variable. Most FT-NK clones express CD3ζ and γ but only some express CD3δ and/or CD3ε. In contrast, FL-NKs express only CD3ζ uniformly, and some express CD3γ but not ε or δ. This would therefore suggest that unlike in humans, where most fetal liver NK clones express transcripts for CD3ε but not CD3δ or γ, the CD3γ transcript probably is expressed first in mice followed by CD3δ and ε transcripts. These cells could therefore have arisen from a population that was at least bipotential (T and NK) or were purely NK cells that expressed CD3 transcripts. It is also of interest that one FL-NK line maintained by the Brooks group secretes IL-2 in spite of the fact that it resembles phenotypically an NK cell (MANOUSSAKA et al. 1997). The lineage potential of these cells in vivo and in vitro is currently under investigation.

2.5 Stromal Cells in NK Cell Development

It is clear that differentiation of NK cells is dependent upon an intact bone marrow environment. Unlike T cells that develop and undergo maturation and selection on thymic epithelial cells, NK cells probably develop on bone marrow stromal cells and probably depend upon cell-cell contact and soluble factors secreted by stromal cells for their differentiation. Because the bone marrow seems critical, NK differentiation in vitro has been studied using long-term bone marrow cultures in which hematopoiesis occurs within the microenvironment of marrow stroma. There are two long-term bone marrow culture systems (LTBMC), both dependent on the development of a complex "stromal microenvironment." In the Dexter LTBMC myelopoiesis is favored although these cultures do maintain transplantable progenitors for T and B cells (DEXTER and TESTA 1980). In contrast, Witte-Whitlock LTBMC sustains B lymphopoiesis (WHITLOCK and WITTE 1982) but not myelopoiesis. If a culture is started under Dexter conditions and switched to Witte-Whitlock condition after several weeks, myelopoiesis declines and B lymphopoiesis ensues, suggesting that the same stromal cells can support both myelopoiesis and lymphopoiesis under different culture conditions. Dexter cultures do not contain mature NK cells nor can they be induced by addition of IL-2. However, they do contain transplantable NK progenitors (Kumar, unpublished data). When Dexter cultures are switched to Witte-Whitlock conditions, IL-2 responsive NK precursors appear in the cultures 7–12 days after switching. These become mature lytic NK cells after the addition of IL-2. However, addition of IL-2 at the time of switch has no effect. This strongly argues against the possibility of the existence of rare, undetectable mature NK cells in these cultures and supports the hypothesis of the existence of an NK progenitor that becomes IL-2 responsive after interaction with the stroma in these switch cultures. POLLACK et al. (1992) have obtained similar but slightly different results. In their system NK1.1^{+} lytic NK cells are produced from these switch cultures without the addition of any exogenous IL-2. It is possible that under the conditions employed by POLLACK et al., the stromal cells produce a factor that can substitute for IL-2 in inducing NK differentiation.

An NK LTBMC has been described using a modified Witte-Whitlock culture system in rats (VAN DEN BRINK et al. 1990). Bone marrow cells were placed in Witte-Whitlock culture media for 4 weeks without any change of media or refeeding. Four weeks after culture initiation the addition of IL-2 generated lytic cells with an NK phenotype. The generation of NK cells depended on the addition of IL-2 and the presence of conditioned media. If IL-2 was added to the culture with fresh media, no NK cell generation was seen. The generation of lytic cells was also dependent on the presence of stromal cells. These data suggest that in these "starvation" cultures NK precursors were selectively enriched, and that these precursors needed IL-2 and some other factor present in the conditioned media to differentiate into mature NK cells. Characterization of the nonadherent population of NK-LTBMC has shown that the NK precursors are concentrated in the CD44$^{-/lo}$ subset that comprise about 10% of "lymphoid " gated cells (DELFINO et al. 1996). When CD44^{lo} cells were sorted from bone marrow of mice treated with 5-fluorouarcil, 30% of the cells were T cells. Culture of post-5-fluorouarcil bone marrow on irradiated LTBMC with IL-2 (after removing the T cells) resulted in the generation of lytic NK cells. The frequency of these cells was estimated by limiting dilution assay to be 1/500.

A long-term culture system to study human NK cell differentiation has also been described (MILLER et al. 1992). Sorted CD34^{+} DR^{-} cells from normal human bone marrow were plated on allogeneic bone marrow stroma with IL-2 for 5 weeks. Cultured cells had a large granular morphology and an NK phenotype (CD56^{+} CD3^{-}) and were able to lyse both K562 and Raji tumor targets. Surprisingly, these cells were CD2^{-} CD16^{-}. It was, however, possible to generate NK cells from an enriched population of progenitors that do not express any myeloid or lymphoid lineage markers. The same group further subdivided this cell population on the basis of expression of CD7 to enrich for NK progenitors (MILLER et al. 1994). Both the CD34^{+} CD7^{+} and CD34^{+} CD7^{-} populations generated CD56^{+} CD3^{-} NK cells following culture in the LTBMC with IL-2 for 5 weeks. However, the CD34^{+} CD7^{+} population showed a greater expansion and cloning efficiency than the CD34^{+} CD7^{-} population, as determined by a limiting dilution assay. This suggests that the CD34^{+} CD7^{+} population is highly enriched for an NK progenitor and a possible intermediate in NK development. Plating of the more primitive CD34^{+} CD7^{-} cells in a transwell system which separates bone marrow stroma and progenitors prevented NK differentiation. In contrast, the more mature CD34$^+$ CD7$^+$ progenitors generated NK cells in the same system. This suggests that primitive but not more mature NK progenitors require direct contact with the stroma for the initial differentiation steps.

We are investigating the ability of the transplantable NK progenitor cells (Ly6$^+$ Lin$^-$ c-kit$^+$ CD43$^+$) to differentiate in vitro in these LTBMCs. Cloned stromal cell lines that have been characterized to produce different cytokines would ideally be used to examine NK development in vitro. There is some evidence that some cloned stromal cell lines support B lymphopoiesis whereas others do not (PIETRAGELI et al. 1988). Addition of different combinations of cytokines to primary as well as cloned stromal cells needs to be attempted to provide a better in vitro system to study NK differentiation.

2.6 Soluble Factors in NK Cell Development

2.6.1 Interleukin-2

While a variety of soluble factors have been implicated in the activation and proliferation of NK cells, little is known about the cytokines that are essential for the development of mature NK cells in the bone marrow. IL-2 is a potent activator of NK cells that causes their expansion and also increases their lytic activity. Unlike T cells which express the high-affinity IL-2 receptor (α, β, and γ subunits), NK cells express the low-affinity IL-2R (β and γ subunits). High IL-2 concentrations (100 U/ml) are therefore required for NK activation and proliferation. IL-2 has been used extensively to induce NK differentiation from bone marrow progenitors and precursors. Mature NK cells can be derived from human bone marrow cultured with IL-2 containing media, after the bone marrow cells have been extensively depleted of mature T and NK cells (YODA et al. 1988; TAGUCHI et al. 1992). To isolate the NK precursor from these T and NK depleted bone marrow cells, expression of IL-2Rα (CD25) and IL-2Rβ (CD122) was studied by flow cytometry. Neither CD25 nor CD122 was observed in these selected cells. Culture with IL-2 for 24 h induced expression of CD25 without detectable expression of CD122 (SHIBUYA et al. 1993). Further analysis revealed that NK cells (CD56$^+$ CD3$^-$) and NK activity were generated only from the CD33$^-$ CD34$^-$ CD25$^+$ cell fraction after culture in IL-2 containing media. This suggests that the NK progenitors are enriched in the CD33$^-$ CD34$^-$ CD25$^+$ population.

A stromal cell independent in vitro system has been established for the generation of NK cells from marrow derived CD34$^+$ human hematopoietic progenitor cells (SHIBUYA et al. 1995). Culture of sorted CD34$^+$ Lin$^-$ cells from adult bone marrow with IL-2 and stem cell factor (SCF) resulted in the generation CD56$^+$ CD3$^-$ NK cells in a dose dependent manner. These cells originated from CD34$^+$ CD33$^+$ Lin$^-$ cells and not from CD34$^+$ CD33$^-$ Lin$^-$ cells. However, on addition of IL-3 the NK differentiation was induced from the latter population although at a lower frequency. Supplementing SCF or SCF and IL-3 for the first 7 days followed by the addition of IL-2 for 21 days resulted in optimal generation of mature CD56$^+$ CD3$^-$ NK cells from these CD34$^+$ populations. These results demonstrate that NK cells arise from CD34$^+$

hematopoietic progenitor cells and show the minimum lymphokine requirement for NK differentiation. Culture of $CD34^+$ Lin^- cells isolated from cord blood with IL-2 and a stromal cell line expressing membrane-bound human SCF can also induce differentiation into NKR-$P1^+$ $CD56^+$ $CD3^-$ cells (BENNETT 1996) that are able to lyse K562 tumor cells.

Several groups have reported that the IL-2 responsive NK precursors in mouse bone marrow are phenotypically distinct from mature NK cells (KOO and MANYAK 1986; KOO et al. 1986; KALLAND 1986; MIGLIORATI et al. 1992). These precursors are $CD25^-$ $ASGM1^-$ $NK1.1^-$ $CD8^-$ Mac-1^-, distinguishing them from mature $ASGM1^+$ $NK1.1^+$ Mac-1^+ NK cells. Attempts to replace this inductive activity of IL-2 with IL-1, IL-3, IFNα/β, and CSF-1 were unsuccessful, suggesting that NK cell maturation requires interaction with IL-2 or some other cytokine with similar activities. The expression of IL-2Rβ on hematopoietic progenitors has been studied in detail by REYA et al. (1996). To determine whether signaling via IL-2Rβ is needed for differentiation of lymphocyte precursors they characterized its expression in fetal liver. A significant fraction of Sca-1^+ Lin^-cells isolated from day 12 murine fetal liver expressed IL-2Rβ (CD122). The majority of $B220^+$ cells in fetal liver expressed CD122. It has been shown that a subpopulation of $B220^+$ $CD19^-$ cells in the bone marrow express NK1.1 and can proliferate and become lytic in response to IL-2 (ROLINK et al. 1996). Together these data suggest that some early NK and B cell precursors express B220 and CD122 and respond to IL-2.

The main source of IL-2 is activated T cells. The lack of a significant number of activated T cells in the bone marrow raises questions about the potential role for IL-2 in NK differentiation in vivo. This doubt is strengthened by the observation that NK development is normal in IL-2 null mice (KUNDIG et al. 1993; SCHORLE et al. 1991). Subsequently it was shown that mice that lack expression of the IL-2Rγ chain are deficient in NK cells, suggesting that while signaling through the IL-2Rγ chain is essential for normal NK development (CAO et al. 1995), IL-2 is not the factor responsible. Human SCID patients with mutations in their IL-2Rγ chains also have a selective lack of T and NK cells (NOGUCHI et al. 1993). Chronic treatment of both fetal and postnatal mice with antibodies to the IL-2Rβ subunit results in a block in NK development (TANAKA et al. 1992, 1993). Transgenic mice which overexpress the IL-2Rβ subunit surprisingly lack NK cells and Thy-1^+ dendritic epidermal cells although development of the other lineages is normal (SUWA et al. 1995). It has been speculated that hyperactivation through the IL-2Rβ subunit perturbs NK development. All these data suggest that an IL-2 independent factor interacts with the IL-2Rβ and γ chains, and that this factor is probably important in NK differentiation. In keeping with this hypothesis, IL-2Rβ knockout mice have been found to lack NK cells or NK activity (SUZUKI et al. 1997). The recently discovered cytokine IL-15 that shares IL-2Rβ with IL-2 seems to meet the requirements of an NK-differentiating factor as discussed below.

2.6.2 Interleukin-12

Another cytokine that has recently been shown to induce NK differentiation in vitro is IL-12. IL-12, initially identified as an NK stimulation factor, has been shown by several groups to modulate hematopoiesis. In vitro IL-12 seems to synergize with different cytokines such as IL-3, IL-11, SCF, granulocyte CSF, and granulocyte-macrophage CSF to induce growth and differentiation (PLOEMACHER et al. 1993a,b; JACOBSON et al. 1993, 1995). In vivo IL-12 actually inhibits hematopoiesis by inducing the production of IFNγ by T and NK cells (GATELY et al. 1994). The role of IL-12 in NK cell differentiation was examined in human cord blood progenitors. Lin^- cells isolated from cord blood were cultured in the presence of feeder cells from Sl/Sl mice expressing membrane-bound human SCF. Addition of IL-2 induced generation of a $CD56^+$ NKR-$P1^+$ population which was inhibited by the addition of IL-12 (BENNETT et al. 1996). This inhibition was not reversed by the addition of either anti-IFNγ or anti-TNFα antibodies. Effects of IL-12 on later stages of NK differentiation were also studied. Culture of Lin^- cord blood cells with SCF and IL-2 generated two distinct populations of NKR-$P1^+$ cells after 30 days in culture. The mature NKR-$P1^+$ $CD56^+$ population lysed K562 targets while the immature NKR-$P1^+$ $CD56^-$ population did not. Culture of the NKR-$P1^+$ $CD56^-$ population with IL-12 induced differentiation into the mature NKR-$P1^+$ $CD56^+$ stage. These cells lysed K562 tumor targets. This suggests a possible role for IL-12 in differentiation of NK cells at later stages. Although mice with a deletion of the p40 chain of IL-12 have been generated, the NK cell number and phenotype in these mice are yet to be characterized (MAGRAM et al. 1996).

2.6.3 Interleukin-15

IL-15 was discovered independently as a proliferation factor for the T cell line CTLL-2 from the supernatants of two cell lines, CV-1/EBNA and HuT-102 (BURTON et al. 1994; GRABSTEIN et al. 1994). This factor also seemed to activate NK cells (BAMFORD et al. 1994). IL-15 shares many features with IL-2. They are both members of the four α helix bundle cytokine family; both utilize the β and γ subunits of the IL-2/IL-15R and also share functional similarity in activating T and NK cells (GRABSTEIN et al. 1994). It was not initially clear why two cytokines with similar properties are produced until further analysis revealed the differences in the cells secreting these cytokines, sites of cytokine production, and regulation of secretion of IL-2 and IL-15. While IL-2 is produced primarily by activated T cells, no IL-15 mRNA has been detected in the T cells as assessed by northern blot analysis. IL-15 message is most abundant in placenta and skeletal muscle, kidney, lung and heart (GRABSTEIN et al. 1994; BAMFORD et al. 1996). In addition, IL-2 secretion seems to be regulated at the level of transcription and message stabilization, whereas IL-15 secretion is controlled at different levels including translation and entry into the secretory pathway (BAMFORD et al. 1996). IL-15 can also activate mast cells by signaling through a receptor system that is independent of the activation system in T cells (TAGAYA et al. 1996). IL-2Rα does not seem to be required for either binding or activation by IL-15 (GIRI et al. 1994). The ability of certain nonlymphoid cell lines to bind IL-15 but not IL-2 suggested the existence of an IL-15 specific receptor subunit, independent of IL-2R (GIRI et al. 1995).

A novel receptor subunit, IL-15Rα, has been identified and cloned (GIRI et al. 1995). This receptor binds IL-15 with greater affinity than IL-2 has for its unique α receptor. Moreover, IL-15Rα is expressed predominantly in T cells, B cells and, more interestingly, on thymic and bone marrow stromal cell lines. The latter observation provided the initial clues to the possible functions of IL-15, especially in NK differentiation. The presence of NK cells in IL-2 null mice along with the lack of NK cells in both IL-2Rγ null mice (CAO et al. 1995) and IL-2Rβ transgenic mice (SUWA et al. 1995) had strongly suggested the existence of another NK differentiating factor that shared the two IL-2R subunits. This has been strengthened further by the lack of NK cells in IL-2Rβ null mice (SUZUKI et al. 1997). The secretion of IL-15 by stromal cell lines and its ability to bind to the low affinity IL-2R indicated that this could potentially be an NK differentiation factor in vivo. IL-15 and IL-15R message have also been found in fetal tissues including fetal liver and thymic epithelium further strengthening the potential role of IL-15 in differentiation of the immune system. The presence of an independent signaling system in mast cells suggests that IL-15 also plays a role in mast cell differentiation and function. In addition to activating T and NK cells, IL-15 also acts as a costimulator with IL-12 for IFNγ secretion by NK cells (CARSON et al. 1994).

To study the potential role of IL-15 in NK cell differentiation we used 17β-estradiol treated mice. In these mice hematopoiesis shifts to the spleen due to the destruction of the marrow environment. NK1.1$^+$ cells isolated from these mice are nonlytic towards YAC-1 targets. Culture of these nonlytic NK1.1$^+$ cells in IL-15 induced lytic activity at concentrations as low as 2 ng/ml; the activity peaked at 20 ng/ml after 24 h in culture (PUZANOV et al. 1996). A lower than normal percentage of NK1.1$^+$ cells isolated from osteopetrotic mice express mature NK markers; for example, B220, Ly-49A, Ly-49G2, Ly-49C, and CD11b (Mac-1). These nonlytic, immature NK1.1$^+$ cells acquired the phenotypic profile of mature NK cells after culture in 20 ng/ml IL-15 for 72 h; even the frequency of cells expressing the Ly-49 family receptors reached control levels. IL-15 also caused a preferential expansion of the NK1.1$^+$ CD3$^-$ population from spleens of these mice compared to the NK1.1$^+$ CD3$^+$ cells. IL-15 seems more effective than IL-2 at activating both immature and mature NK1.1$^+$ cells on a weight/weight basis. These data suggest that IL-15 and not IL-2 is the major differentiation factor for NK cells. However, it is premature to say that the arrest in NK development in osteopetrotic mice is due to the lack of IL-15. The nature of the estradiol-induced defect in NK development is not known. Many factors could be responsible for the phenotype seen, including absence of IL-15, IL-15R, abnormal signaling through the IL-15R, abnormal secretion of IL-15, and inhibition of differentiation by other unknown soluble factors.

Studies in the human system also support the role of IL-15 in differentiation of NK cells. MRÓZEK and colleagues (1996) were able to induce the development of CD56$^+$ CD3$^-$ cells from 21-day cultures of CD34$^+$ hematopoietic progenitor cells in IL-15 or IL-15 and SCF. While IL-15 alone was able to induce the expression of CD56 on these CD34$^+$ cells, SCF and IL-15 together were required for the differentiation and expansion of the $CD56^+$ $CD3^-$ cells. The cells from both types of cultures showed cytolytic activity against K562 targets and produced IFNγ as well as TNFα and granulocyte-macrophage CSF as do mature NK cells. More recently NK cell differentiation has been induced by the culture of cord blood $CD34^+$ cells with a combination of cytokines including IL-15, SCF, IL-2, and IL-7 (CAVAZZANA-CALVO et al. 1996). A combination of SCF, IL-2, and IL-7 was able to induce the proliferation and differentiation of $CD34^+$ $CD7^+$ cord blood cells into mature NK cells with lytic capability. In contrast, a combination of IL-15 and SCF induced NK maturation from a more immature ($CD34^+$ $CD7^-$) population of cord blood cells into $CD56^+$ $CD3^-$ cells. Addition of IL-15 or IL-2 to Lin^- cells isolated from cord blood and cultured on Sl/Sl bone marrow stromal cells transfected with human SCF induced differentiation into $CD56^+$ $CD3^-$ cells (BENNETT 1996).

LECLERCQ et al. (1996) have defined effects of IL-15 on the differentiation of T/NK progenitor cells from the thymus. IL-15 mRNA is detected predominantly in thymic epithelial cells while IL-2 mRNA is detected in thymocytes. Progenitor cells of the phenotype $CD25^-$ $CD44^+$ $Fc\gamma R^+$ $HSA^{-/lo}$ TCR^- $IL\text{-}2R\beta^+$ were either grown in fetal thymic organ cultures or cultured in IL-15 in vitro. The cells grown on fetal thymic organ cultures gave rise to mature T cells while those cultured with IL-15 gave rise to NK cells. These data strongly suggest an important role for IL-15 in NK development in vivo. However, the stage at which IL-15 might play a role is yet to be defined.

We have initiated studies to define the role of IL-15 in the development of murine NK cells from multipotent progenitors. The earliest T-lineage precursor in the murine adult thymus expresses low levels of CD4 and has been shown to be multipotential (WU et al. 1991a,b). "Low CD4 precursor" cells from murine adult thymus were cultured in combinations of SCF, IL-3, IL-6, IL-7, and IL-15. Addition of IL-15 alone did not induce development of $NK1.1^+$ cells from these precursor cells. However, addition of IL-15 along with the other cytokines or addition of IL-15 after culture of these precursors in the other cytokines induced differentiation of the "low CD4 precursor" cells into $NK1.1^+$ cells (Moore and Kumar, unpublished data). Cells phenotypically similar to the earliest thymic precursor, expressing Sca-2 antigen, have been isolated from murine bone marrow (ANTICA et al. 1994). When Lin^- $c\text{-}kit^+$ $Sca\text{-}2^+$ cells from murine bone marrow were cultured with a combination of flt-3 ligand, SCF, IL-6, IL-7, and IL-15, lytic $NK1.1^+$ cells developed (WILLIAMS et al. 1997). It is possible that SCF and possibly other cytokines such as IL-6 and IL-7 are needed for the differentiation of subsets of progenitors to a stage at which IL-15 could drive maturation into lytic NK cells. Further work, especially development of IL-15 and/or IL-15Rα null mice, may provide more definitive answers regarding the role of IL-15 in NK cell differentiation.

3 Natural Killer Cell Receptors

NK cells lyse tumor targets and virally infected cells in a specific manner that has only recently been characterized. Target cell expression of MHC class I molecules is correlated with resistance to NK mediated killing. Currently there are two hypotheses to explain the molecular basis of allospecific recognition and killing by NK cells. The first, stemming from studies of bone marrow transplantation in mice, proposes the positive recognition of nonself antigens by NK cells (BENNETT 1987). These antigens have been called hematopoietic histocompatibility (Hh) antigens, and subsets of NK cells are presumed to express receptors for these determinants. The second hypothesis, the so-called "missing-self" hypothesis (LJUNGGREN and KÄRRE 1990) proposes that NK cells lyse allogeneic targets or class I negative targets because they lack (or are missing) self MHC class I molecules. A corollary of the missing-self hypothesis is that NK cells express two functionally distinct sets of receptors, one that recognizes ligands on the target cells and sends activation signals (positive signal) and another that recognizes ligands on the target cell and sends inhibitory signals (negative signal). The activation signal sends a message to the cell that primes it to lyse the target cell. However, if the target cell expresses the ligand for the inhibitory receptor, this negative signal inhibits lysis of the target, and the cell is spared. The correlation of MHC expression with target resistance tends to argue that the ligand for the inhibitory receptors is MHC class I. This suggests the presence of a receptor for self-MHC on NK cells.

Although neither of the two hypotheses can satisfactorily explain all aspects of NK alloreactivity, the missing-self hypothesis has been strengthened by the recent demonstration of receptors that bind to MHC class I. These receptors belonging to the Ly-49 family (members of which are expressed on subsets of NK cells) have been shown to specifically interact with and receive a negative signal from class I molecules (reviewed in YOKOYAMA 1995; RAULET and HELD 1995; RAULET 1996). Antibodies to the Ly-49 family members or to specific MHC molecules that block this interaction lead to lysis of otherwise resistant syngeneic or allogeneic targets. On the other hand, antibodies that cross-link NK1.1(NKR-P1C) and 2B4 can activate NK cells to kill resistant targets and increase IFNγ secretion and granule exocytosis by NK cells. These surface antigens are expressed on all NK cells and therefore are candidates for the activation molecules. Their ligands, however, are yet to be characterized. Both NKR-P1 and Ly-49 family members are genetically linked on mouse chromosome 6, suggesting the existence of a NK gene complex that could encode both stimulatory and inhibitory NK receptors (YOKOYAMA and SEAMAN 1993).

3.1 Pan-NK Receptors: NKR-P1 Family and 2B4

3.1.1 NKR-P1 Family

The first mouse monoclonal antibody (NK1.1) that defined a cell surface molecule predominantly expressed on NK cells was made by KOO and PEPPARD (1984). Later the mAb 3.2.3 which identifies all rat NK cells was developed (CHAMBERS et al. 1989). Both of these antibodies recognize products of the NKR-P1 gene family and stimulate NK cytotoxicity and degranulation (CHAMBERS et al. 1989). As with antibodies against other cell surface activation molecules, they also mediate redirected lysis of target cells expressing the Fc receptors (CHAMBERS et al. 1989). Cross-linking NKRP-1 leads to an increase in intracellular calcium and stimulates phosphoinositide turnover (RYAN et al. 1991). Based on these observations NKR-P1 has been considered a candidate NK signaling receptor.

The NKR-P1A gene cloned from rat NK cells (GIORDA et al. 1990) is expressed as a disulfide-linked homodimer of 60 kDa. It is a type II integral membrane protein (intracellular aminoterminus) with a single transmembrane domain. The extracellular domain of NKR-P1 has a carbohydrate recognition domain, a common feature of C-type (calcium-dependent) lectins (BEZOUSKA et al. 1994). Murine NKR-P1 belongs to a family of three or more homologous proteins (GIORDA and TRUCCO 1991) These three cDNAs, of different sizes, are correlated with three transcripts found on northern blot analysis. Although the three clones demonstrate considerable homology in their open reading frames, they have divergent 3' untranslated regions of different lengths. These three clones have been named MusNKR-P1 A, B, and C respectively (YOKOYAMA and SEAMAN 1993). The mouse NK1.1 antigen is encoded by NKR-P1C. The NKR-P1B and C gene products are recognized by the mAb 10A7 (Ryan and Kumar, unpublished data). Two groups (GIORDA and TRUCCO 1991; RYAN et al. 1992) working on NKR-P1 isoforms in mice found variants that contained in frame deletions, suggesting that these code for functional proteins.

Some of these deletions have been explained by alternative splicing of a single gene (GIORDA et al. 1992). It has been suggested that these variants lead to receptor diversity (YOKOYAMA and SEAMAN 1993). So far no evidence for this exists. However, it is known that NK cells can express more than one member of the family (Ryan and Kumar, unpublished data). It is also possible that if a single cell expresses more than one isoform, heterodimers of the two proteins can theoretically lead to more diversity (YOKOYAMA and SEAMAN 1993). Expression of NKR-P1 varies between different strains of mice. While NK cells from C57BL/6, NZB, C57BL/10, and CE mice express the NK1.1 antigen, other strains such as BALB/c, AKR, SJL, 129, and DBA/2 do not (GIORDA et al. 1992; SENTMAN et al. 1989a,b). The NK1.1$^-$ strains do contain low levels of transcripts for the other isoforms of NKR-P1. Cloning of the promoter regions from these strains showed a 95%–98% homology, suggesting that the differences in expression are due to strain-specific transactivation factors.

It is interesting to note that most NK1.1$^-$ mouse strains are weaker rejectors of bone marrow transplants than are NK1.1$^+$ strains. Segregation analysis utilizing H-2^b C57BL/6 (NK1.1$^+$) and 129/J (NK1.1$^-$) indicates that the ability to reject allogeneic H-2^d marrow cells cosegregated with NK1.1 expression. However, such segregation analysis is not sufficient to prove that NKR-P1 molecules play a role in marrow allograft rejections because there are several genes in the NK gene complex that cosegregate with NKR-P1. The most direct evidence regarding the role of NKR-P1 in target recognition has come from studies of the rat NKR-P1 molecule. Ethylmethane sulfonate mutants of the rat NK cell line RNK-16 were selected for lack of expression of NKR-P1A (RYAN et al. 1995). The NKR-P1A$^-$ cell line RNK-16.M13 was able to kill many standard tumor targets such as YAC-1 but, unlike the parent cell line, was deficient in the lysis of IC-21 macrophage, B-16 melanoma, and C1498 lymphoma targets. Reexpression of a single member, NKR-P1A, restored lysis of IC-21 but not of B-16 or C1498 target cells. Antibody to NKR-P1A blocked this restored lytic activity, suggesting that NKR-P1A is the molecule responsible for this target recognition. This observation provided direct evidence that NKR-P1 is a target-specific activation receptor. However, given the observation that many strains that are NK1.1$^-$ can lyse a variety targets efficiently, it seems unlikely that NK1.1 is the sole or major triggering molecule on NK cells.

It is possible, however, that other members of the NKR-P1 family act as target specific receptors for certain tumor targets. The role of NK1.1 in hybrid resistance has also been investigated. Hybrid resistance is the term that defines the phenomenon by which lethally irradiated (A×B) F1 hybrid mice can reject parental A or B strain bone marrow cells (BENNETT 1987). This has been shown to be mediated by NK cells. The function of NK1.1 in hybrid resistance was investigated in an in vitro model for hybrid resistance (KUNG and MILLER 1994). Using effector lymphokine-activated killer cells from CB6F1 mice it was shown that mAb PK136 (NK1.1) inhibits killing of either parental targets (C57BL/6 or BALB/c splenic concanavalin A blasts) but does not inhibit killing of YAC-1 cells. Control antibodies produce no inhibition, suggesting that this blocking is specific. Although the possibility that NKR-P1 acts as an adhesion molecule is not ruled out in any of the above cases, the data indicate that it probably is a molecule that can activate NK mediated killing, and that this interaction is target specific.

The role of NK1.1 in ontogeny and differentiation has not been well defined. The earliest work on NK ontogeny was carried out by KOO and colleagues (1982). Using an alloantiserum specific for natural killer cells (NK1.1 antigen) they followed the development of NK1.1$^+$ cells in fetal, neonatal, and adult mice. They detected NK1.1 expression in fetal liver (day 14 gestation) and also in spleens (day 16 gestation) and established that NK1.1 is an early hematopoietic differentiation marker for NK cells. We have detected NK1.1 on murine fetal liver cells at day 16 of gestation (Sivakumar, unpublished data), and we and others have also shown that addition of low doses of IL-2 to fetal liver can give rise to a population of NK1.1$^+$ cells (MANOUSSAKA et al. 1997). The differentiation potential of these fetal-derived NK cells is currently under investigation.

3.1.2 2B4

A panel of monoclonal antibodies against IL-2 propagated NK cells was made to elucidate the molecules involved in non-MHC restricted killing by NK cells (GARNI-

WAGNER et al. 1993). One such mAb 2B4 stained all NK cells and also a subset of activated T cells that exhibited non-MHC restricted lysis (NK-like). It was shown that all non-MHC restricted killing activity in both fresh and cultured spleens is contained within the $2B4^{+}$ population. Also, the mAb 2B4 augmented killing of a variety of FcR^{-} and FcR^{+} targets by IL-2 activated NK cells and non-MHC restricted T cells. As with NK1.1, it also increased secretion of IFNγ and granule exocytosis by IL-2 activated NK cells. This suggests that 2B4 is another signaling receptor on murine NK cells. Cloning of the molecule has revealed that it belongs to the Ig superfamily of proteins, showing homology to murine and rat CD48 human LFA-3 (MATHEW et al. 1993) and to SLAM, a costimulatory molecule expressed on activated human T cells (COCKS et al. 1995). 2B4 has been mapped to mouse chromosome 1. The fetal liver and fetal thymus derived $NK1.1^{+}$ cells (MANOUSSAKA et al. 1997) express 2B4 on their surface and can be activated by 2B4 cross-linking (Sivakumar, unpublished data). These data suggest that, as with NK1.1, 2B4 is expressed early in ontogeny and is functional. The role of 2B4 in NK development and function is being investigated by generation of 2B4 null mice.

3.2 Subset NK Receptors: Ly-49 Family

As stated above, it was initially thought that there is no specificity in NK killing, and that lytic activity of a heterogeneous population of NK cells is not restricted by alloantigens on target cell surfaces. However, observations with class I deficient targets suggested otherwise (KÄRRE et al. 1986; STORKUS et al. 1987). These groups generated class I negative cell lines that showed increased susceptibility to lysis by NK cells. Reconstitution of either a specific MHC class I or β_2-microglobulin gene restored the resistance to NK killing. Normal, untransformed T lymphoblasts derived from class I deficient (β_2-microglobulin knockout) mice showed heightened susceptibility to lysis. Bone marrow from $\beta_2m^{-/-}$ mice fail to engraft into irradiated +/+ congenic host unless NK cells are depleted (BIX et al. 1991). Bone marrow transplants performed in intra-H2 recombinant mice have indicated that the putative Hh-1 determinant mapped to the MHC region, near the H2D locus (REMBECKI et al. 1988). This information raised the possibility that MHC class I antigens inhibit NK cells and thus mediate hybrid resistance.

Supporting evidence was provided with the development of mAb A1 that identifies 20% C57BL/B6 NK cells (YOKOYAMA et al. 1989, 1990). A1 binds to the product of the Ly-49A gene which maps to the NK gene complex on chromosome 6 (YOKOYAMA et al. 1989, 1990). While $Ly\text{-}49^{-}$ cells are able to lyse a number of tumor targets of different H2 haplotypes, Ly-49A cells are unable to lyse targets that are homozygous or heterozygous for $H2^{d}$ and $H2^{k}$ (KARLHOFER et al. 1992). Transfection of susceptible targets with the $H2D^{d}$ gene induced resistance. This resistance was abrogated with mAbs to either Ly-49A or the α_1/α_2 domains of the $H2D^{d}$ molecule, suggesting that NK cells are inhibited specifically by class I antigens. Binding studies revealed that Ly-49A binds to D^{d} and D^{k} (BRENNAN et al. 1994; KANE 1994), and that it has a functional carbohydrate binding domain specific for sugars on D^{d} (DANIELS et al. 1994). In addition to Ly-49A, the Ly-49 gene family is comprised of at least nine members that encode type II integral membrane proteins having lectin superfamily homology (SMITH et al. 1994; BRENNAN et al. 1994). A given NK cell can express more than one Ly-49 molecule on its surface, leading to an overlap of cell populations expressing a different set of Ly-49 family receptors. At present antibodies to five family members – Ly-49A (mAb A1, JR3918, YE 1/48), Ly-49C (NK2.1, 5E6), Ly-49D (12A8, 12A1), Ly-49G2 (4D11), and Ly-49I(5E6) – are available, and different laboratories are investigating the specificity and function of these receptors, a summary of which is given below.

The Ly-49A molecule, as stated above, interacts specifically with α_1/α_2 domains of H-2D^d but not with L^d or K^d (KARLHOFER et al. 1992; SENTMAN et al. 1994). Ly-49G2 (detected by mAb 4D11) is expressed on about 50% of B6 NK cells and has been shown to receive a negative signal from D^d or L^d (MASON et al. 1995). Bone marrow transplantation studies have established that Ly-49G2$^+$ cells from CB6F1 mice are responsible for the rejection of H2^b bone marrow cells but not H2^d bone marrow cells (RAZIUDDIN et al. 1996). Recent studies indicate that mAb 4D11 binds not only to Ly-49G2 but also to Ly-49A, thus complicating the interpretation of some of the earlier data (TAKEI et al. 1997). The 5E6 mAb identifies the product of two genes, Ly-49C (STONEMAN et al. 1995) and Ly-49I (BRENNAN et al. 1996a,b). Approximately 40%–50% of NK cells are 5E6$^+$. Depletion of 5E6$^+$ cells in vivo abrogates the ability of mice to reject H2^d but not H2^b marrow allografts (SENTMAN et al. 1989b).

In vitro studies have shown that the 5E6$^+$ Ly-49A$^-$ cells from (H-2^d×H-2^b) F1 mice are responsible for the lysis of H2^d but not H-2K^b targets (YU et al. 1996). Conversely, the 5E6$^-$Ly-49A$^+$ cells could kill H2^b but not H2^d targets. The resistance of H-2^b targets to lysis by 5E6$^+$ cells could be reversed either by F(ab')2 of 5E6 mAb or anti-H-2K^b, thus suggesting that 5E6$^+$ cells receive negative signals from H-2K^b. These data also provided an explanation of hybrid resistance in the context of the missing-self hypothesis. The fact that 5E6 recognizes both Ly-49C and Ly-49I requires reinterpretation of the functional studies using this antibody. The present status of Ly-49C and Ly-49I in target recognition and in hybrid resistance has been reviewed by GEORGE and colleagues (1997). Recent evidence indicates that unlike the other characterized Ly-49 molecules Ly-49D acts as an activating receptor for NK cells (MASON et al. 1996). The cytoplasmic domain of Ly-49D lacks the V/IxYxxL immunoreceptor tyrosine-based inhibitory motif found in Ly-49A, C, or G2, suggesting that it is not an inhibitory receptor.

3.2.1 Implications of the "Missing-Self" Hypothesis for NK Cell Differentiation

The specific interaction of an Ly-49 molecule with its ligand leads to a negative signal that inhibits target cell lysis. This suggests that the lack of lysis of self targets by NK cells is due to the specific interaction of the self receptor with its MHC class I ligand. During development therefore NK cell precursors and progenitors must "learn" to recognize self and become self-tolerant. A number of different hypotheses have been proposed to explain this phenomenon.

The Receptor Calibration Model

To be functionally competent NK cells should receive just enough negative signals to prevent autoreactivity but not enough to be insensitive to pathologically induced differences in class I expression (e.g., viral infection and tumors). This could be achieved by modulating the level of expression (calibrating) of the self-receptors. The "receptor calibration" model proposed by SENTMAN and colleagues (1995) suggests that NK cells expressing a lower cell surface density of an Ly-49 inhibitory molecule specific for self-MHC class I are selected during development, and that these cells are more sensitive to changes in class I. For example, intensity of expression of Ly-49A in B10.D2 ($H2^d$) and D8 mice ($H2^b$, D^d) is about 50% of the intensity of expression of the same molecule in B6 mice ($H2^b$) (ÖLSSON et al. 1995). This suggests that the level of intensity of Ly-49A is influenced by its self class I antigen ($H2^d$, B10.D2) and more specifically H-$2D^d$ (D8).

Cells of class I deficient Tap and β_2-microglobulin knockout mice are lysed by congenic +/+ NK cells, presumably because they lack self class I molecules. However, NK cells from class I deficient mice do not kill self (class I deficient cells), nor do they reject syngeneic bone marrow grafts (BIX et al. 1991; LIAO et al. 1991; LJUNGGREN et al. 1994). Thus NK cells developing in class I deficient hosts seem to "calibrate" themselves in a manner that prevents autoreactivity. This is further manifested as a ladder effect in the lytic ability of NK cells based on the level of expression of class I in the host in which they develop. For example, C57BL/6 (class I^{hi}) NK cells are able to kill syngeneic T cell blasts from both Tap and β_2-microglobulin knockout mice. It is necessary to point out that there is a greater class I deficiency in $Tap^{-/-}$ mice than in $\beta_2m^{-/-}$ mice. Surprisingly, effectors from $\beta_2m^{-/-}$ mice (class I^{int}) are able to lyse T cell blasts from $Tap^{-/-}$ mice (class I^{lo}) but not vice versa. This strongly suggests that the level of class I not only calibrates the level of expression of the Ly-49 receptors but also regulates the ability of NK cells to recognize the presence or absence of class I on target cells, depending on the environment on which they were "educated."

Altered Repertoire Hypothesis

An alternative hypothesis is that during development MHC molecules influence the Ly-49 repertoire (LIAO et al. 1991; DORFMAN and RAULET 1996). This means that it should be possible to find a different Ly-49 repertoire in different strains of mice based on the MHC haplotype. There is some evidence to support this "altered repertoire hypothesis." Ly-$49A^+$ NK cells receive negative signals from D^d and D^k but not D^b. Thus in H-2^b mice, Ly-$49A^+$ cells may be potentially autoreactive and possibly deleted. However Ly-$49A^+$ cells are found in C57BL/6 ($H2^b$) mice, but they are unable to lyse syngeneic T cell blasts, and thus are tolerant to self. In contrast, however, Ly-$49A^+$ cells from $H2^d$ mice lyse $H2^b$ T cell blasts.

To explain this, it has been proposed that the Ly-$49A^+$ cells from $H2^b$ mice but not $H2^d$ mice are rendered self-tolerant by the expression of other negative signaling receptors on their surfaces, and that the repertoire of receptors expressed by NK cells from these mice differ due to their MHC background. RAULET and colleagues also observed that the frequencies of Ly-49 defined NK cell subsets are influenced by the MHC background. They examined overlapping subsets of NK cells expressing

Ly-49A, C and G2 in different strains of mice (HELD et al. 1996). Firstly, class I deficiency substantially increased the frequency of each subset examined. Secondly, $H2^d$ decreased the frequency of cells expressing the two $H2^d$ receptors, Ly-49A and Ly-49G2. This suggests that during ontogeny NK cells start expressing a random repertoire of receptors and during development the selection of cells expressing at least one self-receptor is favored. Also, selection works against cells that express too many self class I receptors because these cells might be unable to lyse autologous tumor targets in which only a single self class I allele is perturbed. It is also possible that the expression of self MHC receptors is not random but sequential and continues until successful expression of a self receptor occurs.

Gene Regulation

The MHC may also influence the expression of specific members of the Ly-49 family and/or modulate their function. $5E6^+$ cells from (B6×BALB/c) F1 mice behave in a manner identical to B6 $5E6^+$ cells, i.e., they receive a strong negative signal from $H2^b$ and a weak signal from $H2^d$. This means that in these CB6F1 mice NK cells demonstrating BALB type function are somewhat insensitive to perturbations in MHC. Recent data suggest that BALB/c express predominantly Ly-49C while B6 expresses equal frequencies of Ly-49C and Ly-49I (BRENNAN et al. 1996).

3.2.2 Ontogeny of Ly-49 Receptors

In an attempt to understand the regulation of NK cell repertoire during differentiation we are investigating the ontogeny of Ly-49 receptors. We were surprised to find that the fetal thymus and fetal liver derived $NK1.1^+$ cells do not express any Ly-49 molecules on their surface (Ly-49A, C, D, and G2). We have also been unable to detect any transcripts for Ly-49C and other Ly-49 molecules using a set of primers that would amplify most of the Ly-49 members that have been cloned (Sivakumar, unpublished data). This led us to investigate the expression of Ly-49 family members in neonatal mice (C57BL/6, $H2^b$). We were unable to detect Ly-49 surface expression (Ly-49A, C or G2) by flow cytometry until days 6–8 after birth. When first detected, the frequency of Ly-49 expressing cells as a percentage of $NK1.1^+$ cells was significantly lower than in adult mice. It was not until days 20–24 after birth that the frequency of these cells reached adult levels, suggesting that this is a sequential process, and that during development (days 8–24 neonatally) cells slowly begin to express Ly-49 molecules, or that cells that do not express Ly-49 molecules are slowly deleted and a new population of cells expressing Ly-49 family members are generated (SIVAKUMAR et al. 1997).

These observations could suggest (a) that Ly-49 expression requires a mature bone marrow microenvironment, and that fetal cells do not express these molecules because they develop in a fetal liver environment, or (b) that the expression of the Ly-49 repertoire is an intrinsic programmed event that has not been activated in the fetal liver. Preliminary evidence suggests that the former is the case because it has been possible to generate $Ly\text{-}49^+$ cells by transferring fresh fetal liver cells into irradiated, NK cell depleted adult hosts (Sivakumar, unpublished data). This suggests that the marrow environment of the adult host activates the expression of the Ly-49 genes on NK cells derived from fetal liver. Because fetal liver and thymus derived NK cells do not express any Ly-49 molecules, they should not receive any negative signals and therefore should be able to kill almost any target. However, these cells do not kill allogeneic or syngeneic T cell blasts in spite of the fact that they seem to have an intact killing machinery, as evidenced by their ability lyse YAC-1 cells. During ontogeny the ability to kill allogeneic targets is acquired between days 12 and 18 after birth. This could mean either that a certain threshold number of Ly-49 expressing cells is needed for allorecognition, or that Ly-49 molecules are educated during ontogeny to discriminate between self and nonself. An alternative possibility is that fetal and neonatal NK1.1$^+$ cells lack non-Ly-49 receptors that positively recognize alloantigens, and that these are expressed along with the Ly-49 negative signaling molecules. In recent experiments, we have found that fetal liver and fetal thymus derived NK.1$^+$ Ly49$^-$ cells can discriminate between class I^{hi} and class I^{lo} tumor targets; suggesting the existence of non-Ly49 MHC receptors on these cells (SIVAKUMAR et al. 1997).

4 Conclusion

Differentiation of natural killer cells is bone marrow dependent. The factors, both cellular and soluble, that may be instrumental in NK differentiation are yet to be characterized in detail, but significant progress has been made in dissecting the process, both in vivo and in vitro. IL-15 has emerged as the most likely cytokine involved in differentiation of NK cells in vivo. NK killing is no longer considered nonspecific, especially after the discovery of the Ly-49 receptors that bind specific MHC class I molecules and receive negative signals that inhibit target cell lysis. The availability of antibodies to these receptors has led to a better understanding of the specificity and function of these receptors. The Ly-49 repertoire and level of expression is regulated by self class I molecules during development. Fetal NK cells do not express Ly-49 molecules, possibly due to the absence of a bone marrow microenvironment. While IL-15 can substitute for some of the marrow-dependent steps of NK cell differentiation, it has not yet proven sufficient for induction of Ly-49 molecules on Ly-49$^-$precursors. Expression of NK receptors seems to be a sequential process whereby the activating NK receptors are expressed on all NK cells in fetal stages. This is followed by the expression of Ly-49 molecules starting early in neonatal life, reaching adult levels by days 20–24. The ability to recognize alloantigens seems to mature in parallel with expression of the Ly-49 molecules, suggesting that NK cells are probably “selected ” and “educated” during development by the bone marrow environment.

References

Abramson S, Miller RG, Phillips RA (1977) The identification in adult bone marrow of pluripotent and restricted stem cells of the myeloid and lymphoid systems. J Exp Med 145:1567–1579

Akashi K, Kondo M, Weismann IL (1997) A clonogenic common lymphoid precursor in mouse marrow. Blood 90:158a (abstr)

Antica M, Wu L, Shortman K, Scollay R (1993) Intrathymic lymphoid precursor cells during fetal thymus development. J Immunol 151:5887

Antica M, Wu L, Shortman K, Scollay R (1994) Thymic stem cells in mouse bone marrow. Blood 84:111–117

Baccarini M, Hao L, Decker T, Lohmann-Matthes ML (1988) Macrophage precursors as natural killer cells against tumors and microorganisms. Natl Immun Cell Growth Regul 7:316–327

Bamford RN, Grant AJ, Burton JD, Peters C, Kurys G, Goldman CK, Brennan J, Roessler E, Waldmann TA (1994) The IL-2 receptor beta chain is shared by IL-2 and a cytokine, provisionally designated IL-T, that stimulates T cell proliferation and induction of lymphokine-activated killer cells. Proc Natl Acad Sci USA 91:4940–4944

Bamford RN, Battiata AP, Burton JD, Sharma H, Waldmann TA (1996) IL-15/IL-T production by adult T cell leukemia cell line HuT-102 is associated with a human T-cell lymphotropic virus type I region/IL-15 fusion message that lacks many upstream AUGs that normally attenuate IL-15 m RNA translation. Proc Natl Acad Sci USA 93:2897–2902

Bennett IM (1996) Natural killer cell differentiation. Thesis, Thomas Jefferson University

Bennett IM, Zatsepenia O, Zamai L, Azzoni L, Mikheeva T, Perussia B (1996) Definition of a natural killer NKR-P1A$^+$/CD56$^-$/CD16$^-$ functionally immature human NK cell subset that differentiates in vitro in the presence of IL-12. J Exp Med 184:1845–1856

Bennett M (1973) Prevention of marrow allograft rejection with radioactive strontium: evidence for marrow-dependent effector cells. J Immunol 110:510

Bennett M (1987) Biology and genetics of hybrid resistance. Adv Immunol 41:333–445

Bezouska K, Yuen C-T, O'Brien J, Childs RA, Chai W, Lawson AM, Drbal K, Fiserova A, Pospisil M, Feizi T (1994) Oligosaccharide ligands for NKR-P1 protein activate NK cells and cytotoxicity. Nature 327:150–157

Biron CA, van den Elsen P, Tutt MM, Medveczky P, Kumar V, Terhorst C (1987) Murine natural killer cells stimulated in vivo do not express the T cell receptor α, β, γ, T3δ or T3ε genes. J Immunol 139:1704–1710

Bix M, Locksley RM (1995) Natural T cells: cells that co-express NKR-P1 and TCR. J Immunol 95:1020–1022

Bix M, Liao N-S, Zijstra M, Loring J, Jaenisch R, Raulet D (1991) Rejection of class I MHC-deficient hematopoietic cells by irradiated MHC-mismatched mice. Nature 349:329–331

Brecher G, Bookstein N, Redfearn W, Necas E, Pallavicini MG, Cronkite EP (1993) Self-renewal of the long-term repopulating stem cell. Proc Natl Acad Sci USA 90:6028–6031

Brennan J, Mager D, Jeffries W, Takei F (1994) Expression of different members of the Ly-49 family defines distinct natural killer cell subsets and cell adhesion properties. J Exp Med 180:2287–2295

Brennan J, Lemieux S, Douglas Freeman J, Mager DL, Takei F (1996a) Heterogeneity among Ly-49C NK cells: characterization of highly related receptors with differing functions and expression patterns. J Exp Med 184:2085–2090

Brennan J, Mahon G, Mager DL, Jeffries WA, Takei F (1996b) Recognition of class I MHC molecules by Ly-49: specificities and domain interactions. J Exp Med 183:1553–1559

Brooks CG, Georgio A, Jordan RK (1993) The majority of immature fetal thymocytes can be induced to proliferate to IL-2 and differentiate into cells indistinguishable from mature natural killer cells. J Immunol 151:6645–6656

Burton JD, Bamford RN, Peters C, Grant AJ, Kurys G, Goldman CK, Brennan J, Roessler E, Waldmann TA (1994) A lymphokine, provisionally designated IL-T and produced by a human T-cell leukemia line, stimulates T cell proliferation and induction of lymphokine-activated killer cells. Proc Natl Acad Sci USA 91:4935–4939

Cao X, Shores EW, Hu-Li J, Anver MR, Kelsall BL, Russell SM, Drago J, Noguchi M, Grinberg A, Bloom ET, Paul WE, Katz SI, Love PE, Leonard WJ (1995) Defective lymphoid development in mice lacking expression of the common cytokine receptor gamma chain. Immunity 2:223–238

Carlsson L, Candeias S, Staerz U, Keller G (1995) Expression of FcγRIII defines distinct subpopulations of fetal liver B cell and myeloid precursors. Eur J Immunol 25:2308–2317

Carson WE, Giri JG, Lindemann MJ, Linett ML, Ahdieh M, Paxton R, Anderson D, Eisenmann J, Grabstein K, Caligiuri MA (1994) Interleukin (IL) 15 is a novel cytokine that activates human natural killer cells via components of the IL-2 receptor. J Exp Med 94:1395–1403

Cavazzana-Calvo M, Hacien-Bey S, de Saint Basile G, De Coene C, Selz F, Le Deist F, Fischer A (1996) Role of IL-2, IL-7 and IL-15 in natural killer differentiation from cord blood hematopoietic progenitor cells and from γc transduced severe combined immunodeficiency X1 bone marrow cells. Blood 88:3901–3909

Chambers WH, Vujanovic NL, DeLeo AB, Olszowy MW, Hebermann RB, Hiserodt JC (1989) Monoclonal antibody to a triggering structure expressed on rat natural killer cells and adherant lymphokine-activated killer cells. J Exp Med 89:1373–1389

Cocks BG, Chang C-CJ, Carballido JM, Yssel H, de Vries JE, Aversa G (1995) A novel receptor involved in T cell activation. Nature 376:260–263

Colonna M (1996) Natural killer cell receptors specific for MHC class I molecules. Curr Opin Immunol 8:101–107

Cooper MD, Paterson DA, Good RA (1965) Delineation of the thymic and bursal lymphoid systems in the chicken. Nature 205:143

Cudhowicz G, Bennett M (1971) Peculiar immunobiology of bone marrow allografts. I. Graft rejection by irradiated responder mice. J Exp Med 134:83

Cumano A, Paige CJ, Iscove NN, Brady G (1992) Bipotential precursors of B cells and macrophages in murine fetal liver. Nature 356:612–615

Daniels BF, Nakamura MC, Rosen D, Yokoyama WM, Seaman WE (1994) Ly-49A, a receptor for $H2D^d$, has a functional carbohydrate recognition domain. Immunity 1:785–792

Delfino DV, Patrene KD, Lu J, DeLeo A, DeLeo R, Herberman RB, Boggs SS (1996) Natural killer cell precursors in the $CD34^{neg/dim}$ T-cell $receptor^{neg}$ population of the mouse bone marrow. Blood 87:394–2400

Dexter TM, Testa NG (1980) In vitro methods of hematopoiesis and lymphopoiesis. J Immunol Methods 38:177–190

Dorfman JR, Raulet DH (1996) Major histocompatibility complex genes determine natural killer cell tolerance. Eur J Immunol 26:151–155

Dorshkind K, Pollack SB, Bosma MJ, Phillips RA (1985) Natural killer (NK) cells are present in mice with severe combined immunodeficiency (scid). J Immunol 134:3798

Galy A, Travis M, Cen D, Chen B (1995) Human T, B, natural killer and Dendritic cells arise from a comon bone marrow progenitor cell subset. Immunity 3:459–473

Garni-Wagner BA, Purohit A, Mathew PA, Bennett M, Kumar V (1993) Activation of NK cells and non-MHC restricted T cells by a novel cell surface molecule. J Immunol 151:60–70

Gately MK, Warrier RR, Honasoge S, Carvajal DM, Faherty DA, Connaughton SE, Anderson TD, Sarmiento U, Hubbard BR, Murphy M (1994) Administration of recombinant IL-12 to normal mice enhances cytolytic lymphocyte activity and induces production of IFNγ in vivo. Int Immunol 6:157–167

George T, Yu YYL, Liu J, Davenport C, Lemieux S, Stoneman E, Mathew PA, Kumar V, Bennett M (1997) Allorecognition by murine natural killer cells: lysis of T lymphoblasts and rejection of bone marrow grafts. Immunol Rev 155:29–40

Georgiopoulos K, Moore DD, Derfler B (1992) Ikaros, an early lymphoid-specific transcription factor and putative mediator for T cell commitment. Science 92:808–812

Georgopoulos K, Bigby M, Wang JH, Molnar A, Wu P, Winandy S, Sharpe A (1994) The Ikaros gene is required for the development of all lymphoid lineages. Cell 94:143–156

Giorda R, Trucco M (1991) Mouse NKR-P1: a family of genes selectively coexpressed in adherant lymphokine-activated killer cells. J Immunol 91:1701–1708

Giorda R, Rudert WA, Vavassori C, Chambers WH, Hiserodt JC, Trucco M (1990) NKR-P1, a signal transduction molecule on natural killer cells. Science 90:1298–1300

Giorda R, Weisberg EP, Ip TK, Trucco M (1992) Genomic structure and strain-specific expression of the natural killer cell receptor NKR-P1. J Immunol 92:1957–1963

Giri JG, Ahdieh M, Eisenmann J, Shanebeck K, Grabstein K, Kumaki S, Namen A, Park LS, Cosman D, Anderson D (1994) Utilization of the beta and gamma chains of the IL-2 receptor by the novel cytokine IL-15. EMBO J 13:2822–2830

Giri JG, Kumaki S, Ahdieh M, Friend DJ, Loomis A, Shanebeck K, DuBose R, Cosmann D, Park LS, Anderson DM (1995) Identification and cloning of a novel IL-15 binding protein that is structurally related to the alpha chain of the IL-2 receptor. EMBO J 14:3654–3663

Glick B, Whatley S (1967) The presence of immunoglobulin in the bursa of fabricius. Poultry Sci 46 (6):1587–1589

Glimcher L, Shen FW, Cantor H (1977) Identification of a cell surface antigen selectively expressed on the natural killer cell. J Exp Med 77:1–9

Grabstein KH, Eisenmann J, Shanebeck K, Rauch C, Srinivasan S, Fung V, Beers C, Richardson J, Schoenborn MA, Ahdieh M, Johnson L, Alderson MR, Watson JD, Anderson DM, Giri JG (1994) Cloning of a T cell growth factor that interacts with the beta chain of the IL-2 receptor. Science 264:965–968

Hackett J Jr, Bennett M, Kumar V (1985) Origin and differentiation of Natural killer cells. I. Characterization of a transplantable NK cell precursor. J Immunol 134:3731–3738

Hackett J Jr, Tutt M, Lipscomb M, Bennett M, Koo G, Kumar V (1986a) Origin and differentiation of natural killer cells. II. Functional and morphologic studies of purified NK1.1+ cells. J Immunol 136:3124–3131

Hackett J Jr, Bosma G, Bosma M, Bennett M, Kumar V (1986b) Transplantable progenitors of natural killer cells are distinct from those of T and B lymphocytes. Proc Natl Acad Sci USA 83:3427–3431

Haller O, Wigzell H (1977) Suppression of naturla killer cell activity with radioactive strontium: effector cells are bone marrow dependent. J Immunol 118:1503–1506

Haller O, Kiessling R, Orn A, Wigzell H (1977) Generation of natural killer cells: an autonomous function of the bone marrow. J Exp Med 145:1411–1416

Hebermann RB, Nunn ME, Holden HT, Lavrin DH (1975) Natural cytotoxic reactivity of mouse lymphoid cells against syngeneic and allogeneic tumors. II. Characterization of effector cells. Int J Cancer 75:230–239

Held W, Dorfman JR, Wu M-F, Raulet DH (1996) Major histocompatibility complex class I-dependent skewing of the natural killer cell Ly-49 receptor repertoire. Eur J Immunol 26:2286–2292

Ikuta K, Uchida N, Friedman J, Weissman IL (1992) Lymphocyte development from stem cells. Annu Rev Immunol 10:759–783

Jacobsen SE, Veiby OP, Smeland EB (1993) Cytotoxic lymphocyte maturation factor IL-12 is a synergistic growth factor for hematopoietic stem cells. J Exp Med 93:413–418

Jacobson SE, Okkenhaug C, Myklebust J, Veiby OP, Lyman SD (1995) The FLT3 ligand potently and directly stimulates the growth and expansion of primitive bone marrow progenitor cells in vitro: synergisyic interactions with IL-11, IL-12 and other hematopoietic growth factors. J Exp Med 95:1357–1363

Jerne, Nordin (1963) Plaque formation in agar by single antibody producing cells. Science 140:405–408

Kane KP (1994) Ly-49 mediates EL-4 lymphoma adhesion to isolated class I major histocompatibility molecules. J Exp Med 179:1011–1015

Kalland T (1986) Generation of natural killer cells from bone marrow precursors in vitro. Immunology 57:493–498

Karlhofer FM, Ribaudo RK, Yokoyama WM (1992) MHC class I allospecificity of Ly-49^{+} IL-2 activated natural killer cells. Nature 358:66–69

KŠrre K, Ljunggren HG, Piontek G, Kiessling R (1986) Selective rejection of H-2-deficient lyphoma variants suggests alternative immune defence strategy. Nature 319:675–678

Kiessling R, Petranyi G, Klein G, Wigzell H (1975) Genetic variation of in vitro cytolytic activity and in vivo rejection potential of non-immunized semi-syngeneic mice against a mouse lymphoma line. Int J Cancer 15:933–940

Koo GC, Manyak CL (1986) Generation of cytotoxic cells from murine bone marrow by human recombinant IL-2. J Immunol 137:1751–1756

Koo GC, Peppard JR (1984) Establishment of a monoclonal anti-NK1.1 antibody. Hybridoma 3 (3):301–303

Koo GC, Pappard JR, Hatzfeld A (1982) Ontogeny of NK1.1+ natural killer cells. I. Promotion of NK1.1+ cells in fetal, baby and old mice. J Immunol 129:867–871

Koo GC, Dumont FJ, Tutt M, Hackett JJ, Kumar V (1986) The NK1.1^{-} mouse: a model to study differentiation of murine NK cells. J Immunol 137:3742–3747

Kumar V, Ben-Ezra J, Bennett M, Sonnenfeld G (1979) Natural killer cells in mice treated with strontium: normal target-binding cell numbers but inability to kill even after interferon administration. J Immunol 79:1832–1838

Kundig TM, Schorle H, Bachmann MF, Hengartner H, Zinkernagel RM, Horak I (1993) Immune responses in IL-2 deficient mice. Science 262:1059

Kung SKP, Miller RG (1994) The NK1.1 antigen in NK mediated F1 anti-parent killing in vitro. J Immunol 154:1624–1633

Lanier LL, Phillips JH, Hackett J Jr, Tutt M, Kumar V (1986) Natural killer cells: definition of a cell type rather than a function. J Immunol 86:2735–2739

Lanier LL, Chang C, Spits H, Phillips JJ (1992) Expression of cytoplasmic CD3 epsilon proteins in actiavted human adult natural cells and CD3 gamma, epsilon and delta complexes in fetal NK cells. Implications for the relationship of NK and T lymphocytes. J Immunol 92:1876–1880

Lantz CS, Huff TF (1995) Murine c-kit$^+$ Lin$^-$ bone marrow progenitors express FcγRII but do not express FcεRI until mast cell granule formation. J Immunol 154:355–362

Leclercq G, DeBacker V, De Smedt M, Plum J (1996) Differential effects of IL-15 and IL-2 on differentiation of bipotential T/NK progenitor cells. J Exp Med 184:325–336

Li H, Schwinzer R, Baccarini M, Lohmann-Matthes ML (1989) Cooperative effects of colony-stimulating factor I and recombinant interleukin 2 on proliferation and induction of cytotoxicity of macrophage precursors generated from mouse bone marrow cell cultures. J Exp Med 169:973–986

Liao NS, Bix M, Zijlstra M, Jaenisch R, Raulet D (1991) MHC class I deficiency: susceptibility to natural killer (NK) cells and impaired NK activity. Science 253:199–202

Lipinski M, Virelizier JL, Tursz T, Griscelli C (1980) Natural killer and killer cell activities in patients with primary immunodeficiencies or defects in immune interferon production. Eur J Immunol 10:246

Ljunggren HG, KŠrre K (1990) In search of the "missing self": MHC molecules and NK cell recognition. Immunol Today 11:237–244

Ljunggren HG, Van Kaer L, Ploegh HL, Tonegawa S (1994) Altered natural killer cell repertoire in Tap-1 mutant mice. Proc Natl Acad Sci USA 91:6520–6524

MacDonald RH (1995) NK1.1$^+$ T cell receptor-α/β^+ cells: new clues to their origin, specificity and function. J Exp Med 182:633–638

Magram J, Connaughton SE, Warrier RR, Carvajal DM, Wu C, Ferrante J, Stewart C, Sarmiento U, Faherty DA, Gately MK (1996) IL-12 deficient mice are defective in IFNγ production and type 1 cytokine responses. Immunity 4:471–481

Manoussaka M, Georgiou A, Rossiter B, Shrestha S, Toomey JA, Sivakumar PV, Bennett M, Kumar V, Brooks CG (1997) Phenotypic and functional characterization of long-lived NK cell lines of different maturational status obtained from mouse fetal liver. J Immunol 158:112–119

Mason LH, Ortaldo JR, Young HA, Kumar V, Bennett M, Anderson SK (1995) Cloning and functional characteristics of murine large granular lymphocyte-1: a member of the Ly-49 gene family (Ly-49G2). J Exp Med 182:293–303

Mason LH, Anderson SK, Yokoyama WM, Smith HRC, Winkler-Pickett R, Ortaldo JR (1996) The Ly-49D receptor activates murine natural killer cells. J Exp Med 184:2119–2128

Mathew PA, Garni-Wagner BA, Land K, Takashima A, Stoneman E, Bennett M, Kumar V (1993). Cloning and characterization of the 2B4 gene encoding a molecule associated with non-MHC-restricted killing mediated by activated natural killer cells and T cells. J Immunol 151:5328–5337

Migliorati G, Moraca R, Nicoletti I, Riccardi C (1992) IL-2-dependent generation of natural killer cells from bone marrow: role of Mac-1$^-$ NK1.1$^-$ precursors. Cell Immunol 141:323–331

Miller JFAP, Mitchell GF (1969) Thymus and antigen-specific cells. Transplant Rev 1:3

Miller JS, Verfaillie C, McGlave P (1992) The generation of human natural killer cells from CD34+/DR– primitive progenitors in long term bone marrow culture. Blood 80:2182–2187

Miller JS, Alley KA, McGlave P (1994) Differentiation of natural killer (NK) cells from human primitive marrow progenitors in a stroma based long-term culture system: identification of a CD34$^+$ CD7$^+$ NK progenitor. Blood 83:2594–2601

Moore TA, Bennett M, Kumar V (1995) Transplantable NK progenitors in murine bone marrow. J Immunol 154:1653–1663

Moore TA, Bennett M, Kumar V (1996) Murine natural killer cell differentiation: past, present and future. Immunol Res 15 (2):151

Moretta L, Ciccone E, Mingari MC, Biassoni R, Moretta A (1994) Human natural killer cells: origin, clonality, specificity and receptors. Adv Immunol 55:341–380

Mrözek E, Anderson P, Caligiuri M (1996) Role of IL-15 in the development of human CD56$^+$ natural killer cells from CD34$^+$ hematopoietic progenitors. Blood 87:2632–2640

Noguchi M, Yi H, Rosenblatt HM, Filipovich AH, Adelstein S, Modi WS, McBride OW, Leonard WJ (1993) Interleukin-2 receptor gamma chain mutation results in X-linked severe combined immunodeficiency in humans. Cell 93:147–157

Nunn ME, Heberman RB, Holden HT (1977) Natural cell-mediated cytotoxicity in mice against non-lymphoid tumor cells and normal cells. Int J Cancer 20:381–387

Ohara A, Suda T, Tokuyama N, Suda J, Nakayama KI, Miura Y, Nishikawa SI, Nakauchi H (1991) Generation of B lymphocytes from a single hematopoietic progenitor cell in vitro. Int Immunol 3:703–709

Ölsson MY, Kärre K, Sentman CL (1995) Altered phenotype and function of natural killer cells expressing the MHC receptor in mice transgenic for its ligand. Proc Natl Acad Sci USA 92:1649–1653

Perussia B, Starr S, Abraham S, Fanning V, Trinchieri G (1983) Human natural killer cells analyzed by B73.1, a monoclonal antibody blocking Fc receptor functions. I. Characterization of the lymphocyte subset reactive with B73.1. J Immonol 83:2133–2141

Peter HH, Rieger CR, Gendvilis S, Eckert G, Pichler WJ, Stangel W (1982) Spontaneous cell-mediated cytotoxicity (SCMC) in patients with myelodisplastic disorders and immunodeficiency syndromes. Dev Immunol 17:341

Phillips JH, Hori T, Nagler A, Bhat N, Spits H, Lanier L (1992) Ontogeny of human natural killer cells: fetal NK cells mediate cytolytic function and express cytoplasmic CD3ε,δ proteins. J Exp Med 175:1055–1066

Pietrangeli CE, hayashi SI, Kincade PW (1988) Stromal cell lines which support lymphocyte growth: characterization, sensitivity to radiation and responsiveness to growth factors. Eur J Immunol 18:863–872

Ploemacher RE, van Soest PL, Boudewijn A, Neben S (1993a) IL-12 enhances IL-3-dependent multilineage hematopoietic colony formation stimulated by IL-11 or steel factor. Leukemia 93:1374–1380

Ploemacher RE, van Soest PL, Voorwinden H, Boudewijn A (1993b) IL-12 synergizes with IL-3 and steel factor to enhance recovery of murine hematopoietic stem cells in liquid culture. Leukemia 93:1381–1388

Pollack SB, Tsuji J, Rosse C (1992) Production and differentiation of NK lineage cells in long-term bone marrow cultures in the absence of exogenous growth factors. Cell Immunol 139:352–362

Puzanov IJ, Bennett M, Kumar V (1996) IL-15 can substitute for the marrow microenvironment in the differentiation of natural killer cells. J Immunol 157:4282–4285

Raulet DH (1996) Recognition events that inhibit and activate natural killer cells. Curr Opin Immunol 8:372–377

Raulet DH, Held W (1995) Natural killer cell receptors: the offs and ons of NK cell recognition. Cell 82:697–700

Raziuddin A, Longo DL, Mason L, Ortaldo JR, Murphy WJ (1996) Ly-49 G2+ NK cells are responsible for the mediating rejection of H2b bone marrow grafts. Int Immunol 8:1833–1839

Rembicki RM, Kumar V, David CS, Bennett M (1988) Bone marrow cell transplants involving intra-H-2 recombinant inbred mouse strains. J Immunol 141:2253–2260

Renard V, Ardouin L, Malissen M, Milon G, Lebastard M, Gillet A, Malissen B, Vivier E (1995). Normal development and function of natural killer cells in $CD3\varepsilon^{\Delta5/\Delta5}$ mutant mice. Proc Natl Acad Sci USA 92:7545–7549

Reya T, Yang-Snyder JA, Rothenberg EV, Carding S (1996) Regulated expression and function of CD122 (IL-2Rβ) during lymphoid development. Blood 87:190–201

Rodewald HR, Moingeon P, Lucich JL, Dosiou C, Lopez P, Reinherz EL (1992) A population of early fetal thymocytes expressing FcγRII/III contains precursors of T lymphocytes and natural killer cells. Cell 69:139–148

Rolink A, ten Boekel E, Melchers F, Fearon DT, Krop I, Andersson J (1996) A subpopulation of $B220^+$ cells in murine bone marrow does not express CD19 and contains natural killer cell progenitors. J Exp Med 183:187–194

Rosenberg EB, Heberman RB, Levine PH, Halterman R, McCoy JL, Wunderlich JR (1972) Lymphocyte cytotoxicity reactions to leukemia-associated antigens in identical twins. Int J Cancer 9:648–657

Rosenau W, Moon HD (1964) The specificity of the cytolytic effect of sensitized lymphoid cells in vitro. J Immunol 93:910

Ryan JC, Niemi EC, Goldfien R, Hiserodt JC, Seaman WE (1991) NKR-P1, an activating molecule on natural killer cells, stimualtes phosphoinositide turnover and rise in intracellular calcium. J Immunol 147:3244–3250

Ryan JC, Turck J, Niemi EC, Yokoyama WM, Seaman WE (1992) Molecular cloning of the NK1.1 antigen, a member of the NKR-P1 family of natural killer cell activation molecules. J Immunol 149:1631–1635

Ryan JC, Niemi EC, Nakamura MC, Seaman WE (1995) NKR-P1A is a target specific receptor that activates natural killer cell cytotoxicity. J Exp Med 181:1911–1915

Sánchez MJ, Muench MO, Roncarolo MG, Lanier L, Phillips JH (1994) Identification of a common T/natural killer cell progenitor in human fetal thymus. J Exp Med 180:569–576

Schorle H, Holtschke T, Hunig T, Schimpl A, Horak I (1991) Development and function of T cells in mice rendered IL-2 deficient by gene targeting. Nature 352:621–624

Seaman WE, Gindhart TD, Greenspan JS, Blackman MA, Talal N (1979) Natural killer cells, bone and bone marrow: studies in estrogen-treated mice and in congenitally osteopetrotic (mi/mi) mice. J Immunol 79:2541–2547

Sentman CL, Kumar V, Koo GC, Bennett M (1989a) Effector cell expression of NK1.1, a natural killer cell-specific molecule, and ability of mice to reject bone marrow allografts. J Immunol 142:1847–1853

Sentman CL, Hackett J, Kumar V, Bennett M (1989b) Identification of a subset of murine natural killer cells that mediates rejection of Hh-1^d but not Hh-1^b bone marrow grafts. J Exp Med 170:191–202

Sentman CL, …lsson MY, Salcedo M, Hšglund P, Lendahl U, Kärre K (1994) H-2 allele-specific protection from NK cell lysis in vitro for lymphoblasts but nto tumor targets. J Immunol 153:5482–5490

Sentman CL, …lsson MY, KŠrre K (1995) Missing self recognition by natural killer cells in MHC class I transgenic mice. A 'receptor calibration' model for how effector cells adapt to self. Semin Immunol 7:109–119

Shibuya A, Kojima H, Shibuya K, Nagayoshi K, Nagasawa T, Nakauchi H (1993) Enrichment of IL-2-responsive natural killer cell progenitors in human bone marrow. Blood 81:1819–1826

Shibuya A, Nagayoshi K, Nakamura K, Nakauchi H (1995) Lymphokine requirement for the generation of natural killer cells from $CD34^+$ hematopoietic progenitor cells. Blood 85:3538–3546

Sivakumar PV, Bennett M, Kumar V (1997) Fetal and neonatal $NK1.1^+$ $Ly\text{-}49^-$ cells can distinguish between MHC class I^{hi} and class I^{lo} target cells – evidence for a Ly-49 independent negative signaling receptor. Eur J Immunol (in press)

Smith HRC, Karlhofer FM, Yokoyama WM (1994) The Ly-49 multigene family expressed by IL-2-activated natural killer cells. J Immunol 153:1068–1079

Spangrude GJ, Heimfeld S, Weissman IL (1988) Purification and characterization of mouse hematopoietic stem cells. Science 241:58–62

Stechschulte DJ, Sharma R, Dileepan KN, Simpson KM, Aggarwal J, Clancey J Jr, Jilka RL (1987) Effect of the mi allele on mast cells, basophils, natural killer cells and osteoclasts in C57BL/6 mice. J Cell Physiol 132:565–570

Stoneman E, Bennett M, An J, Chestnut KA Wakeland EK, Scheerer J, Siciliano MJ, Kumar V, Mathew PA (1995) Cloning and characterization of 5E6 (Ly-49C), a receptor molecule expressed on a subset of murine natural killer cells. J Exp Med 182:305–313 [erratum, J Exp Med 183:2705]

Storkus WJ, Howell DN, Salter RD, Dawson JR, Cresswell P (1987) NK susceptibility varies inversely with target cell class I HLA antigen expression. J Immunol 138:1657–1659

Suwa H, Tanaka T, Kitamura F, Shiohara T, Kuida K, Miyasaka M (1995) Dysregulated expression of the IL-2Rβ-chain abrogates development of NK cells and $Thy1.1^+$ dendritic epidermal cells in transgenic mice. Int Immunol 7:1441–1449

Suzuki H, Duncan GS, Takimoto H, Mak TW (1997) Abnormal development of intestitial intraepithelial lymphocytes and perepheral natural killer cells in mice lacking the IL-2Rβ chain. J Exp Med 185:499–505

Sykes M, Harty MW, Karlhofer FM, Pearson DA, Szot G, Yokoyama WM (1993) Hematopoietic cells and radioresistent host elements influence natural killer cell differentiation. J Exp Med 178:223–229

Tagaya T, Bamford RN, DeFilippis AP, Waldmann TA (1996) IL-15: a pleiotropic cytpkine with diverse receptor/signaling pathways whose expression is controlled at multiple levels. Immunity 4:329–336

Taguchi K, Shibuya A, Inazawa Y, Abe T (1992) Suppressive effect of GM-CSF on the generation of natural killer cells in vitro. Blood 79:3227

Takasugi M, Mickey MR, Terasaki PI (1973) Reactivity of lymphocytes from normal persons on cultured tumor cells. Cancer Res 33:2898–2902

Takei F, Brennan J, Magar D (1997) The Ly-49 family: genes, proteins and recognition of class I MHC. Immunol Rev 155:67–77

Tanaka T, Takeuchi Y, Shiohara T, Kitamura F, Nagasaka Y, Hamamura K, Yagita H, Miyasaka M (1992) In utero treatment with monoclonal antibody to the IL-2Rβ chain completely abrogates development of Thy1.1^{+} dendritic epidermal cells. Int Immunol 4:487

Tanaka T, Kitamura F, Nagasaka Y, Kuida K, Suwa H, Miyasaka M (1993) Selective long-term elimination of natural killer cells in vivo by an anti-IL-2Rβ chain monoclonal antibody in mice. J Exp Med 178:1103

Trinchieri G (1989) Biology of natural killer cells. Adv Immunol 47:187–375

Trinchieri G, Santoli D, Koprowski H (1978) Spontaneous cell-mediated cytotoxicity in humans: role of interferon and immunoglobulins. J Immunol 120:1849–1855

Tutt MM (1988) Regulation and differentiation of murine natural killer cells. Thesis, University of Texas Southwestern Medical Center, Dallas

van den Brink MR, Boggs SS, Herberman RB, Hiserodt JC (1990) The generation of natural killer (NK) cells from NK precursors in rat long-term bone marrow cultures. J Exp Med 172:303–313

Wang B, Biron CA, She J, Higgins K, Sunshine MJ, Lacy E, Lonberg N, Terhorst C (1994) A block in both early T lymphocyte and natural killer cell development in transgenic mice with high-copy numbers of the human CD3E gene. Proc Natl Acad Sci USA 91:9402–9406

Whitlock CA, Witte ON (1982) Long term culture of B lymphocytes and their precursors from murine bone marrow. Proc Natl Acad Sci USA 79:3608

Williamd NS, Moore TA, Schatzle JD, Puzanov IJ, Sivakumar PV, Zlotnik A, Bennett M, Kumar V (1997) Generation of lytic NK1.1^{+} Ly-49^{-} cells from multipotent bone marrow progenitors in a stroma-free culture: definition of cytokine requirements and developmental intermediates. J Exp Med 186:1609–1614

Wu L, Antica M, Johnson GR, Scollay R, Shortman K (1991a) Developmental potential of the earliest precursor cells from the adult thymus. J Exp Med 174:1617

Wu L, Scollay R, Egerton M, Pearse M, Spangrude GJ, Shortman K (1991b) CD4 expressed on earliest T-lineage precursor cells in the adult murine thymus. Nature 349:71

Yoda Y, Kawakami Z, Shibuya A, Abe T (1988) Characterization of natural killer cells cultured from human bone marrow cells. Exp Hematol 16:712

Yokoyama WM (1995) Natural killer cell receptors specific for MHC class I molecules. Proc Natl Acad Sci USA 92:3081–3085

Yokoyama WM, Seaman WE (1993) The Ly-49 and NKR-P1 gene families encodong lectin-like receptors on natural killer cells: the NK gene complex. Annu Rev Immunol 11:613–635

Yokoyama WM, Jacobs LB, Kanagawa O, Shevach EM, Cohen DI (1989) A murine lymphocyte antigen belongs to a superfamily of type II integral membrane proteins. J Immunol 143:1379

Yokoyama WM, Kehn PJ, Cohen DI, Shevach EM (1990) Chromosomal location of the Ly-49 (A1,YE1/48) multigene family. Genetic association with the NK1.1 antigen. J Immunol 145:2353–2360

Yu YYL, George T, Dorfmann JR, Roland J, Kumar V, Bennett M (1996) The role of Ly-49A and 5E6 (Ly-49C) molecules in hybrid resistence mediated by murine natural killer cells against normal T cell blasts. Immunity 4:67–76

D. Role of NK Cells in Infections and Tumors

Control of Infections by NK Cells

C.H. TAY, E. SZOMOLANYI-TSUDA, and R.M. WELSH

1 Introduction

The natural immune system consists of preexisting or rapidly inducible effector components as a first line of defense against pathogens to which the host has not previously been exposed. Such a system is necessary as the B and T cell specific responses to any pathogen require the selective expansion of high-affinity antigen-specific clones which take several days to develop. An unimpeded replication of a virus producing 10^5 progeny per cell could potentially infect all of the cells in the

Department of Pathology, University of Massachusetts Medical Center, 55 Lake Avenue North, Worcester, MA 01655, USA

host after only three or four replication cycles. Without the natural immune system holding infections in check, pathogens could overwhelm the host before the T and B cell responses become effective.

Natural killer (NK) cells, which provide an early host response to viral, parasitic, and bacterial infections, are important components of the natural immune system. NK cells have now been shown to provide resistance to some of these infections as and to play roles in tumor surveillance and in the regulation of hematopoiesis (STORKUS and DAWSON 1991; WELSH and VARGAS-CORTES 1992; BELLONE et al. 1993; SCOTT and TRINCHIERI 1995). NK cells have a large granular lymphocyte morphology, with their granules containing the membrane pore-forming molecule, perforin, and a group of serine proteases known as granzymes (O'SHEA and ORTALDO 1992). NK cells do not express the T cell receptor/CD3 complex or immunoglobulins on their cell surfaces and do not rearrange their B and T cell antigen receptor genes, but NK cells do express a variety of NK cell specific receptors encoded by genes found within the distal portion of mouse chromosome 6 and on human chromosome 12p13.2, in a region now known as the NK gene complex (YOKOYAMA 1993, 1995). Many of these NK cell receptors have MHC class I molecules as their ligands (GUMPERZ and PARHAM 1995; RAULET and HELD 1995; COLONNA 1996). NK cells can secrete a number of cytokines, including interferon gamma (IFN-γ), tumor necrosis factor alpha (TNF-α), granulocyte/macrophage colony stimulating factors (GM-CSF), and interleukin 1 (IL-1) (TRINCHIERI 1989). Several recent reviews have detailed previous work documenting the activation of NK cells by pathogens and their roles in controlling those infections (WELSH and VARGAS-CORTES 1992; SCOTT and TRINCHIERI 1995; BRUTKIEWICZ and WELSH 1995). This review focuses on the mechanisms by which NK cells may control these infections and reviews evidence that such control may be mediated by cytotoxic mechanisms or by cytokines, acting either directly on infected cells or by modulating immune system functions and altering the nature of the specific immune response.

2 NK Cells and Virus Infections

The importance of NK cells in the regulation of viral infections has been most definitively shown with the murine cytomegalovirus (MCMV) infection of mice. Genetic resistance of mice to MCMV maps to a single gene within the NK gene complex (SCALZO et al. 1990, 1992). Intraperitoneally inoculated adult C57BL/6 mice depleted of NK cells with antisera to asialo GM_1 (aGM_1) or with monoclonal antibodies (mAbs) to NK1.1 have enhanced virus replication in the spleen, lung, and liver (BUKOWSKI et al. 1984; WELSH et al. 1991, 1994). Suckling mice are very sensitive to MCMV until the third week of life, at which time the NK cell response develops to maturity (BOOS and WHEELOCK 1971; KIESSLING et al. 1975). Adoptive transfer experiments using adult splenocyte populations or purified culture-derived NK cells showed that NK cells protect suckling mice from MCMV (BUKOWSKI et al. 1985). NK cells were also shown to inhibit MCMV replication in mice with severe combined immunodeficiency (SCID), demonstrating the function of these cells in an environment devoid of T and B cells (WELSH et al. 1991, 1994). However, NK cells in SCID mice are incapable of completely eradicating MCMV, even at limiting dilutions of the virus, indicating that T and/or B cells are ultimately necessary for clearance (BRUBAKER 1993). This is consistent with the concept that NK cells inhibit the spread of infection, allowing time for specific immune responses to develop. In humans the importance of NK cells was highlighted in our institution by a patient who had a complete and selective NK cell immunodeficiency; this patient had unusually severe cases of human cytomegalovirus (HCMV) infection and other herpes virus infections (BIRON et al. 1989).

How NK cells control MCMV and other viral infections in vivo has until recently been a poorly understood phenomenon. Recent work has suggested that NK cells can control MCMV infections via two different mechanisms, by the secretion of antiviral cytokines such as IFN-γ or alternatively by the direct lysis of virus-infected cells. As MCMV is the most well-studied NK-sensitive virus, most of the discussion on the mechanisms utilized by NK cells in the regulation of virus infections is focused on this virus.

2.1 Activation of NK Cells During Virus Infections

When a virus infects a host, virus-infected cells are stimulated to produce IFN-α and IFN-β, which induce the NK cells to proliferate and increase their cytotoxic potential (WELSH 1978; BIRON and WELSH 1982; BIRON et al. 1984). In mice the levels of NK cell activation and blastogenesis parallel the IFN-α/β levels (WELSH 1978; BIRON and WELSH 1982), and direct injections of purified IFN-β into mice induce NK cell activation and proliferation (BIRON et al. 1984). Mice treated with antibodies to IFN-α/β (GIDLUND et al. 1978) or mice whose IFN-α/β receptors have been inactivated by genetic recombination (MULLER et al. 1994) generate a poor NK cell response to viral infections (BIRON 1994). These activated NK cells respond to chemotactic factors and migrate into areas of virus-infected tissue, such as the liver (MCINTYRE and WELSH 1986; NATUK and WELSH 1987a; NATUK et al. 1989), where they are presumed to mediate their antiviral activities.

NK cells from virus-infected C57BL/6 mice have both high cytolytic activity and the potential to produce antiviral cytokines. They express transcripts for IFN-γ, but the translation of these transcripts into the IFN-γ protein is dependent on additional factors. ORANGE and BIRON (1996b) studied the differences in the cytokine responses in mice infected with the NK-sensitive virus MCMV and in mice infected with lymphocytic choriomeningitis virus (LCMV), which is very resistant to NK cells (BUKOWSKI et al. 1983). Both infections induced type I IFNs and the cytolytic activation of NK cells, and in both infections NK cells expressed mRNA for IFN-γ. However, only in the MCMV infection did the NK cells synthesize and secrete the IFN-γ protein. The IFN-γ production during MCMV infection was linked to the fact that MCMV but not LCMV is a good inducer of IL-12 in vivo (ORANGE and BIRON 1996a). IL-12 is a pleiotropic cytokine produced by macrophages and was shown in these studies to be required for the production of IFN-γ by NK cells early in the infection. Antibodies to IFN-γ or IL-12 did not affect NK cell cytolytic activity, a result consistent with the concept that IFN-α/β rather than IFN-γ activates NK cells at the early stages of infection (ORANGE et al. 1995).

Another cytokine that plays a role in the activation of NK cells is TNF-α. Data generated using anti-TNF-α treated, MCMV-infected normal mice suggest that TNF-α can synergize with IL-12 to induce the production of IFN-γ by NK cells. TNF-α can also inhibit the effects of IFN-α/β on NK cells by negatively influencing NK cell blastogenesis and the induction of NK cell cytotoxicity (ORANGE and BIRON 1996b).

2.2 Antiviral Functions of NK Cell Produced Cytokines

A suggestion that NK cell produced cytokines are important in controlling virus infections came initially from studies using athymic nude mice infected with a vaccinia virus (VV)–IL-2 recombinant (KARUPIAH et al. 1990). IL-2 is a strong activator (KURIBAYASHI et al. 1981) as well as a chemotactic factor (NATUK and WELSH 1987b) for NK cells. This cytokine also has the ability to induce NK cells to produce IFN-γ (YOUNG and ORTALDO 1987). Administration of either anti-IFN-γ antibodies or anti-aGM$_1$ antiserum into the VV–IL-2 recombinant-infected nude mice exacerbated the infection, suggesting that the production of IFN-γ by the NK cells in the nude mice was controlling the infection (KARUPIAH et al. 1990). A role for NK cell produced IFN-γ in an unmodified system has since been established with MCMV (ORANGE et al. 1995). Depletion of IFN-γ or IL-12 with mAbs increased the incidence of MCMV-induced hepatitis and virus replication in the liver (ORANGE et al. 1995; ORANGE and BIRON 1996a; TAY and WELSH 1997). A role for IFN-γ in the NK cell mediated regulation of MCMV was further demonstrated in IFN-γ receptor knockout (IFN-γR$^{0/0}$) 129 mice reconstituted with C57BL/6 bone marrow cells, which give rise to high NK cell activity normally effective against MCMV. NK cells in these bone marrow chimeras failed to restrict MCMV replication in the IFN-γR$^{0/0}$ livers but did restrict the virus replication in IFN-γ receptor-intact chimeric controls (TAY and WELSH 1997).

One of the ways in which IFN-γ can exert its antiviral effects is by inducing the expression of the gene for inducible nitric oxide synthase (iNOS) in cells such as macrophages, Kupffer cells, and hepatocytes (NATHAN 1992). NOS in turn catalyzes the production of a free radical gas, nitric oxide (NO), from the guanidine nitrogen of L-arginine. NO production by NOS has been shown both in vivo and in vitro to inhibit the replication of VV, ectromelia virus, and herpes simplex virus type 1 (HSV-1) (KARUPIAH et al. 1993; HARRIS et al. 1995). Recently it was also shown that mice treated with an inhibitor to NOS, N^{ω}-methyl-L-arginine (L-NMA), had greatly enhanced MCMV synthesis in the liver by 3 days postinfection (TAY and WELSH 1997).

The other antiviral cytokine that NK cells can secrete to control viral infections is TNF-α. An early report provided some evidence that TNF-α and lymphotoxin produced by cloned human NK cell lines can have antiviral cytotoxicity, and that human recombinant TNF-α can selectively induce the lysis of cells infected with vesicular stomatitis virus, HCMV, Theiler's murine encephalomyelitis virus, or HSV-1- (PAYA et al. 1988). In vivo $CD4^+$ T cell dependent TNF-α production has been shown to participate in the inhibition of MCMV replication (PAVIC et al. 1993), and in vitro this cytokine can synergize with IFN-γ to inhibit MCMV late protein production (LUCIN et al. 1994). The role of NK cell produced TNF-α in the regulation of MCMV is not clear, as E26 mice, which do not have any T or NK cells, produce normal levels of TNF-α 2–3 days after MCMV infection (ORANGE and BIRON 1996b). This means that NK cells are not a primary or required source for the production of TNF-α, which can be made at high levels by macrophages and other cell types. Nevertheless, it is possible the NK cell produced TNF-α feeds back onto its own regulatory pathway and synergizes with IL-12 to stimulate the production of more IFN-γ. In the liver macrophage/Kupffer cell produced IL-12 and TNF-α might act on the NK cells to stimulate the production of IFN-γ, which in turn stimulates the macrophages, Kupffer cells, and hepatocytes to produce NO to control MCMV replication in that organ.

2.3 Role of NK Cell Cytotoxicity in the Regulation of Virus Infections

Evidence suggesting that a cytotoxic mechanism is involved in the control of MCMV comes from studies with beige mice and perforin knockout (perforin 0/0) mice. Beige mice, whose NK cells are deficient in cytotoxic function, control MCMV infection poorly (SHELLAM et al. 1981; BUKOWSKI et al. 1984). However, the beige mutation confers a lysosomal defect affecting many types of leukocytes, and it is possible that these other defects influence the ability of the beige mouse to control the infection. More interpretable data have been generated in perforin 0/0 mice, whose NK cells lack cytotoxic function. In the early phase of MCMV infection MCMV replicates to substantially higher titers in the spleens of perforin 0/0 mice than in perforin wild-type (+/+) controls. This suggests that NK cells utilize a cytotoxic mechanism to control splenic MCMV replication (TAY and WELSH 1997).

2.4 Distinct Organ-Dependent Mechanisms for the Control of MCMV Infection

Evidence provided above supports the conclusions that either cytokine production or direct cytotoxicity by NK cells can control MCMV infection, but the relative importance of these effector mechanisms differs with the target organ. We have examined MCMV infections in the perforin 0/0 mice, IFN-$\gamma R^{0/0}$ mice, and in normal mice treated with anti-IFN-γ mAbs and iNOS inhibitors and have come to the conclusion that NK cells control MCMV infection predominantly by a perforin-dependent, IFN-γ-independent mechanism in the spleen and by a perforin-independent, IFN-γ-dependent mechanism in the liver (TAY and WELSH 1997). Three days after the infection MCMV titers in the spleens of perforin 0/0 mice were higher than in perforin +/+ mice, but no elevation of liver titers was found in perforin 0/0 mice. NK cell depletion of MCMV-infected perforin 0/0 mice resulted in an increase in liver

Table 1. Use of various mechanisms in the spleen and liver by NK cells in the regulation of MCMV (adapted from TAY and WELSH 1997)

Group/treatment	Control	Increase in PFU MCMV/organ	
		Spleen	Liver
Perforin 0/0	Perforin +/+	+++++	±
Perforin 0/0 + anti-NK1.1	Perforin 0/0	±	+++
C57BL/6 + anti-NK1.1	C57BL/6	+++++	+++
C57BL/6 + anti-IFN-γ	C57BL/6	±	+++
C57BL/6 + anti-IFN-γ + anti-NK1.1	C57BL/6	+++++	+++
C57BL/6→129 + anti-NK1.1	C57BL/6→129	++++	+++
C57BL/6IFN-γR$^{0/0}$ + anti-NK1.1	C57BL/6→IFN-γR$^{0/0}$	+++++	±
Perforin 0/0IFN-γR$^{0/0}$ + anti-NK1.1	Perforin 0/0→IFN-γR$^{0/0}$	±	±
C57BL/6 + L-NMA	C57BL/6	±	+++
C57BL/6 + L-NMA	C57BL/6 + D-NMA	±	+++

Group/treatment is compared with the control group, and the relative increase in MCMV titers is depicted as +. The symbo ± is used to depict nonsignificant changes in virus titers. MCMV titers were measured 3 days postinfection. Age-matched mice were infected i.p. with 10^4 PFU MCMV. Mice were either left untreated or were treated with anti-NK1.1 antibodies i.v. 1 day prior to infection. Anti-IFN-γ Abs were given i.p. on days 0, 1, and 2 of the infection. *N*-Methyl-L-arginine or *N*-methyl-D -arginine were given i.v. on days 0, 1, and 2 of the infection.

viral titers but not in splenic titers (TAY and WELSH 1997). By mAb depletion of IFN-γ in C57BL/6 mice and by using IFN-γR$^{0/0}$ mice rendered chimeric with C57BL/6 bone marrow cells we found that IFN-γ inhibits MCMV replication in the liver but not in the spleen (TAY and WELSH 1997). Similarly, an inhibitor of iNOS, L-NMA, which prevents the production of IFN—induced NO, enhanced MCMV synthesis in the liver but not in the spleen (TAY and WELSH 1997). These results suggest that NK cells in C57BL/6 mice exert their effects predominantly through a perforin-mediated mechanism in the spleen and through an IFN-γ-induced NO mechanism in the liver. This utilization of different mechanisms by NK cells in the regulation of MCMV is summarized in Table 1. Just as NK cells use different mechanisms to control viruses in different organs, their efficacy in certain organs varies considerably. It is noteworthy that NK cells do not effectively control MCMV replication in the lungs after intranasal inoculation of the virus. The lungs of beige mice or normal mice depleted of NK cells with antibodies had similar MCMV titers as normal controls (BUKOWSKI et al. 1984).

2.5 *Cmv-1* and the Genetic Resistance of Mice to MCMV

Scalzo et al. have shown that there is a non-MHC linked resistance gene to MCMV that maps very closely to the *NK1.1* locus within the NK gene complex (SCALZO et al. 1990, 1992, 1995b). *Cmv-1* confers resistance to MCMV in the spleen but not in the liver (SCALZO et al. 1990). The effects of *Cmv-1* are mediated through NK1.1$^+$ cells, and mice that have the gene (*Cmv-1^r*) have lower splenic MCMV titers than strains of mice that do not have the gene (*Cmv-1^s*) (SCALZO et al. 1992). However, the viral titers in the livers of the different strains of mice are similar. This organ-dependent genetic resistance parallels the function of perforin, which is needed to control MCMV in the spleens of mice, but *Cmv-1* and perforin are on different chromosomes. *Cmv-1^s* BALB/c mice, when made congenic with the *Cmv-1^r* C57BL/6 NK gene complex, have their resistance to MCMV changed from a *Cmv-1^s* phenotype to a *Cmv-1^r* phenotype (SCALZO et al. 1995a).

The mapping of *Cmv-1* within the NK gene complex suggests that its yet to be identified gene product may be a receptor molecule associated with the cytotoxic function of NK cells. It is possible that *Cmv-1* encodes a receptor that recognizes MCMV-infected cells or even MCMV itself. It is interesting to note that a genetic susceptibility of mice to ectromelia virus has also been mapped within the NK gene complex, close to the *Cmv-1* locus, suggesting that *Cmv-1* or closely related gene(s) also regulate other viral infections (DELANO and BROWNSTEIN 1995).

2.6 Rationale for the Different Mechanisms Utilized by NK Cells in the Regulation of MCMV

The documentation of a *Cmv-1^r*, perforin-dependent mechanism controlling MCMV replication in the spleen leads to the suggestion that MCMV-infected splenocytes are lysed by NK cells. Surprisingly little information has been available concerning the direct cytotoxicity of MCMV-infected targets by NK cells. An early report of MCMV-infected fibroblasts being lysed by NK cells in overnight cytotoxicity assays could be accounted for by activation of the NK cells in the assays rather than by a selective lysis of MCMV-infected cells (LEE and KELLER 1982). Studies designed to examine the intrinsic sensitivity of MCMV-infected fibroblasts to NK cells in short-term assays that precluded additional NK cell activation failed to find any indication of increased sensitivity of these target cells to lysis (BUKOWSKI and WELSH 1985a). However, most demonstrations of natural targets for NK cells in vivo and virtually all the studies on the specificity of NK receptor interactions with MHC class I molecules have been limited to cells of hematopoietic lineage, especially lymphocytes or lymphoma cells (BRUTKIEWICZ and WELSH 1995). It is thus possible that studies on the NK cell sensitivity of MCMV-infected targets had not used the most relevant target. Three days after infection normal mice infected with MCMV have a 100-fold more virus in the spleen than do T and B cell deficient SCID mice, suggesting that the T and/or B cells are the primary targets of MCMV infection in the spleen (WELSH et al. 1991). Our recent studies using infective center assays have shown directly that low percentages (0.001%–0.1%) of splenic T and B cells from 3 day MCMV-infected C57BL/6 mice harbor the virus (Tay and Welsh, unpublished). It is therefore possible that, in the early regulation of MCMV, NK cells control MCMV in the spleen by lysing the lymphocytes.

The lysis of a virus-infected cell requires that the NK cell bind to and be triggered by the target cell. However, if the virus replication can be inhibited by the cytokines produced by activated NK cells, the effector cell may not have to come into contact with the virus-infected target. Target cells in the spleen may be good targets for NK cell recognition and lysis, but hepatocytes, which constitute the major fraction of liver cells infected by MCMV, may either not stimulate the NK cells appropriately or else not respond to the lytic signals delivered by NK cells. Nevertheless, their sensitivity to NK cell produced factors such as IFN-γ would render them susceptible to the antiviral functions of NK cells.

This strategy has a few advantages from the viewpoint of the host. The dissipation of IFN-γ in the liver would allow the antiviral cytokine to reach a maximum number of infected hepatocytes in the shortest amount of time, and this method of virus control may be more efficient than a direct cytotoxic mechanism. Hepatitis B virus (HBV)-transgenic mice adoptively reconstituted with virus-specific CTL produce IFN-γ and TNF-α that selectively degrade the HBV nucleocapsid particles and their replicating genomes and destabilize the viral RNA. Direct lysis of the hepatocytes by the CTLs is sufficiently minimal that the host is spared from adverse immunopathological effects brought on by the destruction of the hepatocytes (GUIDOTTI et al. 1996). The same phenomenon may be happening here with regards to MCMV. Rather than destroying the hepatocytes that are harboring the virus the production of IFN-γ may also be selectively destroying the virus without causing much damage to the cells themselves.

2.7 MHC Class I Expression and Virus Infections

The mapping of the *Cmv-1* locus within the NK gene complex raises the possibility that the NK receptor molecules interact with virus-infected targets. In both the human and mouse systems most of the cloned NK cell receptors interact with and receive negative signals from MHC class I molecules (STORKUS and DAWSON 1991; YOKOYAMA 1995). The ability of in vivo stimulated NK cells to lyse allogeneic targets and target cells that do not express MHC class I molecules was in fact initially used to differentiate virus-induced NK cell mediated killing from CTL-mediated lysis (KIESSLING and WELSH 1980; WELSH 1978; WELSH et al. 1979). The "missing-self hypothesis" proposes that the susceptibility of target cells to NK cell mediated lysis is inversely proportional to the amount of class I molecules on the target cell surface (LJUNGGREN and KARRE 1990; SENTMAN et al. 1995). LJUNGGREN et al. showed that tumor cells that are class I negative are rejected by the NK cells in their syngeneic host, and that the induction of MHC class I on the cell surfaces after transfection of β_2-microglobulin (β_2m) into β_2m negative [β_2m (–/–)] mutant tumor cells restores the tumorigenic potential (GLAS et al. 1992). They also showed that the IFN-mediated resistance of cells to NK cell mediated lysis is in part due to the presence of class I molecules, as YAC-1 lymphoma β_2m (–/–) variants could only be protected by IFNs after transfection and expression of β_2m, which allowed for transport of class I molecules in stable form to the cell surface (LJUNGGREN et al. 1990). As the interaction between the NK cell receptors and MHC class I molecules may have an inhibitory effect on the engaged NK cells, and because some virus infections markedly alter MHC class I expression, it has been speculated that virus-induced modifications of MHC class I expression on target cells render the cells susceptible to NK cell killing (STORKUS and DAWSON 1991; BRUTKIEWICZ and WELSH 1995). Although an unambiguous link between virus-induced class I alterations and sensitivity to NK cells has to date not been made, the potential connection compels us to briefly review this area.

2.7.1 Virus-Induced Downregulation of MHC Class I Molecules

Some viruses quantitatively alter the expression of MHC class I antigens by directly downregulating cell surface expression and/or by interfering with the ability of IFNs to upregulate class I molecules (BRUTKIEWICZ and WELSH 1995). During virus infections in vivo the induced IFN-α/β not only activates the NK cells but also transcriptionally induces the expression of MHC class I on many of the cells in the infected host (BUKOWSKI and WELSH 1985b, 1986). This upregulation of class I expression renders the uninfected host cells resistant to NK cell mediated lysis and more susceptible to allospecific CTL (HANSSON et al. 1980; BUKOWSKI and WELSH 1986). It has been suggested that an impairment of IFN-induced protection in virus-infected cells leaves these cells susceptible to attack by the highly activated NK cells, while the uninfected cells in the host would be protected from such attack (SANTOLI and KOPROWSKI 1979; TRINCHIERI and SANTOLI 1978; BUKOWSKI and WELSH 1986). A downregulation of class I molecules or an inhibition of IFN-induced upregulation of class I molecules on infected cells undoubtedly helps the virus to escape the immune surveillance by T cells, as T cells require the interactions between the viral peptide presented on MHC class I molecules with their cell surface T cell receptors to be activated. Whether these alterations directly influence their susceptibility to NK cells in the context of a viral infection in vivo is a question under investigation.

2.7.2 Mechanisms of Virus-Induced Downregulation of MHC Class I Expression

Different viruses have evolved various mechanisms to quantitatively reduce cell surface MHC class I expression, presumably in their attempt to escape CTL-mediated lysis. Blocks in class I heavy-chain transcription, class I assembly or class I transport are some of the mechanisms described to date. HCMV infection affects the stability of class I heavy chains (WARREN et al. 1994; BEERSMA et al. 1993; YAMASHITA et al. 1994). The HCMV glycoproteins US2 and US11 downregulate MHC class I molecules by misdirecting class I molecules from the endoplasmic reticulum to the cytosol for degradation by proteosomes (JONES et al. 1995; WIERTZ et al. 1996a,b; HENGEL et al. 1996). This shunting of class I molecules out of the ER effectively prevents any form of class I from being expressed on the cell surface. MCMV prevents antigen presentation by blocking the transport of peptide-loaded MHC class I molecules into the medial-Golgi compartment (DEL VAL et al. 1992). This block is carried out by MCMV's early gene products, and, in contrast to HCMV, these gene products also downregulate the synthesis of class I molecules but have no discernible effect on the rate of class I degradation (CAMPBELL and SLATER 1994; THALE et al. 1995). MCMV also inhibits the ability of IFN to upregulate class I expression (CAMPBELL and SLATER 1994). In HSV-1-infected cells class I molecules are not transported to the cell surface early in infection under conditions where class I synthesis remains normal (HILL et al. 1994). This class I deficiency is due to the HSV-1 immediate early gene product, ICP47, which blocks the presentation of viral and endogenous peptides to the CTL by physically associating with the transporter associated with antigen presentation (TAP), efficiently blocking the transport of peptides by TAP into the ER (FRUH et al. 1995; HILL et al. 1995). This block in peptide transport into the ER prevents normal MHC class I complexes to form and thus not be expressed on the cell surface.

Human immunodeficiency virus 1 (HIV-1) has been reported to downregulate class I antigens in a CD4$^+$ T cell line. The defect in the expression of class I is not due to a block in the transport or the assembly of class I molecules but is instead due to HIV-1 tat protein-induced reduction in class I heavy chain transcription (SCHEPPLER et al. 1989). In Burkitt's lymphoma cells or Epstein-Barr virus (EBV)-transformed lymphoblastoid cell lines there is a selective downregulation in the expression of one of several class I alleles (MASUCCI et al. 1987, 1989; IMREH et al. 1995). Mutational analyses reveal that the internal glycine-alanine repeat of EBNA1, an EBV nuclear protein, has the ability to inhibit antigen processing and MHC class I presentation (LEVITSKYAYA et al. 1995). Adenovirus subgroups B–E prevent the expression of class I complexes by binding the E3 19-kDa glycoprotein to class I molecules and retaining them in the ER (WOLD and GOODING 1991; HERMISTON et al. 1993). The E1A protein of adenovirus subgroup A, as with HIV-1's tat protein, interferes primarily through the downregulation of class I heavy-chain mRNA transcription (SHEMESH et al. 1991; FRIEDMAN and RICCIARDI 1988). A summary of MHC class I downregulation by viruses is shown in Table 2.

2.7.3 Effects of Virus-Induced Downregulation of MHC Class I Molecules on NK Cell Mediated Lysis

Although it is well-established that viral infections downregulate class I expression, it has not yet been clearly shown that this affects the sensitivity of virus-infected cells to NK cells. A correlation between MHC class I downregulation by different strains of adenovirus and susceptibility of adenovirus-infected cells to NK cell mediated lysis was made in one report, but no further work has supported this claim (DAWSON et al. 1989). Cells infected by an adenovirus E3 mutant, which lacks the gene that retains class I molecules in the ER, express normal levels of class I molecules on the cell surface that can be further upregulated by treatment with IFN-γ, similarly to normal uninfected cells (ROUTES 1992). However, despite the high levels of class I molecules on the cell surfaces of IFN-γ-treated, E3 mutant infected cells, these cells

Table 2. Virus-induced downregulation of MHC class I molecules

Virus	Gene(s) involved	Effects on MHC class I	References
HCMV	US2, US11	Shunts class I heavy chain into the cytoplasm	JONES et al. 1995; WIERTZ et al. 1996a,b; HENGEL et al. 1996; WIERTZ et al. 1996.
MCMV	Early gene(s)	Downregulation of class I synthesis and prevention of transport out of the ER	DEL VAL et al. 1992; CAMPBELL and SLATER 1994; THALE et al. 1995
HSV	ICP47	Prevents peptide translocation into the ER	FRUH et al. 1995; HILL et al. 1994
HIV-1	tat	Downregulation of class I heavy chain mRNA transcription	SCHEPPLER et al. 1989
EBV	EBNA1	Inhibits antigen processing and expression of HLA-A11 allele	MASUCCI et al. 1987, 1989; IMREH et al. 1995; LEVITSKAYA et al. 1995
Adenovirus subgroups B–E	E3	Retention of class I heavy chain in the ER	WOLD et al. 1991; HERMISTON et al. 1993
Adenovirus subgroup A	E1A	Downregulation of class I heavy chain mRNA transcription	FRIEDMAN and RICCIARDI 1988; SHEMESH et al. 1991.

remain more susceptible to NK cell mediated lysis than do untreated E3 mutant infected cells and uninfected cells. HIV-infected cells have enhanced sensitivity to lysis by NK cells, but the link has not yet been made between this enhanced sensitivity to lysis and the HIV tat-induced downregulation of class I molecules (RUSCETTI et al. 1986; BANDYOPADHYAY et al. 1990). It is noteworthy that HIV-infected individuals have fewer NK cells than normal subjects, and that these NK cells have defective NK cell cytolytic activity (ULLUM et al. 1995; BONAGURA et al. 1992; HU et al. 1995). Therefore even though HIV-infected targets may be susceptible to NK cell mediated lysis, NK cells in these individuals would have poor ability to lyse the targets. It is possible that this HIV-induced defective natural immunity contributes to the host's susceptibility to opportunistic infections and the reactivation of herpes viruses thought to be controlled by NK cells (BIRON et al. 1989; ULLUM et al. 1995).

Substantial work has indicated that human fibroblasts infected with HCMV or HSV-1 are more susceptible to NK cell mediated lysis than uninfected cells (CHING and LOPEZ 1979; BORYSIEWICZ et al. 1985). Evidence that this is related to class I molecules is confined to one report showing that increased sensitivity of HSV-1-infected targets to NK cells was limited to cells expressing class I molecules and not to a class I negative cell line, which was quite sensitive to lysis even when uninfected (KAUFMAN et al. 1992). It has been speculated that the downregulation of class I molecules by HSV-1 has clinical significance in gestating mothers infected with the virus. HSV infections can sometimes be deleterious to the unborn child, as there is an association between the HSV-1 infection and spontaneous fetal loss (ZDRAVKOVIC et al. 1994). Human trophoblasts do not express the classical MHC class I molecules but instead express the nonclassical class I molecule HLA-G, as well as a HLA-C-like molecule, HLA-C_{JED} (SCHUST et al. 1996). The interaction of HLA-G molecules and the p58 NK cell receptor proteins on cloned human NK cells has an inhibitory effect on NK cell mediated lysis (PAZMANY et al. 1996). Recently it has been shown that HSV-1 ICP47 blocks the intracellular transport of HLA-G, thereby preventing the expression of HLA-G on the cell surface of extravillous cytotrophoblast cell lines (SCHUST et al. 1996). It has been speculated that this prevention of HLA-G molecules from expressing on the cell surface is linked to spontaneous fetal loss during HSV-1 infection, as the extravillous cytotrophoblasts would not be protected from maternal NK cell mediated lysis. More information is required to evaluate this hypothesis.

2.7.4 Qualitative Alterations in MHC Class I Molecules Associated with Insertion of Viral Peptides

A second mechanism by which viruses might alter MHC class I expression is by the insertion of virus-encoded peptides into the class I peptide-binding groove. Studies using site-directed mutagenesis on human MHC class I molecules and with MHC-congenic strains of mice suggest that human and mouse NK cells interact with the class I molecules near the antigen peptide-binding groove and the surrounding α-helices, specifically the α_1 and α_2 domains, which cradle the peptide (KARLHOFER et al. 1994; KURAGO et al. 1995). Indeed, cloned NK cells have been shown to be inhibited by self peptides in the context of self MHC molecules (MALNATI et al. 1995; CORREA and RAULET 1995). This work suggests that the self peptides presented by the class I molecules may be important in the inhibition of NK cell lysis and lead to the hypothesis that the insertion of foreign (i.e., viral) peptides into the peptide-binding groove interferes with this interaction and render a virus-infected cell sensitive to NK cell killing.

Studies on the sensitivity of target cells to lysis by NK cells after treatment of targets with immunodominant viral peptides for CTL have led to conflicting results. One study suggested that an influenza virus peptide enhances the susceptibility of concanavalin A induced lymphoblasts to syngeneic NK cells (CHADWICK et al. 1992). A second conflicting report showed that under conditions that would sensitize target cells to CTL killing, immunodominant T-cell peptides from several viruses including influenza failed to sensitize these target cells to NK cell mediated lysis (BRUTKIEWICZ and WELSH 1995). Studies using the Ly-$49A^+$ NK cell subset and TAP-mutant RMA-S cells transfected with H-$2D^d$ showed that any of a variety of peptides that enable the H-$2D^d$ molecule to form a stable complex on the cell surface delivers a negative signal to Ly-$49A^+$ NK cells (CORREA and RAULET 1995). A recent report showed that empty MHC class I molecules which can be stably expressed on RMA-S cell surfaces at 26°C are sufficient to confer protection to the target cells, implying that polymorphic structures on the class I molecules and not the peptides interact with the NK cells (MANDELBOIM et al. 1996). It is thus likely that when peptides do alter the sensitivity of targets to NK cells it is not because they are recognized by NK cells per se, but because they either change the conformation of the class I molecule or destabilize it on the cell surface.

Whether the insertion of immunodominant or even nonimmunodominant peptides into MHC class I during a viral infection alters the negative signal to NK cells and renders a virus-infected target preferentially susceptible to NK cell mediated lysis remains unclear. As VV-infected target cells become sensitive to lysis by VV-specific CTL, the infected targets have a period in time when they display enhanced sensitivity to NK cell mediated lysis and markedly reduced sensitivity to killing by allospecific CTL, even though the quantitative expression of class I antigens remains high. It has been suggested that the replacement of endogenous peptides presented by the MHC molecules by foreign VV-encoded peptides abrogate the abilities of class I molecules to be recognized properly by either allospecific CTL or NK cells (BRUTKIEWICZ et al. 1992). In a second, similar study HSV-1 infection was found to enhance the NK cell sensitivity of class I deficient C1R cells transfected with class I genes but to have no effect on the NK cell sensitivity of nontransfected cells (KAUFMAN et al. 1992). This enhanced sensitivity occurred under conditions where class I expression remained high on the cell surface, leading again to the speculation that viral peptides replace endogenous peptides in the expressed class I molecules. While suggestive, neither of these studies formally proved the hypotheses.

2.7.5 β_2m (–/–) Mice: An In Vivo Model to Study the Role of MHC Class I Molecules in the Regulation of Virus Infections by NK Cells

The role of class I molecules in the NK cell mediated control of the NK-sensitive MCMV has been examined in β_2m (–/–) mice. Cells from the β_2m (–/–) mice do not express class I α-chain detectable by conformation-dependent or conformation-independent antibodies on their plasma membranes. In this in vivo system where detectable cell surface MHC class I expression is not induced, sensitivity to NK cells by MCMV and the resistance to NK cells by LCMV are unchanged (TAY et al. 1995). Adult mice depleted of NK cells synthesized considerably more MCMV in their spleens (TAY et al. 1995). This suggests that the regulation of virus infections by NK cells is carried out through mechanisms that are not dependent on the recognition of class I molecules, and that the downregulation of MHC antigens by some viruses may be inconsequential regarding the ability of NK cells to regulate the infection.

2.8 Other Potential Recognition Systems Between NK Cells and Virus-Infected Targets

There undoubtedly are many NK cell ligands that remain undefined and could play a role in NK cell interactions with virus-infected targets. An earlier study with human NK cell clones showed that some clones lysed targets infected with varicella zoster virus, HCMV, or VV while others did not, suggesting the possibility of some NK subset selectivity in recognizing virus-infected targets (MASON et al. 1993). Recent studies using cloned human NK cells have shown similar selectivity against human herpes virus 6 (HHV-6) infected cells (MALNATI et al. 1993), but the ability of the NK clones to lyse these infected cells is thought not to depend on MHC class I expression, as there was little difference in class I levels between HHV-6 infected and uninfected cells (MALNATI et al. 1993). These results suggest that other cell surface elements can restrict NK cell recognition. The mouse NK receptor Ly-49A is a C-type lectin that has a functional carbohydrate-recognition-domain, and the rat NKR-P1 can bind to oligosaccharide ligands (DANIELS et al. 1994; BEZOUSKA et al. 1994). NK cell receptors may therefore recognize the carbohydrate or sugar motifs on the class I molecules or even on other proteins. Substantial earlier work had indicated that purified glycoproteins from mumps, measles, influenza, and other viruses can augment the cytolytic activity of NK cells in vitro and in vivo (CASALI et al. 1981; HARFAST et al. 1980; ARORA et al. 1984; ARORA and HOUDE 1988); it is not known whether these glycoproteins or their sugar moieties interact with the defined NK receptor molecules.

Cell surface molecules other than MHC class I may act as NK cell triggering molecules. Costimulatory molecules expressed on the target cells may activate NK cells to lyse the target. NK cells have long been implicated in the outgrowth of B cells transformed by EBV, and EBV has recently been shown to upregulate the costimulatory molecule CD80 (B7-1) on infected cells (MONTEL et al. 1995). In fact this upregulation of B7-1 molecules on EBV-infected cells enhances their susceptibility to lysis by a human NK variant cell line that expresses CD28 (MONTEL et al. 1995). A recent article suggests that mouse NK cells can be activated by B7-1 (CHAMBERS et al. 1996), but this activation is reported not to occur through B7-1/CD28 or B7-1/CTLA-4 interactions, implicating a third receptor for B7-1. Interestingly, the presence of MHC class I molecules on the target cells does not inhibit their susceptibility to NK cell killing as long as the targets express B7-1. These results suggest that B7-1 expressed on virus-infected cells triggers the NK cells to lyse the virus-infected targets, and that the expression of class I molecules is inconsequential to the outcome.

2.9 Role of NK Cells in Humoral Immunity During Virus Infections

As discussed above, NK cells can provide resistance to viral infections in the absence of acquired immune responses, and such resistance can be mediated by perforin-dependent mechanisms or by antiviral effects of cytokines such as IFN-γ and by cytokine-induced products, such as NO. As some NK cell produced cytokines, notably IFN-γ, TNF-α, and GM-CSF, have immunomodulatory properties, NK cells have the potential to influence specific B and/or T cell responses. In fact, several reports suggest that NK cells play an important role in T cell independent (TI) humoral immunity. Polysaccharides present in bacterial cell walls are TI antigens (MOND et al. 1995), and recent work has indicated that virus infections can also induce TI antibody responses (SZOMOLANYI-TSUDA and WELSH 1996). Our studies with polyomavirus-infected immunodeficient mice suggest that NK cells provide helper factors for B cells during this antiviral Ig response.

Antibody responses to soluble proteins normally require the cooperation of T and B cells. During this process T cell receptor (TCR) α/β^+, $CD4^+$ T cells that had been activated by antigens provide signals to B cells. Surface determinants such as CD40L induced on the activated T cells make contact with molecules such as CD40 expressed on B cells. Activated T cells also secrete cytokines, and the specific combination of secreted cytokines is a major determinant of the antibody isotype produced (NOELLE et al. 1989; ABBAS et al. 1993). The requirement for T cell help, however, is not absolute, as TI antigens can elicit humoral immune responses in the absence of T cells (MOND et al. 1995). It has been long suspected that during TI antibody responses, "non-T helper" cells contribute the signals necessary for B cell activation, differentiation, isotype switching, and antibody secretion. An obvious candidate for this role is the NK cell, which makes cytokines such as IFN-γ, TNF-α, and GM-CSF that can act on B cells.

Several laboratories have demonstrated that NK cells can deliver help to B cells in vitro (BURNS et al. 1975; BRENNER et al. 1987; YUAN et al. 1992; SNAPPER and MOND 1993; SNAPPER et al. 1993, 1994; WILDER et al. 1996). SNAPPER et al. developed an in vitro polyclonal model system to study B cell activation through the antigen receptor and the resulting Ig production in response to TI antigens (SNAPPER and MOND 1993; MOND et al. 1995). Anti-Ig antibodies conjugated to high molecular weight dextran (anti-Ig-dextran) were used to simulate TI antigens, which are usually large molecules with highly repetitive epitopes. In this system small, resting B cell-enriched mouse spleen cells were capable of TI antibody production in response to anti-Ig-dextran in the presence of IL-1 and IL-2, but highly purified B cells did not show any detectable Ig production in the same type of experiments. Addition of aGM_1^+ spleen cells or in vitro activated and culture-purified NK cell populations to these B cell cultures restored the Ig secretion, strongly suggesting that NK cells provide help for B cells (TUTT et al. 1987; SNAPPER et al. 1993). The effect of NK cells in this system was mediated by soluble factors and was shown to be dependent on IFN-γ and GM-CSF (SNAPPER et al. 1996). In the absence of added IL-1 and IL-2 NK cells failed to stimulate the Ig response unless they were previously activated. This indicates that the Ig production by B cells in this in vitro system requires antigen stimulation and cytokine-producing, activated NK cells. The repetitive nature of the antigen seems to play a crucial role in this process, as only B cells that were activated through multivalent membrane Ig cross-linking with anti-Ig-dextran were stimulated to Ig secretion. Unconjugated anti-Ig treatment resulted in B cell activation as measured by increase in B cell size and upregulation of MHC class II expression but did not stimulate B cells to secrete Ig even in the presence of activated NK cells (SNAPPER et al. 1994). Other laboratories have demonstrated that IL-5, together with IL-2 can activate murine NK cells to induce Ig secretion in vitro in B cells not stimulated through the antigen receptor (YUAN et al. 1992; WILDER et al. 1996). In these experiments soluble factors produced by activated NK cells were essential for the stimulatory effect on Ig production.

Recently obtained in vivo data in mice strongly support the idea that NK cells play a physiological role in TI antibody responses to pathogens. WILDER et al. (1996) demonstrated that poly I:C treatment of mice, which activates NK cells, leads to the enhancement of IgG2a responses to a classical TI antigen, TNP. Depletion of the NK cells with anti-NK1.1 antibodies before poly I:C treatment prevented this enhancement, indicating that the increased IgG2a secretion to TNP is NK cell dependent.

Direct evidence that NK cells can stimulate antiviral antibody production comes from studies in immunodeficient mice infected with polyoma virus (PyV). PyV was shown to replicate to high levels and to induce a severe acute myeloproliferative disease in SCID mice, resulting in their death by 16 days postinfection (SZOMOLANYI-TSUDA et al. 1994). Transfers of nonimmune B cell populations into these mice protected them from the disease and controlled viral synthesis. Mice lacking T cells (TCR α/β knockout or TCR α/β/γ/δ knockout) controlled the infection, did not contract disease, and synthesized relatively high levels of IgG (predominantly IgG2a) antibody specific to PyV. Transfer of this antibody into SCID mice protected them from the disease and controlled the spread of virus. These results indicate that PyV infection induces a protective TI IgG2a response in T cell deficient mice (SZOMOLANYI-TSUDA and WELSH 1996). Earlier reports showing antiviral antibody production in nude mice (BURNS et al. 1975) and a recent report showing that CD40 knockout mice can mount detectable IgG2a responses to several virus infections, such as Pichinde virus and LCMV, even when depleted of their $CD4^+$ T cells (BORROW et al. 1996), suggest that antiviral IgG2a production in the absence of T cell help may be a general phenomenon. The highly repetitive nature of virus antigens might be an important factor in this process, as it allows extensive cross-linking of the antigen receptors on B cells, similar to the "classical" TI antigens, such as bacterial polysaccharides, Ficoll, or TNP.

In addition, virus infections lead to activation of several cell types and to the induction of a wide variety of non-T cell derived cytokines, which may provide the necessary stimuli for B cells and enable them to secrete antibodies. The role of NK cells in the TI IgG2a response to PyV infection was tested by comparing the antibody production of T cell knockout mice to that of E26 mice, which are deficient in both T and NK cells (WANG et al. 1994, 1996). PyV capsid antigen-specific enzyme-linked immunosorbent assays showed no detectable IgG2a in the sera of mice deficient in both T and NK cells, whereas mice lacking T cells but containing NK cells produced a significant amount of virus-specific IgG2a (Fig. 1). Although these mice are on different genetic backgrounds, these results suggest that in the absence of T cells NK cells have the ability to stimulate the production of protective antiviral antibodies by B cells. Unpublished data by Q. Vos mentioned in a recent review article (SNAPPER and MOND 1996) suggest that NK cells also enhance IgG3 responses to bacterial polysaccharides. IgG3 is an isotype regulated by IFN-γ and the IgG3 produced in the T and NK cell deficient E26 mice immunized with killed *Streptococcus pneumoniae* was only 10% of the responses observed in normal euthymic, or athymic nude mice.

The collaboration of NK cells and B cells during virus infection might be a very complex process. Virus-activated NK cells can produce IFN-γ. This IFN-γ production might be further increased by interaction of NK cells with activated B cells. It has been shown that in vitro coculture of activated B cells with NK cells induces the production of IFN-γ by the NK cells (MICHAEL et al. 1988, 1991). IFN-γ is a major "switch factor," promoting isotype switch to IgG2a production (COLLINS and DUNNICK 1993). The ability of activated NK cells to promote IgG2a production by secreting IFN-γ may thus explain the preferential increase in IgG2a levels observed

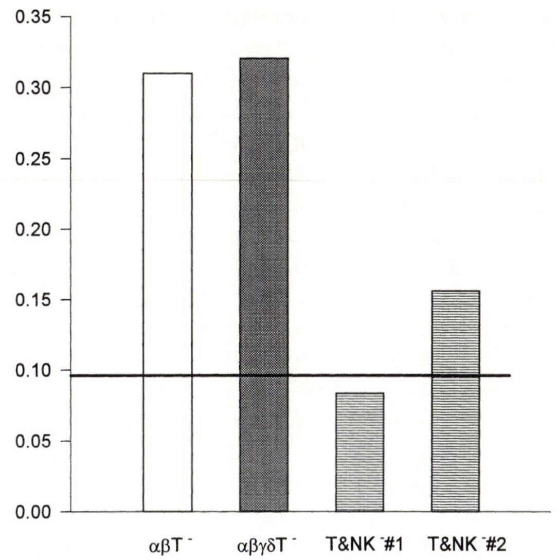

Fig. 1. IgG2a response to PyV in immunodeficient mice. PyV major capsid protein VP1-specific IgG2a levels in serum samples of day 14 PyV-infected TCR$\beta^{0/0}$ ($\alpha\beta T^-$), TCR$\beta\delta^{0/0}$ ($\alpha\beta\gamma\delta T^-$) and two CD3ε transgenic E26 mice (T and NK^-) were measured by IgG2a isotype-specific enzyme-linked immunosorbent assays. Data obtained with 1:200 dilutions of the serum samples are shown in this representative experiment. *Bold horizontal line*, background value obtained with negative control sera. The T cell knock-out mice were on the 129×C57BL/6 background, whereas the E26 mice were on the CBA background

after most virus infections (COURTELIER et al. 1988). The dominance of antiviral IgG2a may be advantageous for the host defense, as IgG2a is a good mediator of antibody-dependent cellular cytotoxicity (ADCC) (HERLYN and KOPROWSKI 1982), and, perhaps not coincidentally, NK cells are major effector cells for ADCC.

The B cell "helper" function provided by NK cells might make an important contribution to generating efficient humoral responses to virus infections not only in T cell deficient mice but in normal, immunocompetent hosts as well. TI antibody responses can be induced before T cells become activated by antigens presented on antigen-presenting cells. Although the magnitude of TI antiviral antibody production may be very low at this early stage of infection, the small amount of antibody produced might still diminish virus spread before the onset of T cell dependent immune mechanisms.

3 NK Cells as Effector Cells Against Parasitic Infections

In vivo and in vitro evidence has indicated that NK cells can contribute to the early resistance against *Toxoplasma gondii, Leishmania major*, and *Schistosoma mansoni* infections by producing IFN-γ, which stimulates microbicidal activity in macrophages. To date there is little evidence of direct NK cell mediated killing of parasites or parasite-infected cells. *T. gondii* infected IFN-γ knockout mice or C57BL/6 mice treated with anti-IFN-γ antibodies have good NK cell activity but cannot control the infection, whereas beige mice deficient in NK cell cytotoxic activity can control the parasitic infection (JOHNSON and SAYLES 1995). The first example of a protozoan stimulating the production of T cell independent IFN-γ was shown using *T. gondii* (SHER et al. 1993). In vitro studies showed that SCID mouse splenocytes exposed to live tachyzoites of *T. gondii* or just to soluble parasitic extracts can be stimulated to produce high levels of IFN-γ (SHER et al. 1993). This IFN-γ production was abolished when spleen cells from SCID mice were first treated with anti-aGM_1 antisera, suggesting that it is the NK cells that are the source of the IFN-γ. In vivo the depletion of IFN-γ or NK cells in *T. gondii* infected SCID mice abrogated the resistance to the parasite, adding further evidence that NK cell produced IFN-γ is essential in the regulation of *T. gondii* (GAZZINELLI et al. 1993). The protection afforded by NK cells in the early resistance to *T. gondii* was examined in β_2m (–/–) mice (DENKERS et al. 1993). Depletion of NK1.1$^+$ cells in β_2m (–/–) mice enhanced the growth of the parasite, whereas the depletion of CD4$^+$ or CD8$^+$ T cells had no effect on this early resistance. As in the MCMV infection, NK cell produced IFN-γ during *T. gondii* infection requires the help of macrophage-produced IL-12 and TNF-α (GAZZINELLI et al. 1993).

IFN-γ produced by NK cells also contributes to the early innate resistance to *L. major* and *S. mansoni*. In vivo depletion of NK cells in C57BL/6 mice with anti-NK1.1 antibodies reduced the amount of IFN-γ produced, resulting in enhanced growth of *L. major* (LASKAY et al. 1993; SCHARTON-KERSTEN and SCOTT 1995). In *S. mansoni* infected C3H and C57BL/6 mice the depletion of NK cells or IFN-γ resulted in increased parasitic burden and granuloma formation (WYNN et al. 1994).

In addition to providing resistance to parasites during the early phase of infection, NK cells can also modulate the adaptive immune response. The depletion of NK cells, IFN-γ, or IL-12 from *S. mansoni* infected C3H or C57BL/6 mice resulted in the skewing of the initial Th1 response to a Th2 response (OSWALD et al. 1994; WYNN et al. 1994). The same principle was true for *L. major* infected mice, as the removal of NK cells decreased IFN-γ levels and promoted IL-4 production, leading to higher parasitic burden and lesion development (SCHARTON and SCOTT 1993). Depletion of aGM_1^+, CD3$^-$ cells or IL-12 in the genetically resistant C3H mice infected with *L. major* abrogated NK cell produced IFN-γ, causing the mice to mount a Th2 response rather than the usual Th1 response (SCHARTON-KERSTEN et al. 1995; SCHARTON-KERSTEN and SCOTT 1995). BALB/c mice cannot control *L. major* infection because they are genetically predisposed to mount a Th2 response to the parasite. Administration of IL-12 promoted CD4$^+$ Th1 development in *L. major*-infected BALB/c mice, and these Th1 cells failed to develop if the NK cells were depleted at the time of infection (AFONSO et al. 1994).

NK cells are not always a determining factor in modulating Th1 versus Th2 responses, as removal of NK cells in *Candida albicans* infected C57BL/6 mice or in *L. major* infected C3H mice still allowed for the development of a Th1 response (ROMANI et al. 1993; SCHARTON-KERSTEN and SCOTT 1995). However, there still was an increase in parasite burden in the *L. major* infected C3H mice because the Th1 response was delayed (SCHARTON-KERSTEN and SCOTT 1995). Both C57BL/6 and C3H mice are naturally high NK strains, and it is possible their high NK cell activity predispose them to mount a Th1 instead of a Th2 response. The inability of BALB/c mice to mount a Th1 response may be because BALB/c mice have low NK cell activity, and their NK cells are poor producers of IFN-γ (SCHARTON and SCOTT 1993;

AFONSO et al. 1994). It would be interesting to determine whether BALB/c mice made congenic with either the C3H or C57BL/6 NK gene complex would have a Th1 response instead of a Th2 response to *L. major* infection.

4 NK Cells as Effector Cells Against Bacterial Infections

NK cells have been reported to have the capacity to be directly bactericidal and to lyse bacterially infected cells in vitro, but the more likely way in which NK cells control bacterial infections in vivo is by producing cytokines that activate the macrophages to degrade the bacteria. Purified human NK cells when mixed with *Salmonella typhimurium* have been shown to inhibit the outgrowth of the bacterial colonies (GARCIA-PENARRUBIA et al. 1989). Macrophages when exposed to bacteria or bacterial products are stimulated to produce NK cell activating cytokines such as IFN-α/β, IL-12, and TNF-α, which in turn activate the NK cells to kill NK-sensitive targets (WOLF et al. 1976; WOLD and GOODING 1991; GUO et al. 1992). Direct incubation of NK cells with fixed bacteria can also activate the NK cells to kill NK-sensitive targets (TARKKANEN et al. 1986). NK cells have been shown to lyse cells infected with *S. typhimurium*, *Mycobacterium avium* complex, or *Shigella flexneri* in vitro (KLIMPEL et al. 1986; KATZ et al. 1990; GRIGGS and SMITH 1994). However, experimental evidence in vivo has suggested that NK cell produced cytokines are probably more important than the cytotoxic potential of NK cells in the control of bacterial infections. *Listeria monocytogenes*, *M. avium*, and *S. typhimurium* infection in mice can stimulate the production of IFN-γ by NK cells, and this stimulation, as with viruses and parasites, requires factors produced by macrophages (RAMARATHINAM et al. 1993; TRIPP et al. 1993; APPELBERG et al. 1994). *L. monocytogenes* infection in SCID mice induces the production of TNF-α and IL-12 from macrophages, and these cytokines subsequently activate the NK cells to produce IFN-γ (TRIPP et al. 1993). Neutralization of IL-12, the cytokine that induces the production of IFN-γ, decreases the resistance to *Listeria* in SCID mice, indicating the importance of NK cell produced IFN-γ in the regulation of this intracellular bacterial infection (TRIPP et al. 1994).

IFN-γ-mediated resistance to mycobacterial or listerial infections may involve the production of NO by macrophages and other cells (GLESCH and KAUFMANN 1991; BECKERMAN et al. 1993). iNOS-deficient mice cannot control *L. monocytogenes* replication (MACMICKING et al. 1995). The production of NO in *L. monocytogenes* infected SCID mice is dependent on NK cell produced IFN-γ, and inhibitors of NO synthase, N^G-monomethyl arginine, or aminoguanidine inhibited the production of NO and increased the titers of listeria in these mice (BECKERMAN et al. 1993).

Even though there is strong evidence that the depletion of NK cell produced IFN-γ increases the susceptibility of immunodeficient mice to *L. major* infection, several studies using normal mice have ironically suggested that the depletion of NK cells *increases* host resistance to the bacteria. Depletion of NK cells in C57BL/6 mice by anti-NK1.1 mAb increased the resistance *to L. monocytogenes* (TAKADA et al. 1994).

This result is surprising as IFN-γ has been shown to be important for the control of the listerial infection, and anti-NK1.1 treatment decreases the number of IFN-γ producing cells (TEIXEIRA and KAUFMANN 1994). The explanation for this may reside in competition between host effector functions. One study suggests that NK cells inhibit the proliferation of γδ T cells that play a role in the enhanced clearance of *L. monocytogenes* in the early stage of infection (TAKADA et al. 1994), and a second study has shown that the presence of NK cells inhibits the accumulation of neutrophils in bacterially infected lesions (NEWTON et al. 1992).

5 Conclusions

It is now clear that NK cells can participate in host resistance to viruses, parasites, and intracellular bacteria, that they can be mediators of natural or "innate" immunity in the absence of T and B cells, and that they can influence specific immune responses by directing shifts in the Th1/Th2 ratios and by altering antibody isotype production by B cells (Fig. 2). To date many of the activities of NK cells have been attributed to their ability to secrete cytokines, most notably IFN-γ, which can establish an antiviral and antimicrobial state in infected cells, in part by inducing iNOS, which generates

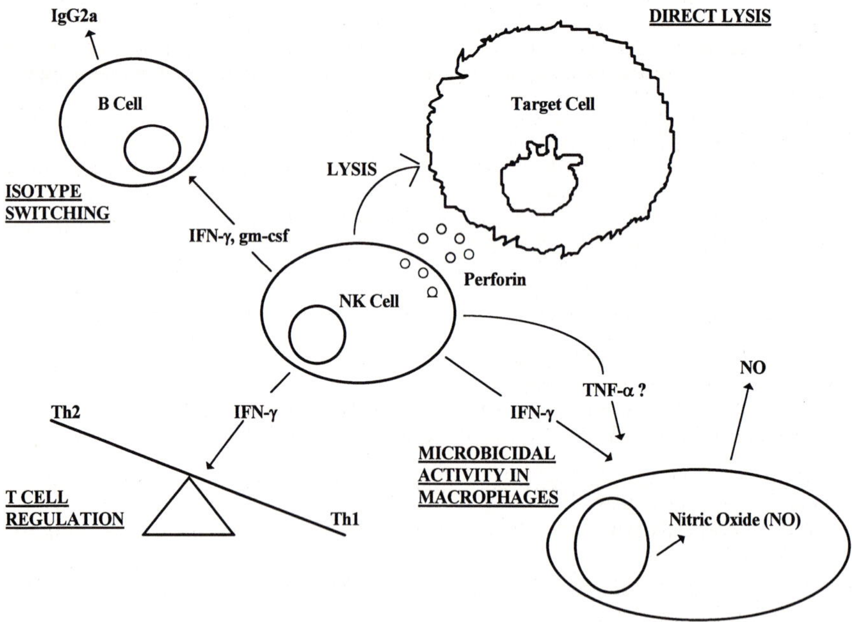

Fig. 2. Function of NK cells in the regulation of infections

the antimicrobial metabolite NO. IFN-γ can suppress the development of Th2 cells and augment the expansion of Th1 cells. In addition, it is an antibody switch factor that stimulates B cells to produce IgG2a, an antibody isotype that can be engaged by the Fc receptors on the NK cell. For IFN-γ to be made by NK cells the pathogen must induce from macrophages the synthesis of IL-12, which enhances the translation of the NK cell IFN-γ mRNA into protein. The ability of NK cells to lyse in vitro target cells harboring intracellular pathogens suggests that the cytotoxic function of NK cells also play a role in the control of these infections, but the evidence for this is restricted to the control of MCMV in the spleen, which is deficient in mice lacking perforin. The control of MCMV and ectromelia virus synthesis in the mouse spleen maps within the complex of genes that encode receptors on NK cells. This might suggest the presence of an NK cell receptor molecule that recognizes and facilitates the lysis of virus-infected splenocytes, but this still needs to be resolved. Although many viral infections can downregulate or otherwise alter class I MHC expression, the role of class I molecules in the control of infections by NK cells remains undefined. Clarification of these issues should soon be forthcoming.

References

Abbas AK, Burstein HJ, Bogen SA (1993) Determinants of helper T cell-dependent antibody production. Semin Immunol 5:441–447

Afonso LCC, Scharton TM, Vieira LQ, Wysocka M, Trinchieri G, Scott P (1994) The adjuvant effect of interleukin-12 in a vaccine against Leishmania major. Science 263:235–237

Appelberg R, Castro AG, Pedrosa J, Silva RA, Orme IM, Minoprio P (1994) Role of gamma interferon and tumor necrosis factor alpha during T-cell-independent and -dependent phases of mycobacterium avium infection. Infect Immun 62:3962–3971

Arora DJS, Houde M (1988) Purified glycoproteins of influenza virus stimulate cell-mediated cytotoxicity in vivo. Nat Immun Cell Growth Regul 7:287–296

Arora DJS, Houde M, Justewicz DM, Mandeville R (1984) In vitro enhancement of human natural cell-mediated cytotoxicity by purified influenza virus glycoproteins. J Virol 52:839–845

Bandyopadhyay S, Ziegner U, Campbell DE, Miller DS, Hoxie JA (1990) Natural killer cell-mediated lysis of T cell lines chronically infected with HIV-1. Clin Exp Immunol 79:430–435

Beckerman KP, Rogers HW, Corbett JA, Schreiber RD, McDaniel ML, Unanue ER (1993) Release of nitric oxide during T cell-independent pathway of macrophage activation. J Immunol 150:888–895

Beersma MFC, Bijlmakers MJE, Ploegh HL (1993) Human cytomegalovirus down-regulates HLA class I expression by reducing the stability of class I H chains. J Immunol 151:4455–4464

Bellone G, Valiante NM, Viale O, Ciccone E, Moretta L, Trinchieri G (1993) Regulation of hematopoiesis in vitro by alloreactive natural killer cell clones. J Exp Med 177:1117–1125

Bezouska K, Yuen C-T, O'Brien J, Childs RA, Chai W, Lawson AM, Drbal K, Fiserova A, Pospisil M, Feizi T (1994) Oligosaccharide ligands for NKR-P1protein activate NK cells and cytotoxicity. Nature 372:150–157

Biron CA (1994) Cytokines in the generation of immune responses to, and resolution of, virus infection. Curr Opin Immunol 6:530–538

Biron CA, Welsh RM (1982) Blastogenesis of natural killer cells during viral infections in vivo. J Immunol 129:2788–2798

Biron CA, Sonnenfeld G, Welsh RM (1984) Interferon induces natural killer cell blastogenesis in vivo. J Leukoc Biol 35:31–37

Biron CA, Byron KS, Sullivan JS (1989) Severe herpes virus infections in an adolescent without natural killer cells. N Engl J Med 320:1731–1735

Bonagura VR, Cunningham-Rundles SL, Schuval S (1992) Dysfunction of natural killer cells in human immunodeficiency virus-infected children with or without Pneumocystis carinii pneumonia. J Pediatr 121:195–201

Boos J, Wheelock EF (1971) Correlation of survival from MCMV infection with spleen cell responsiveness to concanavalin A. Proc Soc Exp Biol Med 149:443–446

Borrow P, Tishon A, Lee S, Xu J, Greval IS, Oldstone MBA, Flavell RA (1996) CD40L-deficient mice show deficits in antiviral immunity and have impaired memory $CD8^+$ CTL response. J Exp Med 183:2129–2142

Borysiewicz LK, Rodgers B, Morris S, Graham S, Sissons JGP (1985) Lysis of human cytomegalovirus infected fibroblasts by natural killer cells: demonstration of an interferon-independent component requiring expression of early viral proteins and characterization of effector cells. J Immunol 134:2695–2701

Brenner MK, Vyakarnam A, Reittie JE, Wimperis JZ, Grob JP, Hoffbrand AV, Prentice HG (1987) Human large granular lymphocytes induce immunoglobulin synthesis after bone marrow transplantation. Eur J Immunol 17:43–47

Brubaker JO (1993) Studies on the natural killer cell-mediated resistance to murine cytomegalovirus infection. Thesis, Worcester Polytechnic Institute

Brutkiewicz RR, Welsh RM (1995) Major histocompatibility complex class I antigens and the control of viral infections by natural killer cells. J Virol 69:3967–3971

Brutkiewicz RR, Klaus SJ, Welsh RM (1992) Window of vulnerability of vaccinia virus-infected cells to natural killer (NK) cell-mediated cytolysis correlates with enhanced NK cell triggering and is concomitant with a decrease in H-2 class I antigen expression. Nat Immun 11:203–214

Bukowski JF, Welsh RM (1985a) Inability of interferon to protect virus-infected cells against lysis by natural killer (NK) cells correlates with NK cell-mediated antiviral effects in vivo. J Immunol 135:3537–3541

Bukowski JF, Welsh RM (1985b) Interferon enhances the susceptibility of virus-infected fibroblasts to cytotoxic T cells. J Exp Med 161:257–262

Bukowski JF, Welsh RM (1986) Enhanced susceptibility to cytotoxic T lymphocytes of target cells isolated from virus-infected or interferon-treated mice. J Virol 59:735–739

Bukowski JF, Woda BA, Habu S, Okumura K, Welsh RM (1983) Natural killer cell depletion enhances virus synthesis and virus-induced hepatitis in vivo. J Immunol 131:1531–1538

Bukowski JF, Woda BA, Welsh RM (1984) Pathogenesis of murine cytomegalovirus infection in natural killer cell-depleted mice. J Virol 52:119–128

Bukowski JF, Warner JF, Dennert G, Welsh RM (1985) Adoptive transfer studies demonstrating the antiviral effect of natural killer cells in vivo. J Exp Med 161:40–52

Burns WH, Billups LC, Notkins AL (1975) Thymus dependence of viral antigens. Nature 256:654–656

Campbell AE, Slater JS (1994) Down-regulation of major histocompatibility complex class I synthesis by murine cytomegalovirus early gene expression. J Virol 68:1805–1811

Casali P, Sissons JGP, Buchmeier MJ, Oldstone MBA (1981) In vitro generation of human cytotoxic lymphocytes by viral glycoproteins induce nonspecific cell-mediated cytotoxicity without release of interferon. J Exp Med 154:840–855

Chadwick BS, Sambhara SR, Sasakura Y, Miller RG (1992) Effect of class I MHC binding peptides on recognition by natural killer cells. J Immunol 149:3150–3156

Chambers BJ, Salcedo M, Ljunggren H-G (1996) Triggering of natural killer cells by the costimulatory molecule CD80 (B7-1). Immunity 5:311–317

Ching C, Lopez C (1979) Natural killing of herpes virus type-1-infected target cells: normal human responses and influence of anti-viral antibody. Infect Immun 26:49–56

Collins JT, Dunnick WA (1993) Germline transcripts of the murine immunoglobulin gamma2a gene: structure and induction by IFN-gamma. Int Immunol 5:885–891

Colonna M (1996) Natural killer cell receptors specific for MHC class I molecules. Curr Opin Immunol 8:101–107

Correa I, Raulet DH (1995) Binding of diverse peptides to MHC class I molecules inhibits target cell lysis by activated natural killer cells. Immunity 2:61–71

Courtelier J-P, Jos TM, Van der Logt JT, Hessen FWA, Vink A, Van Snick J (1988) Virally induced modulation of murine IgG antibody subclasses. J Exp Med 168:2373–2378

Daniels BF, Nakamura MC, Rosen SD, Yokoyama WM, Seaman WE (1994) Ly-49A, a receptor for $H\text{-}2D^d$, has a functional carbohydrate recognition domain. Immunity 1:785–792

Dawson JR, Storkus WJ, Patterson EB, Cresswell P (1989) Adenovirus inversely modulates target cell class I MHC antigen expression and sensitivity to natural killing. In: Ades EW, Lopez C (eds) Natural killer cells and host defense. Karger, Basel, pp 156–159

del Val M, Hengel H, Hacker H, Hartlaub U, Ruppert T, Lucin P, Koszinowski UH (1992) Cytomegalovirus prevents antigen presentation by blocking the transport of peptide-loaded major histocompatibility complex class I molecules into the medial-golgi compartment. J Exp Med 176:729–738

Delano ML, Brownstein DG (1995) Innate resistance to lethal mousepox is genetically linked to the NK gene complex on chromosome 6 and correlates with early restriction on virus replication by cells with an NK phenotype. J Virol 69:5875–5877

Denkers EY, Gazzinelli RT, Martin D, Sher A (1993) Emergence of $NK1.1^+$ cells as effectors of IFN-gamma dependent immunity to Toxoplasma gondii in MHC class I-deficient mice. J Exp Med 178:1465–1472

Friedman DJ, Ricciardi RP (1988) Adenovirus type 12 E1A gene represses accumulation of MHC class I mRNAs at the level of transcription. Virology 165:303–305

Fruh K, Ahn K, Djaballah H, Sempe P, van Endert PM, Tampe R, Peterson PA, Yang Y (1995) A viral inhibitor of peptide transporters for antigen presentation. Nature 375:415–418

Garcia-Penarrubia P, Koster FT, Kelley RO, McDowell TD, Bankhurst AD (1989) Antibacterial activity of human natural killer cells. J Exp Med 169:99–113

Gazzinelli RT, Hieny S, Wynn TA, Wolf S, Sher A (1993) Interleukin 12 is required for the T-lymphocyte-independent induction of interferon gamma by an intracellular parasite and induces resistance in T-cell-deficient hosts. Proc Natl Acad Sci USA 90:6115–6119

Gidlund M, Orn A, Wigzell H, Senik A, Gresser I (1978) Enhanced NK activity in mice injected with interferon and interferon inducers. Nature 273:759–761

Glas R, Sturmhoffel K, Hammerling GJ, Karre K, Ljunggren H (1992) Restoration of a tumorigenic phenotype by β_2-microglobulin transfection to EL-4 mutant cells. J Exp Med 175:843–846

Glesch IEA, Kaufmann SHE (1991) Mechanisms involved in mycobacterial growth inhibition by gamma interferon-activated bone marrow macrophages: role of reactive nitrogen intermediates. Infect Immun 59:3213–3218

Griggs ND, Smith RA (1994) Natural killer cell activity against uninfected and Salmonella typhimurium-infected murine fibroblast L929 cells. Nat Immun 13:42–48

Guidotti LG, Ishikawa T, Hobbs MV, Matzke B, Schreiber R, Chisari FV (1996) Intracellular inactivation of the hepatitis B virus by cytotoxic T lymphocytes. Immunity 4:25–36

Gumperz JE, Parham P (1995) The enigma of the natural killer cell. Nature 378, 245–248

Guo Y, Niesel DW, Ziegler HK, Klimpel GR (1992) Listeria monocytogenes activation of human perpheral blood lymphocytes: induction of non-major histocompatibility complex-restricted cytotoxic activity and cytokine production. Infect Immun 60:1813–1819

Hansson M, Kiessling R, Andersson B, Welsh RM (1980) Effect of interferon and interferon inducers on the NK sensitivity of normal mouse thymocytes. J Immunol 125:2225–2231

Harfast B, Orvell C, Alsheikhly A, Andersson T, Perlmann P, Norrby E (1980) The role of viral glycoproteins in mumps virus-dependent lymphocyte-mediated cytotoxicity in vitro. Scand J Immunol 11:391–400

Harris N, Buller RML, Karupiah G (1995) Gamma interferon-induced, nitric oxide-mediated inhibition of vaccinia virus replication. J Virol 69:910–915

Hengel H, Flohr T, Hammerling GJ, Koszinowski UH, Momburg F (1996) Human cytomegalovirus inhibits peptide translocation into the endoplasmic reticulum for MHC class I assembly. J Gen Virol 77:2287–2296

Herlyn D, Koprowski H (1982) IgG2a monoclonal autobodies inhibit human tumor growth through interaction with effector cells. Proc Natl Acad Sci USA 79:4761–4765

Hermiston TW, Tripp RA, Sparer T, Gooding LR, Wold WSM (1993) Deletion mutation analysis of the adenovirus type 2 E3-gp 19 K protein: identification of sequences within the endoplasmic reticulum luminal domain that are required for class I antigen binding and protection from adenovirus-specific cytotoxic T lymphocytes. J Virol 67:5289–5298

Hill A, Jugovic P, York I, Russ G, Bennink J, Yewdell J, Ploegh H, Johnson D (1995) Herpes simplex virus turns off the TAP to evade host immunity. Nature 375:411–415

Hill AB, Barnett BC, McMichael AJ, McGeoch DJ (1994) HLA class I molecules are not transported to the cell surface in cells infected with herpes simplex virus types 1 and 2. J Immunol 152:2736–2741

Hu PF, Hultin LE, Hausner MA, Hirji K, Jewett A, Bonavida B, Detels R, Giogi JV (1995) Natural killer cell immunodeficiency in HIV disease is manifest by profoundly decreased numbers of CD16$^+$ CD56$^+$ cells and expansion of a population of CD16dim D56$^-$ cells with low lytic activity. J AIDS Hum Retrovirol 10:331–40

Imreh MP, Zhang Q, De Campos-Lima PO, Imreh S, Krausa P, Browning M, Klein G, Masucci MG (1995) Mechanisms of allele-selective down-regulation of HLA class I in Burkitt's lymphoma. Int J Cancer 62:90–96

Johnson LL, Sayles PC (1995) Strong cytolytic activity of natural killer cells is neither necessary nor sufficient for preimmune resistance to Toxoplasma gondii infection. Nat Immunol 14:209–215

Jones TR, Hanson LK, Sun L, Slater JS, Stenberg RM, Campbell AE (1995) Multiple independent loci within the human cytomegalovirus unique short region down-regulate expression of major histocompatibility complex class I heavy chains. J Virol 69:4830–4841

Karlhofer FM, Hunziker R, Reichin A, Margulies DH, Yokoyama WM (1994) Host MHC class I molecules modulate in vivo expression of a NK cell receptor. J Immunol 153:2407–2416

Karupiah G, Blanden RV, Ramshaw IA (1990) Interferon gamma is involved in the recovery of athymic nude mice from recombinant vaccinia virus/interleukin 2 infection. J Exp Med 172:1495–1503

Karupiah G, Xie Q-W, Buller RML, Nathan C, Duarte C, MacMicking JD (1993) Inhibition of viral replication by interferon gamma-induced nitric oxide synthase. Science 261:1445–1448

Katz P, Yeager H Jr, Whalen G, Evans M, Swartz RP, Roecklein J (1990) Natural killer cell-mediated lysis of Mycobacterium-avium complex-infected monocytes. J Clin Immunol 10:71–77

Kaufman DS, Schoon RA, Leibson PJ (1992) Role of major histocompatibility complex class I in regulating natural killer cell-mediated killing of virus-infected cells. Proc Natl Acad Sci USA 89:8337–8341

Kiessling R, Welsh RM (1980) Killing of normal cells by activated mouse natural killer cells: evidence for two patterns of genetic regulation of lysis. Int J Cancer 25:611–615

Kiessling R, Klein E, Pross H, Wigzell H (1975) 'Natural' killer cells in the mouse. II. Cytotoxic cells with specificity for mouse Moloney leukemia cells. Characteristic of the killer cell. Eur J Immunol 5:117–121

Klimpel GR, Niesel DW, Klimpel KD (1986) Natural cytotoxic effector cell activity against Shigella flexneri-infected HeLa cells. J Immunol 136:1081–1086

Kurago ZB, Smith KD, Lutz CT (1995) NK cell recognition of MHC class I: NK cells are sensitive to peptide-binding groove and surface a-helical mutations that affect T cells. J Immunol 154:2631–2641

Kuribayashi K, Gillis S, Kern DE, Henney CS (1981) Murine NK cells cultures: effects of interleukin-2 and interferon on cell growth and cytotoxic reactivity. J Immunol 126:2321–2327

Laskay T, Rollinghoff M, Solbach W (1993) Natural killer cells participate in the early defense against Leishmania major infection in mice. Eur J Immunol 23:2237–2241

Lee GD, Keller R (1982) Natural cytotoxicity to murine cytomegalovirus-infected cells mediated by mouse lymphoid cells: role of interferon in the endogenous natural cytotoxicity reaction. Infect Immun 35:5–12

Leibson PJ (1995) MHC-recognizing receptors: they're not just for T cells anymore. Immunity 3:5–8

Levitskyaya J, Coram M, Levitsky V, Imreh S, Steigerwald-Mullen PM, Klein G, Kurilla MG, Masucci MG (1995) Inhibition of antigen processing by the internal repeat region of the Epstein-Barr virus nuclear antigen-1. Nature 375:685–688

Ljunggren H, Sturmhoffel K, Wolpert E, Hammerling GJ, Karre K (1990) Transfection of β_2-microglobulin restores IFN-mediated protection from natural killer cell lysis in YAC-1 lymphoma variants. J Immunol 145:380–386

Ljunggren H-G, Karre K (1990) In search of the 'missing self': MHC molecules and NK cell recognition. Immunol Today 11:237–243

Lucin P, Jonjic S, Messerle M, Polic B, Hengel H, Koszinowski UH (1994) Late phase inhibition of murine cytomegalovirus replication by synergistic action of interferon-gamma and tumor necrosis factor. J Gen Virol 75:10–110

MacMicking JD, Nathan C, Hom G, Chartrain N, Fletcher DS, Trumbauer M, Stevens K, Xie QW, Sokol K, Hutchinson N (1995) Altered responses to bacterial infection and endotoxic shock in mice lacking inducible nitric oxide synthase. Cell 81:641–650

Malnati MS, Lusso P, Ciccone E, Moretta A, Moretta L, Long EO (1993) Recognition of virus-infected cells by natural killer cell clones is controlled by polymorphic cell elements. J Exp Med 178:961–969

Malnati MS, Peruzzi M, Parker KC, Biddison WE, Ciccone E, Moretta A, Long EO (1995) Peptide specificity in the recognition of MHC class I by natural killer cell clones. Science 267:1016–1018

Mandelboim O, Reyburn HT, Vales-Gomez M, Pazmany L, Colonna M, Borsellino G, Strominger JL (1996) Protection from lysis by natural killer cells of group 1 and 2 specificity is mediated by residue 80 in human histocompatibility leukocyte antigen C alleles and also occurs with empty major histocompatibility complex molecules. J Exp Med 184:913–922

Mason PD, Sissons JGP, Borysiewicz LK (1993) Heterogeneity amongst natural killer cells revealed by limiting dilution culture; selectivity against virus-infected and tumor cell targets. Immunology 80:625–632

Masucci MG, Torsteinsdottir S, Colombani J, Braubar C, Klein E, Klein G (1987) Down-regulation of class I HLA antigens and of the Epstein-Barr virus-encoded latent membrane protein in Burkitt lymphoma lines. Proc Natl Acad Sci USA 84:4567–4571

Masucci MG, Stam NJ, Torsteinsdottir S, Neefjes JJ, Klein G, Ploegh HL (1989) Allele-specific down-regulation of MHC class I antigens in Burkitt lymphoma lines. Cell Immunol 120:396–400

McIntyre KW, Welsh RM (1986) Accumulation of natural killer and cytotoxic T large granular lymphocytes in the liver during virus infection. J Exp Med 164:1667–1681

Michael A, Hackett JJ, Bennett M, Kumar V, Yuan D (1988) Regulation of B lymphocytes by natural killer cells Role of IFN-gamma. J Immunol 142:1095–1101

Michael A, Shao A, Yuan D (1991) Productive interactions between B and natural killer cells. Nat Immun Cell Growth Regul 10:71–82

Mond JJ, Lees A, Snapper CM (1995) T cell-independent antigens type 2. Annu Rev Immunol 13:655–698

Montel AH, Morse PA, Brahmi Z (1995) Upregulation of B7 molecules by the Epstein-Barr virus enhances susceptibility to lysis by a human NK-like cell line. Cell Immunol 160:101–114

Muller U, Steinhoff U, Reis LFL, Hemmi S, Pavlovic J, Zinkernagel RM, Aguet M (1994) Functional role of type I and type II interferons in antiviral defense. Science 264:1918–1921

Nathan C (1992) Nitric oxide as a secretory product of mammalian cells. FASEB J 6:3051–3064

Natuk RJ, Welsh RM (1987a) Accumulation and chemotaxis of natural killer/large granular lymphocytes at sites of virus replication. J Immunol 138:877–883

Natuk RJ, Welsh RM (1987b) Chemotactic effect of human recombinant interleukin 2 on mouse activated large granular lymphocytes. J Immunol 139:2737–2743

Natuk RJ, Bukowski JF, Brubaker JO, Welsh RM (1989) Antiviral effect of lymphokine-activated killer cells: chemotaxis and homing to sites of virus infection. J Virol 63:4969–4971

Newton DWJ, Runnels HA, Kearns RJ (1992) Enhanced splenic bacterial clearance and neutrophilia in anti-NK11-treated mice infected with Pseudomonas aeruginosa. Nat Immun 11:335–344

Noelle RJ, McCann J, Marshall L, Bartlett WC (1989) Cognate interactions between helpher T cells and B cells Contact-dependent, lymphokine-independent induction of B cell cycle entry by activated helper T cells. J Immunol 143:1807–1814

O'Shea J, Ortaldo JR (1992) The biology of natural killer cells: insights into the molecular basis of function. In: Lewis CE, McGee JO (eds) The natural killer cell. IRL, Oxford, pp 2–40

Orange JS, Biron CA (1996a) An absolute and restricted requirement for IL-12 in natural killer IFN-gamma production and antiviral defense. J Immunol 156:1138–1142

Orange JS, Biron CA (1996b) Characterization of early IL-12, IFN-$\alpha\beta$, and TNF effects on antiviral state and NK cell responses during murine cytomegalovirus infection. J Immunol 156:4746–4756

Orange JS, Wang B, Terhorst C, Biron CA (1995) Requirement for natural killer cell-produced interferon gamma in defense against murine cytomegalovirus infection and enhancement of this defense pathway by interleukin 12 administration. J Exp Med 182:1045–1056

Oswald IP, Caspar P, Jankovic D, Wynn TA, Pearce EJ, Sher A (1994) IL-12 inhibits Th2 cytokine responses induced by eggs of Schistosoma mansoni. J Immunol 153:1707–1713

Pavic I, Polic B, Crnkovic I, Lucin P, Jonjic S, Koszinowski UH (1993) Participation of endogenous tumour necrosis factor a in host resistance to cytomegalovirus infection. J Gen Virol 74:2215–2223

Paya CV, Kenmotsu N, Schoon RA, Leibson PJ (1988) Tumor necrosis factor and lymphotoxin secretion by human natural killer cells leads to anti-viral cytotoxicity. J Immunol 141 1989–1995

Pazmany L, Mandelboim O, Vales-Gomez M, Davis DM, Reyburn HT, Strominger JL (1996) Protection from natural killer cell-mediated lysis by HLA-G expression on target cells. Science 274:792–795

Ramarathinam L, Niesel DW, Klimpel GR (1993) Salmonella typhimurium induces IFN-gamma production in murine splenocytes. J Immunol 150:3973–3981

Raulet DH, Held W (1995) Natural killer cell receptors: the offs and ons of NK cell recognition. Cell 82:697–700

Romani L, Mencacci A, Cenci E, Spaccapelo R, Schiaffella E, Tonnetti L, Puccetti P, Bistoni F (1993) Natural killer cells do not play a dominant role in $CD4^+$ subset differentiation in Candida albicans-infected mice. Infect Immun 61:3769–3774

Routes JM (1992) IFN increases class I MHC antigen expression on adenovirus-infected human cells without inducing resistance to natural killer cell killing. J Immunol 149:2372–2377

Ruscetti FW, Mikovits JA, Kalyanaraman VS, Overton R, Stevenson H, Stromberg K, Herberman RB, Farrar WL, Ortaldo JR (1986) Analysis of effector mechanisms against HTLV-1- and HTLV-III/LAV-infected lymphoid cells. J Immunol 136:3619–3624

Santoli D, Koprowski H (1979) Mechanisms of activation of human natural killer cells against tumor and virus-infected cells. Immunol Rev 44:125–163

Scalzo AA, Fitzgerald NA, Simmons A, La Vista AB, Shellam GR (1990) Cmv-1, a genetic locus that controls murine cytomegalovirus replication in the spleen. J Exp Med 171:1469–1483

Scalzo AA, Fitzgerald NA, Wallace CR, Gibbons AE, Cheng Smart Y, Burton RC, Shellam GR (1992) The effect of the Cmv-1 resistance gene, which is linked to the natural killer cell gene complex, is mediated by natural killer cells. J Immunol 149:58196589

Scalzo AA, Lyons PA, Fitzgerald NA, Forbes CA, Shellam GR (1995a) The BALBB6-Cmv-1^r mouse: a strain congenic for Cmv-1 and the NK gene complex. Immunogenetics 41:148–151

Scalzo AA, Lyons PA, Fitzgerald NA, Forbes CA, Yokoyama WM, and Shellam GR (1995b) Genetic mapping of Cmv-1 in the region of mouse chromosome 6 encoding NK gene complex-associated loci Ly49 and musNKR-P1. Genomics 27:435–441

Scharton TM, Scott P (1993) Natural killer cells are a source of interferon gamma that drives differentiation of $CD4^+$ T cell subsets and induces early resistance to Leishmania major in mice. J Exp Med 178:567–577

Scharton-Kersten T, Scott P (1995) The role of the innate immune response in Th1 cell development following Leishmania major infection. J Leukoc Biol 57:515–522

Scharton-Kersten T, Afonso LCC, Wysocka M, Trinchieri G, Scott P (1995) Interleukin 12 is required for natural killer cell activation and subsequent T helper cell development in experimental leishmaniasis. J Immunol 154:5320–5330

Scheppler JA, Nicholson JKA, Swan DC, Ahmed-Ansari A, McDougal JS (1989) Down-modulation of MHC-I in a $CD4^+$ T cell line, CEM-E5, after HIV-1 infection. J Immunol 143:2858–2866

Schust DJ, Hill AB, Ploegh HL (1996) Herpes simplex virus blocks intracellular transport of HLA-G in placentally derived human cells. J Immunol 157:3375–3380

Scott P, Trinchieri G (1995) The role of natural killer cells in host-parasite interactions. Curr Opin Immunol 7:34–40

Sentman CL, Olsson MY, Karre K (1995) Missing self recognition by natural killer cells in MHC class I transgenic mice A 'receptor calibration' model for how effector cells adapt to self. Semin Immunol 7:109–119

Shellam GR, Allan JE, Papadimitriou JM, Bancroft GJ (1981) Increased susceptibility to cytomegalovirus infection in beige mutant mice. Proc Natl Acad Sci USA 78:5104–5108

Shemesh J, Rotem-Yehudar R, Ehrlich R (1991) Transcriptional and postranscriptional regulation of class I major histocompatibility complex genes following transformation with human adenoviruses. J Virol 65:5544–5548

Sher A, Oswald IP, Hieny S, Gazzinelli RT (1993) Toxoplasma gondii induces a T-independent IFN-gamma response in natural killer that requires both adherent accessory cells and tumor necrosis factor-alpha. J Immunol 150:3982–3989

Snapper CM, Mond JJ (1993) Towards a comprehensive view of immunoglobulin class switching. Immunol Today 14:15–17

Snapper CM, Mond JJ (1996) A model for induction of T cell-independent humoral immunity in response to polysaccharide antigens. J Immunol 157:2229–2233

Snapper CM, Yamaguchi H, Moorman MA, Sneed R, Smoot D, Mond JJ (1993) Natural killer cells induce activated murine B cells to secrete Ig. J Immunol 151:5251–52600

Snapper CM, Yamaguchi H, Moorman MA, Mond JJ (1994) An in vitro model for T cell-independent induction of humoral immunity. A requirement for NK cells. J Immunol 152:4884–4892

Snapper CM, Rasa FR, Moorman MA, Jin L, Shanebeck K, Klinman DM, Kehry MR, Mond JJ, Maliszewski CR (1996) IFN-gamma is a potent inducer of Ig secretion by sort-purified murine B cells activated through the mIg, but not the CD40 signalling pathway. Int Immunol 8:877–885

Storkus WJ, Dawson JR (1991) Target structures involved in natural killer (NK): characteristics, distribution, and candidate molecules. Crit Rev Immunol 10:393–416

Szomolanyi-Tsuda E, Welsh RM (1996) T cell-independent antibody-mediated clearance of polyomavirus in T cell-deficient mice. J Exp Med 183:403–411

Szomolanyi-Tsuda E, Dundon PL, Joris I, Schultz LD, Woda BA, Welsh RM (1994) Acute, lethal, natural killer cell-resistant myeloproliferative disease induced by polyomavirus in severe combined immunodeficient mice. Am J Pathol 144:359–371

Takada H, Matsuzaki G, Hiromatsu K, Nomoto K (1994) Analysis of the role of natural killer cells in Listeria monocytogenes infection: relation between natural killer and T-cell receptor gamma/delta T cells in the host defence mechanism at the early stage of infection. Immunology 82:106–112

Tarkkanen J, Saksela E, Lanier LL (1986) Bacterial activation of human natural killer cells. Characteristics of the activation process and identification of the effector cell. J Immunol 137:2428–2433

Tay CH, Welsh RM (1997) Distinct organ-dependent mechanisms for the control of murine cytomegalovirus infection by natural killer cells. J Virol 71:267–275

Tay CH, Welsh RM, Brutkiewicz RR (1995) NK cell response to viral infections in β_2-microglobulin-deficient mice. J Immunol 154:780–789

Teixeira HC, Kaufmann SHE (1994) Role of NK1.1$^+$ cells in experimental listeriosis. J Immunol 152:1873–1882

Thale R, Szepan U, Hengel H, Gegina G, Lucin P, Koszinowski UH (1995) Identification of the mouse cytomegalovirus genomic region affecting major histocompatibility complex class I molecule transport. J Virol 69:6098–6105

Trinchieri G (1989) Biology of natural killer cells. Adv Immunol 47:187–376

Trinchieri G, Santoli D (1978) Antiviral activity induced by culturing lymphocytes with tumor derived or virus-transformed cells. Enhancement of natural killer activity by interferon and antagonistic inhibition of susceptibility of target cells to lysis. J Exp Med 147:1314–1333

Tripp CS, Wolf SF, Unanue ER (1993) Interleukin 12 and tumor necrosis factor alpha are costimulators of interferon gamma production by natural killer cells in severe combined immunodeficiency mice with listeriosis, and interleukin 10 is a physiologic antagonist. Proc Natl Acad Sci USA 90:3725–3729

Tripp CS, Gately MK, Hakimi J, Ling P, Unanue ER (1994) Neutralization of IL-12 decreases resistance to Listeria in SCID and CB-17 mice. J Immunol 152:1883–1887

Tutt MM, Schuler W, Kuziel WA, Tucker PW, Bennett M, Bosma MJ, Kumar V (1987) T cell receptor genes do not rearrange or express functional T cell transcripts in natural killer cells of SCID mice. J Immunol 138:2338–2347

Ullum H, Gotzsche PC, Victor J, Dickmeiss E, Skinhoj P, Pedersen BK (1995) Defective natural immunity: an early manifestation of human immunodeficiency virus infection. J Exp Med 182:789–799

Wang B, Biron CA, She J, Higgins K, Sunshine M, Lacy E, Lonberg N, Terhorst C (1994) A block in both early T lymphocyte and natural killer cell development in transgenic mice with high copy numbers of the human CD3E gene. Proc Natl Acad Sci USA 91:9402–9406

Wang B, Hollander GA, Nichogiannopoulou A, Simpson SJ, Orange JS, Gutierrez-Ramos JC, Burakoff SJ, Biron CA, Terhorst C (1996) Natural killer cell development is blocked in the context of aberrant T lymphocyte ontogeny. Int Immunol 8:939–949

Warren AP, Ducroq DH, Lehner PJ, Borysiewicz LK (1994) Human cytomegalovirus-infected cells have unstable assembly of major histocompatibility complex class I complexes and are resistant to lysis by cytotoxic T lymphocytes. J Virol 68:2822–2829

Welsh RM (1978) Cytotoxic cells induced during lymphocytic choriomeningitis virus infection of mice. I. Characterization of natural killer cell induction. J Exp Med 148:163–181

Welsh RM, Vargas-Cortes M (1992) Natural killer cells in viral infection. In: Lewis CE, McGee JO (eds) The natural killer cell. The natural immune system. IRL, Oxford, pp 107–150

Welsh RM, Zinkernagel RM, Hallenbeck LA (1979) Cytotoxic cells induced during lymphocytic choriomeningitis virus infction of mice. II. Specificities of the natural killer cells. J Immunol 122:475–481

Welsh RM, Brubaker JO, Vargas-Cortes M, O'Donnell CL (1991) Natural killer (NK) cell response to virus infections in mice with severe combined immunodeficiency. The stimulation of NK cells and the NK cell-dependent control of virus infections occur independently of T and B cell functions. J Exp Med 173:1053–1063

Welsh RM, O'Donnell CL, Shultz LD (1994) Antiviral activity of NK1.1$^+$ natural killer cells in C57BL/6 SCID mice infected with murine cytomegalovirus. Nat Immun 13:239–245

Wiertz EJHJ, Jones TR, Sun L, Bogyo M, Geuze HJ, Ploegh HL (1996a) The human cytomegalovirus US11 gene product dislocates MHC class I heavy chains from the endoplasmic reticulum to the cytosol. Cell 84:769–779

Wiertz EJHJ, Tortorella D, Bogyo M, Yu J, Mothes W, Jones TR, Rapoport TA, Ploegh HL (1996b) Sec61-mediated transfer of a membrane protein from the endoplasmic reticulum to the proteasome for destruction. Nature 384:432–438

Wilder JA, Koh CY, Yuan D (1996) The role of NK cells during in vivo antigen-specific antibody responses. J Immunol 156:146–152

Wold WSM, Gooding LR (1991) Region E3 of adenovirus: a cassette of genes involved in host immunosurveillance and virus-cell interactions. Virology 184:1–8

Wolf SA, Tracey DE, Henney DS (1976) Induction of 'natural killer' cells by BCG. Nature 262:584–586

Wynn TA, Eltoum I, Oswald IP, Cheever AW, Sher A (1994) Endogenous interleukin 12 (IL-12) regulates granuloma formation induced by eggs of Schistosoma mansoni and exogenous IL-12 both inhibits and prophylactically immunizes against egg pathology. J Exp Med 179:1551–1561

Yamashita Y, Shimokata K, Saga S, Mizuno S, Tsurumi T, Nishiyama Y (1994) Rapid degradation of the heavy chain of class I major histocompatibility complex antigens in the endoplasmic reticulum of human cytomegalovirus-infected cells. J Virol 68:7933–7943

Yokoyama WM (1993) The Ly-49 and NKR-P1 gene families encoding lectin-like receptors on natural killer cells: the NK gene complex. Annu Rev Immunol 11:613–635

Yokoyama WM (1995) Natural killer cell receptors. Curr Opin Immunol 7:110–120

Young HA, Ortaldo JR (1987) One-signal requirement for interferon-gamma production by human large granular lymphocytes. J Immunol 139:724–727

Yuan D, Wilder JA, Dang T, Bennett M, Kumar V (1992) Activation of B lymphocytes by NK cells. Int Immunol 4:1373–1380

Zdravkovic M, Aboagye-Mathiesen G, Zachar V, Mosborg-Petersen P, Toth FD, Liu X, Ebbesen P (1994) In vitro cytotoxic activity of cord blood NK cells against herpes simplex virus type-1 infected purified human term villous cytotrophoblast. Viral Immunol 7:133–140

Natural Killer Cells and Tumor Therapy

T.L. WHITESIDE[1], N.L. VUJANOVIC[2], and R.B. HERBERMAN[3]

1 Introduction

Natural killer (NK) cells are a morphologically and functionally distinct subset of lymphocytes endowed with the ability spontaneously to kill virally infected and a wide variety of tumor cells but spare most normal cells (WHITESIDE and HERBERMAN 1995; VUJANOVIC et al. 1996). Recent studies indicate that NK cells are capable of mediating the killing of tumor cells by several distinct mechanisms, of secreting a broad spectrum of cytokines, and of extravasating as well as entering tissue sites, including premalignant or malignant tissues (WHITESIDE and HERBERMAN 1995; VUJANOVIC et al. 1996). NK cells are also known to be highly responsive to many biological agents, including cytokines such as interleukin (IL)-2 or IL-12 and interferons (IFNs), and rapidly to increase their cytolytic, secretory, proliferative, and

[1]Departments of Pathology and Otolaryngology, School of Medicine, and Cancer Institute, University of Pittsburgh, W1041 Biomedical Science Tower, 211 Lothrop Street, Pittsburgh, PA 15213-2582, USA

[2]Department of Pathology, School of Medicine, and Cancer Institute, University of Pittsburgh, W1041 Biomedical Science Tower, 211 Lothrop Street, Pittsburgh, PA 15213-2582, USA

[3]Departments of Pathology and Medicine, School of Medicine, and Cancer Institute, W1041 Biomedical Science Tower, 211 Lothrop Street, University of Pittsburgh, Pittsburgh, PA 15213-2582, USA

other functions upon stimulation with these agents (Vujanovic et al. 1996; Herberman et al. 1992).

A subset of IL-2 activated NK cells described by us recently comprises effector cells endowed with a set of phenotypic and functional characteristics that facilitate antitumor activities in tissues. These NK cells are referred to as A-NK cells, with the "A" signifying activation and adherence, both of which are necessary for isolation of A-NK cells from human peripheral blood lymphocytes (Vujanovic et al. 1993a) or from rodent splenocytes (Vujanovic et al. 1987). A-NK cells mediate potent antitumor activity, and based on extensive preclinical in vitro and in vivo experiments they have been selected for therapy of patients with cancer (Vujanovic et al. 1994b). In this chapter we summarize evidence for the role of activated NK cells in elimination of tumors or tumor metastases, highlighting their therapeutic potential, and then review the results of therapy with NK cells in patients with advanced cancer.

For several years our goal has been to develop a novel and effective strategy for immunotherapy of tumor metastases using NK cells. Two general strategies for the therapeutic use of NK cells have been considered. One involves upregulation of antitumor activity of endogenous NK cells, while the other depends on adoptive transfer of ex vivo activated NK cells. Both strategies have been evaluated experimentally in animal models of tumor metastasis and in human clinical trials. Of the two, activation of endogenous NK cells with biological response modifiers (BRMs) such as cytokines or with other agents seems to be conceptually more appealing. Its therapeutic efficacy depends, however, on the ability of the activating agents to mobilize a sufficient number of endogenous NK cells to the sites of metastasis and to achieve and maintain the level of activation necessary for eradication of these metastases. In tumor-bearing hosts, both these requirements might be difficult to achieve, as discussed below. Adoptive immunotherapy (AIT) with in vitro activated NK cells depends on the successful reconstitution of tumor-bearing hosts with effector cells, which are expected to reach the sites of metastasis and eliminate tumor cells without disturbing normal cells present in the microenvironment. In both circumstances NK cells are perceived as killers and tumor cells as victims, and the derived therapeutic benefits are thought to be the result of direct interactions between the two protagonists. In reality, the mechanisms responsible for the elimination of metastases by NK cells are much more complex, may not require direct contact of effector with target cells, and almost certainly involve active participation of tumor cells in determining the fate of antitumor effector cells in situ and even at sites distant from the tumor.

2 Antitumor Functions of Endogenous NK Cells

For many years NK cells have been recognized as effector cells responsible for the elimination of blood-borne metastases, and a considerable body of literature has accumulated in support of this concept (Whiteside and Herberman 1995; Vujanovic et al. 1996). Thus NK cells appear to serve as the earliest cellular effector mechanism against dissemination of blood-borne tumor cells. Early studies have shown that NK cells can rapidly eliminate tumor cells from the blood stream or from lungs in experimental animals (RICCARDI et al. 1980; BARLOZZARI et al. 1983). Several years ago GORELIK and HERBERMAN (1986) demonstrated that removal of NK cells from mice with surgically resected B16 melanoma resulted in uncontrolled metastasis and death of the animals. On the other hand, adoptive transfer of purified large granular lymphocytes to immunosuppressed rodents restores the resistance to metastasis (BARLOZZARI et al. 1983). In humans, NK activity appears to be important in control of metastases since patients with cancer who have low NK activity at diagnosis tend to develop metastases more frequently than those with normal levels of NK activity (WHITESIDE and HERBERMAN 1994). In patients with congenital or acquired immunodeficiencies, including the absence or defective function of NK cells, such as X-linked severe combined immunodeficiency (mutation of the γ chain of IL-2 receptor), Chediak-Higashi syndrome, AIDS, and posttransplant immunosuppression develop at a relatively high frequency certain types of malignancies, particularly lymphomas, leukemias, and Kaposi's sarcomas, (ROSEN et al. 1995; HO et al. 1988; ULLUM et al. 1995).

In addition, low NK activity has been reported in patients with preleukemic disorders (PROSS and LOTZOVA 1993) and in those with leukemia. Decreases in the level of NK activity often precede or accompany relapses following periods of therapy-induced remission (MATERA and GIANCOTTI 1983). Not only in patients with hematological malignancies but also in those with solid tissue cancers, levels of NK activity have been documented to decrease in concert with disease progression, and patients with advanced metastases often have abnormalities in NK cell function and/or NK cell numbers (INTRONA and MONTAVANI 1983; ZEIGLER et al. 1981). In several instances of familial cancer (e.g., familial melanoma or breast carcinoma), it has been shown that not only affected but also unaffected family members have low NK activity (STRAYER et al. 1984, 1986), an indication that the level of NK activity might be important as a predictive factor for cancer development. Together these observations suggest that endogenous NK cells play a role in the control of dissemination of cancer metastasis and in prevention of metastasis development (reviewed by WHITESIDE and HERBERMAN 1994).

3 Endogenous NK Cells in Tumors and Metastases

NK cells represent about 10% of circulating lymphocytes (WHITESIDE et al. 1990), and they also account for a substantial but variable proportion of tissue-resident lymphocytes. For example, in humans NK cells are found in the liver, lungs, spleen, lymph nodes, placenta, and intestine (reviewed by VUJANOVIC et al. 1996). In the normal liver close to 50% of liver-associated lymphocytes (LALs) are NK cells (WHITESIDE et al. 1990), which exhibit phenotypic and functional characteristics of precursors for a subset of activated NK cells, namely, A-NK cells (VUJANOVIC et al. 1993a,b). LALs have been shown to express CD69, CD25, and HLA-DR activation antigens and to have a higher level of expression of various adhesion molecules than NK cells in the peripheral blood (HATA et al. 1992). LALs have also been shown to mediate high levels of NK activity in vitro and to respond to exogenous IL-2 by rapid adherence to solid surfaces and extensive proliferation. While LALs are found largely in sinusoids, they are also detectable by immunostaining in the liver parenchyma (Garcia-Barcina et al. 1995). During inflammation, following tissue injury (e.g., in the early stages of liver regeneration) or a viral infection, the number of NK cells has been found to increase dramatically in the liver (Vujanovic et al. 1995b).

It is reasonable to hypothesize that cytokine cascades induced by the inflammatory processes regulate NK cell accumulation in the liver and other tissues. In support of this hypothesis, studies of Biron et al. in mice clearly delineate the hierarchy of cytokines involved in control of accumulation of tissue-infiltrating lymphocytes, including NK cells, during infection with lymphocytic choriomeningitis and murine cytomegalovirus (Biron et al. 1996). Also, a role for exogenous cytokines and other BRMs in the recruitment of NK cells into various organ sites, including liver, has been well documented in the literature (Wiltrout et al. 1984, 1989). Thus Basse and colleagues (1993) observed that the treatment of normal mice with poly I:C is followed by an increase in the number of NK cells in most organs. It has been reported that TNF-α plays an important role in the recruitment of NK cells into liver parenchyma following treatment with a BRM and suggested that TNF-α induced alterations of NK-endothelial cell interactions contribute to the entry of NK cells into tissues (Pilaro et al. 1994).

In tumor-bearing hosts, the administration of BRMs such as poly I:C or of cytokines induces accumulation of endogenous NK cells at tumor sites and metastases (Basse et al. 1993) whereas few NK cells are seen in established metastases of B16 melanoma not treated with a BRM (P.H. Basse, unpublished data). In human solid tumors tumor-infiltrating NK cells are either not detectable or are present in only a small number, as assessed by immunostaining of cryostat tumor sections with anti-CD56 or anti-CD16 antibodies (Vujanovic et al. 1996). In contrast, using the same antibodies for flow cytometry of tumor-infiltrating lymphocytes (TIL) it has been possible to show that NK cells represent a small but significant proportion of TILs in various solid tumors, including breast, ovarian, renal, head, and neck carcinomas and melanomas (Vujanovic et al. 1996; Lai et al. 1996).

In addition, our preliminary data indicate that a large majority of tumor-infiltrating human NK cells express a marker characteristic of pre-A-NK cells, termed ANK-1 (Vujanovic et al. 1993b). The ANK-1 epitope, which is recognized by the antibody produced in our laboratories, appears to be a 240-kDa isoform of neural cellular adhesion molecules (N-CAM) and is expressed on a subset of circulating NK cells (30%) capable of rapid adherence to solid substrates in the presence of IL-2 (Vujanovic et al. 1993a, 1995a). The antibody works well on cryostat tissue sections and in flow cytometry assays, and the immunostaining results indicate that in comparison to peripheral blood NK cells, ANK-1^+ NK cells are variably but significantly enriched (3- to 15-fold) in tumor tissues (N.L. Vujanovic, unpublished data). These results suggest that endogenous NK cells are able to reach tumor sites and are consistently found, albeit in small numbers, in human and experimental murine metastases.

Little is known about antitumor functions of tumor-infiltrating NK cells. As indicated above, most studies of NK cell functions in tumor-bearing hosts have been performed with circulating NK cells in humans and spleen-derived NK cells in

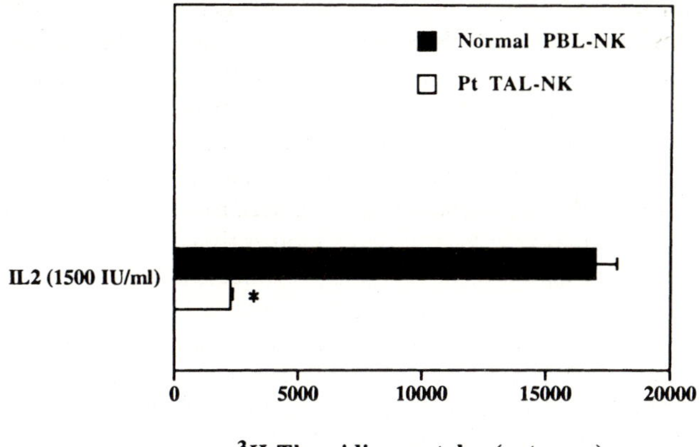

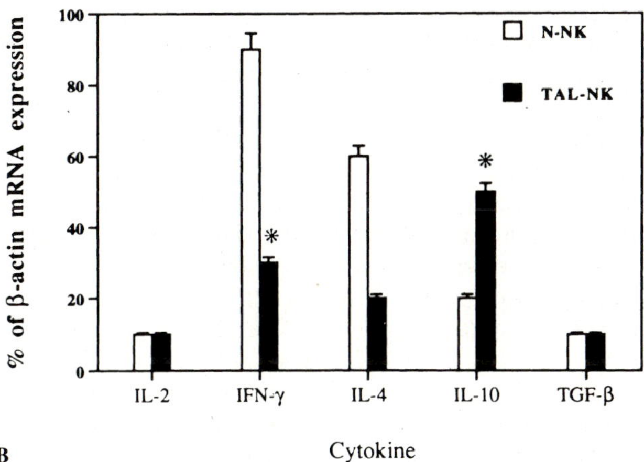

Fig. 1. A Proliferative response to IL-2 of NK cells purified from peripheral blood lymphocytes (*PBL-NK*) of normal donors (n=4) or from ovarian ascites of patients with advanced ovarian carcinoma (n=4). * p<0.001 between response of patients' vs. normal donors' NK cells. *TAL*, Tumor-associated lymphocytes. Proliferation of NK cells was measured in 3-day [^{3}H]thymidine incorporation assays. (Reproduced with permission from LAI et al. 1996) **B** Expression of mRNA for various cytokines in NK cells purified from PBL of normal donors (n=4) or TAL of patients with ovarian carcinoma (n=4). Results are from semiquantitative RT-PCR and represent means ± SEM of the ratio between each cytokine and β action mRNA expression. * p<0.05 in mRNA expression between N-NK vs. TAL-NK. (Reproduced with permission from RABINOWICH et al. 1996a)

rodents. Recently we have been able to purify NK cells from ascites obtained from women with ovarian cancer in numbers sufficient for phenotypic and functional studies (LAI et al. 1996). These NK cells were found to be defective in proliferative responses to IL-2 and the ability to produce IFN-γ, as compared to normal circulating NK cells (Fig. 1). Furthermore, defective expression of several signaling molecules,

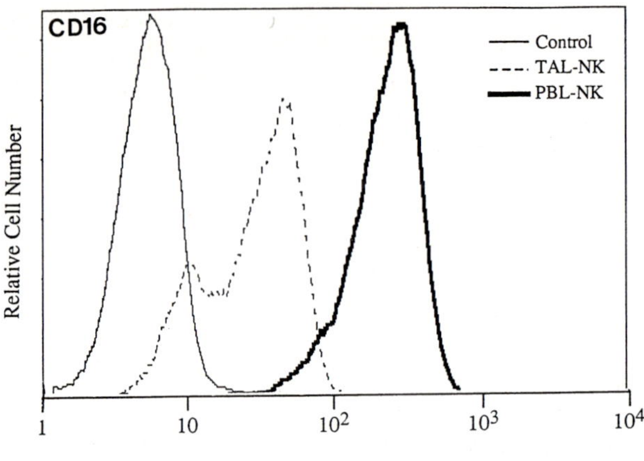

Fig. 2. Expression of FcγRIII (CD16) on the surface of NK cells purified from PBL of a normal donor or from TAL of a patient with ovarian carcinoma. Control is isotype-matched IgG. Note decreased expression of CD16 on the patient's NK cells. Representative data of seven experiments with cells of different individuals. (Reproduced with permission from LAI et. 1996)

including the ζ chain associated with FcγRIII and $p56^{lck}$, was detected in NK cells obtained from ovarian ascites but not normal NK cells. Expression of FcγRIII on patients' NK cells was significantly decreased (Fig. 2), as measured by flow cytometry relative to that in normal NK cells (LAI et al. 1996).

These abnormalities were also observed in peripheral blood NK cells of patients with ovarian carcinoma (LAI et al. 1996; RABINOWICH et al. 1996a). Similar observations have been made by KIESSLING and collaborators, who studied NK cells in patients with colon carcinoma (MATSUDA et al. 1995). We have reported earlier that NK activity of TIL freshly isolated from human solid tumors was nearly absent but was induced by incubation of these cells in the presence of IL-2 (WHITESIDE 1993). Likewise, proliferative and signaling defects observed in human tumor-associated NK cells were repaired by exposure of NK cells to IL-2 in vitro or by administering high-dose IL-2 therapy to patients with metastatic melanoma (RABINOWICH et al. 1996b). In aggregate, these findings suggest that endogenous NK activity is compromised in tumor-bearing hosts but can be restored by immunotherapy.

While the evidence for tumor-induced immunosuppression and defective NK cell functions in patients with metastases is strong, as reviewed above, a controversy has developed with respect to the presence or extent of immunosuppression in murine hosts. OCHOA and colleagues have reported both decreased ζ chain expression and defective NFκ-B-mediated signaling in mice bearing advanced metastases (MIZOGUCHI et al. 1992). In contrast, LEVEY and SRIVASTAVA (1995) demonstrated no ζ chain defects in murine hosts with metastases from various tumor cell lines, therefore concluding that immune cells are functionally normal in tumor-bearing mice. Using in vitro 4-h ^{51}Cr release or ^{125}I-UdR release cytotoxicity assays and in vivo clearance assays with radiolabeled NK-sensitive tumor cell targets, others have demonstrated that endogenous NK cells in the liver or lung can mediate considerable antitumor cytotoxic activity (RICCARDI et al. 1980; GORELIK and HERBERMAN 1986; VUJANOVIC et al. 1995b; WILTROUT et al. 1985). Earlier studies utilizing NK depleting procedures also indicated an important role of NK cells in the processes of formation and elimination of metastases. Thus in animals treated with cyclophosphamide, β-estradiol, corticosteroids, urethane, anti-asialo-GM1 (ASGM1) or anti-NK1.1 antibodies, all of which eliminate circulating NK cells, clearance of intravenously injected tumor cells was depressed, and the number of metastases in the lungs or liver was significantly increased (RICCARDI et al. 1980; GORELIK and HERBERMAN 1986; VUJANOVIC et al. 1995b). Both normal levels of clearance of tumor cells and formation of lung metastases were completely restored in NK cell-depleted mice or rats by adoptive transfer of normal murine splenocytes containing NK cells or of highly purified rat NK cells, respectively, but not by intravenous injections of thymocytes or peritoneal macrophages (RICCARDI et al. 1980; GORELIK and HERBERMAN 1986; BARLOZZARI et al. 1985). Also, pretreatment of mice with high doses of anti-ASGM1 antibody, which eliminates circulating and splenic NK cells, facilitates establishment of experimental tumors and formation of metastases.

The data accumulated so far indicate that endogenous NK cells play an important role in tumor surveillance (reviewed by WHITESIDE and HERBERMAN 1995) and control of metastasis dissemination not only in the circulation but also in tissues. Once the tumor is established, it might subvert antitumor functions of NK cells, especially the subset of NK cells found at the sites of metastasis. Administration of BRMs or cytokines appear to be effective in reversing tumor-induced suppression of endogenous NK cells.

4 Upregulation of Antitumor Functions of Endogenous NK Cells

The potential of endogenous NK cells for prevention of metastasis formation and for elimination of existing metastases has been explored in various experimental tumor models. The rationale for these studies is based on the evidence reviewed above that NK cells are present in metastases but are not functionally competent, and that treatment with BRMs can induce activation and accumulation of endogenous NK cells in various organs, including those involved by metastases. Indeed, a series of studies performed by BASSE et al. (1993) demonstrated that administration of poly I:C to mice bearing established (12d) hepatic metastases of B16 melanoma resulted in significantly increased infiltration of ASGM1$^+$ NK cells in the liver, development of necrotic foci around these cells, and significantly decreased tumor burden (BASSE et al. 1993). These results indicate that the recruitment and accumulation of NK cells in metastases, which accompany the administration of BRMs to animals bearing established (day 9–12) B16 melanoma, might result in the destruction of tumor cells by mechanisms that involve killing by necrosis (BASSE et al. 1993).

NK cell proliferation in vitro and their cytotoxicity depend on the presence of IL-2. NK cells constitutively express IL-2R and are able to rapidly respond to IL-2 stimulation (CALIGIURI et al. 1990). It has been rationalized that delivering exogenous IL-2 to tumor-bearing animals should upregulate endogenous NK activity, leading to tumor rejection. However, therapy of mice bearing 3-day established lung or liver metastases with a moderate dose of IL-2 ($\sim 6\times 10^3$ IU) was not effective in elimination of metastases. On the other hand, antimetastatic effects were observed when a high-dose (60×10^3 IU) IL-2 therapy was used (BASSE et al. 1994). These data suggest that induction of antimetastatic activity of endogenous NK cells in situ or their recruitment from the bone marrow requires the delivery of high concentrations of exogenous IL-2.

With the advent of gene transfer technology it has become possible to transduce tumor cells or tissue cells such as fibroblasts with the IL-2 gene and upon selection of stable transfectants producing IL-2 to transfer these cells to experimental animals. BUBENIK and colleagues (1988) were the first to transfer genetically modified, IL-2-secreting fibroblasts to tumor-bearing mice and to document tumor regression resulting from this form of therapy. Numerous other investigators have successfully transduced tumor cells with the IL-2 gene and confirmed therapeutic effectiveness of this type of gene transfer (GANSBACHER et al. 1994; ZIER et al. 1994). The great majority of these studies have focused attention on T cells as effectors of antimetastatic activity in animals injected with genetically engineered IL-2-secreting cells (GANSBACHER et al. 1994; ZIER et al. 1994).

To determine effects of this form of therapy on NK cells we used two different xenograft models of human tumors growing in nude mice (NAGASHIMA et al. 1997a,b). The animals were injected subcutaneously with 10×10^6 squamous cell carcinoma cells to establish subcutaneous tumors or intrasplenically with 5×10^6 gastric carcinoma cells to establish liver metastases (NAGASHIMA et al. 1997a,b). Three types of tumor cells were injected each to groups of ten animals: (a) parental, nontransduced tumor cells; (b) *lacZ*-gene transduced tumor cells (control), and (c) tumor cells transduced with the IL-2 gene and producing more than 10 ng IL-2 per 10^5 cells/48 h. In both the subcutaneous tumor and liver metastasis models, transduced tumor cells initially grew as well as parental tumor cells. Within 4–5 days of their injection, however, IL-2-secreting tumors or tumor metastases became surrounded by mononuclear cells (Fig. 3a), and stopped progressing, while parental tumor or metastases were not infiltrated at all and continued to enlarge (NAGASHIMA et al. 1997a,b). Immunoperoxidase staining indicated that the infiltrating cells consisted of murine NK cells (NK1.1$^+$) and macrophages (Fig. 3b). Regression of the subcutaneous squamous cell carcinoma tumors and of liver metastases were observed in animals injected with tumor cells secreting IL-2 (NAGASHIMA et al. 1997a,b). We have confirmed that these tumor cells secreted IL-2 in vivo by measuring its level in the liver tissue as well as in the circulation (NAGASHIMA et al. 1997b). Mice with liver metastases secreting IL-2 failed to develop ascites and survived significantly longer (50 days) than those injected with parental tumor cells (days). The histological appearance of metastases or subcutaneous tumors established with IL-2-producing tumor cells was consistent with necrosis and apoptosis of tumor cells, presumably mediated by infiltrating NK cells or macrophages.

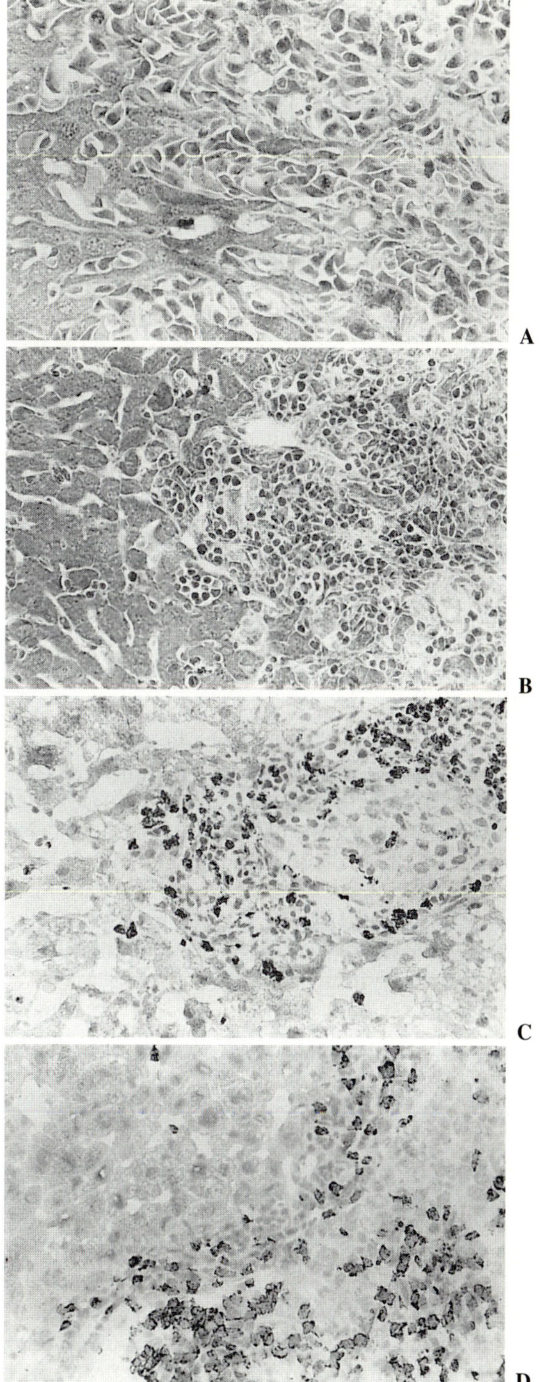

Fig. 3A–D. Histological or immunohistological findings in the liver of nude mice injected intrasplenically with parental or IL-2 gene transduced HR cells. **A** Liver metastases formed by parental HR cells. H&E staining, ×1000 **B** Liver metastases formed by IL-2 gene-transduced HR cells, H&E staining. Note numerous mononuclear cells. **C**,**D** Mononuclear cells around a liver metastasis formed by IL-2 gene-transduced HR cells stained with anti-mouse NK 5E6 mAb (**C**) or anti-mouse macrophage Mac-3 mAb (**D**). ×1000 (Reproduced with permission from NAGASHIMA et al. 1997b)

The remarkable thing about these experiments is that all nude mice were treated with anti-ASGM1 antibody throughout the experiment to eliminate circulating NK cells and to enable establishment and growth of tumors or metastases. However, locally secreted IL-2 induced influx of NK cells from the bone marrow or tissue sites, indicating that the antibody given at the dose of 0.2 mg/mouse did not deplete NK cell precursors or NK cells residing in tissues. Furthermore, IL-2 released locally at a sustained high level was able to induce tumor or metastasis regression in these animals, while therapy with exogenous IL-2 (60×10^3 IU twice daily for 5 days given i.p.) was ineffective in arresting growth or metastases of 3-day established tumor/metastases in the same animal models (Whiteside et al. unpublished data).

In humans high-dose IL-2 given as intravenous bolus injections three or four times a day or 24-h continuous infusions (18×10^6 IU/m^2) was shown to induce partial or complete responses in a proportion (20%–30%) of patients with metastatic melanoma or renal cell carcinoma (ROSENBERG et al. 1989). However, it remains undetermined why only some patients respond to this therapy, and the mechanism(s) responsible for tumor regression during systemic high-dose IL-2 therapy is not understood. The contribution of endogenous NK cells to a favorable response is not altogether clear. In vivo generation of lymphokine-activated killer (LAK) activity in the peripheral blood of patients treated with intravenous IL-2 has been reported (SONDEL 1989), but it is not correlated with clinical responses. On the other hand, continuous long-term infusion to cancer patients of low doses of IL-2 (2×10^5 U/m^2 per day) resulted in selective activation and in vivo expansion of circulating CD56^{bright} CD16$^-$ cells (CALIGIURI 1992). This subset of NK cells has been shown by CALIGIURI et al. to respond to low dose of IL-2 by proliferation in vitro, due to expression of high-affinity (α, β, γ) IL-2R [41]. However, in vivo expansion of circulating CD56^{bright} NK cells did not lead to appreciable clinical responses (SOIFFER et al. 1992). We interpret these results to indicate that this subset of endogenous NK cells, while able to kill tumor cell targets in vitro, is not as effective in extravasation and infiltration of tumor tissues as A-NK cells, which require high doses of IL-2 for optimal in vivo activity.

Exogenous IL-2 has also been delivered locally to the tumor site both in experimental animals and patients with cancer (SACCHI et al. 1991; WHITESIDE et al. 1993). The rationale for this therapeutic approach has been a desire to activate local effector cells, induce influx of additional effector cells to the tumor, and avoid toxicites associated with systemic IL-2 therapy. Various strategies have been used to deliver IL-2 to sites of tumor or metastases, including direct injections into or around the tumor (SACCHI et al. 1991), slow-release pumps implanted into tissues or delivery via lysosomes (ANDERSON et al. 1992). To the best of our knowledge, responses have been achieved using this strategy in some animal models of tumor growth (ANDERSON et al. 1992); locoregional delivery of exogenous IL-2 alone has not produced satisfactory clinical responses in patients with cancer (WHITESIDE et al. 1993).

On the other hand, there is emerging evidence that survival of patients with advanced metastatic disease may be prolonged following locoregional therapy with IL-2 (EDWARDS et al. 1997). Some of these studies found NK activity to be increased in the peripheral blood and documented in vivo LAK generation, but neither of these were correlated to clinical results, which were modest. In our hands, locoregional delivery of IL-2 to 36 patients with inoperable head and neck cancer during a phase

I dose-escalating trial resulted in one partial response (WHITESIDE et al. 1993). We did, however, demonstrate significant accumulation of activated NK cells at the tumor site and their activation by immunostaining of tumor sections and significant elevations in the number as well as the level of NK activity in the circulation of all patients participating in this trial (WHITESIDE et al. 1993). Thus local and systemic effects on NK cells were observed, but they did not lead to tumor shrinkage. Lack of therapeutic effects in this and other clinical trials with locoregionally delivered IL-2 may be due to excessive tumor burden present at the time of therapy or to inadequate (too little, too short) doses of IL-2 delivered.

Evidence for activation of endogenous NK cells during IL-2 therapy without accompanying clinical responses has introduced considerable skepticism about the role of NK cells in control of cancer. It has also led to re-evaluation of strategies for effective delivery of cytokines and other BRMs in order to optimally upregulate endogenous NK activity. Such a re-evaluation appears in order on the basis of work in animal models of metastasis, gene therapy experiments, and observations that some patients expected to die of metastatic disease within months survive for 5 or more years after IL-2 therapy (EDWARDS et al. 1997). Lessons from gene therapy experiments similar to those described above suggest that sustained activation of endogenous NK cells by IL-2 may be necessary to achieve clinical responses. This might require high doses of IL-2 administered over a period of time to facilitate effector cell extravasation, migration in tissues, localization to the tumor, and maintenance of effector cell function in the environment that is basically immunosuppressive. Alternatively, to avoid systemic toxicities of high-dose IL-2 sustained local release of IL-2 can be engineered by gene therapy or by various liposomal formulations. Clinical trials are in progress, implementing these strategies. It will be important to monitor events in tissue, especially at sites of metastases, to determine the nature, state of activation, numbers of infiltrating effector cells, and changes in the tumor microenvironment that occur during therapy to achieve a better understanding of the mechanisms responsible for therapeutic effects, if they are observed.

IL-2 is certainly not the only BRM that can be used for activation of endogenous NK cells. We have selected IL-2 as an example, because it is known to be necessary for activation, growth, and functions of NK cells, and because it has been extensively used in experimental and clinical trials. Other cytokines, including IL-12 and IFNs alone or in combination with IL-2, as well as other BRMs (e.g., OK432) have been investigated for the ability to upregulate antitumor functions of endogenous NK cells (e.g., NAUME et al. 1992; NASTALA et al. 1994; KIRKWOOD et al. 1997a). It is interesting to note that all of the above agents are effective in vitro in upregulating NK activity and generating LAK activity, using cells from animals with established metastases or patients with advanced cancer (reviewed in by WHITESIDE and HERBERMAN 1990). However, in human clinical trials, none, perhaps with the exception of IFN-α administered in the adjuvant setting (COLE et al. 1996), has been shown to prolong patient survival.

A phase II dose seeking trial of IFN-γ given at one of seven different doses spanning a log 3 range for at least 3 months to patients with metastatic melanoma was recently completed at our institution (KIRKWOOD et al. 1997b). Immunological studies performed on a subset of patients in this trial demonstrated durable and significant immunomodulatory activity of low doses (0.1–0.9 mg/m^2 per day) of IFN-γ on the NK cell number and activity as well as on T cell subsets (KIRKWOOD et al. 1997b). We have obtained no evidence of antitumor activity in this trial, however (KIRKWOOD et al. 1997b). Also, in a phase IB trial of picibanil (OK432) performed in patients with resected high-risk melanoma, we obtained evidence that higher numbers of $CD16^+$ cells and NK activity in the peripheral circulation correlated with disease relapse and death (KIRKWOOD et al. 1997a). These data should not be interpreted to mean that endogenous NK cells are not involved or important in achieving therapeutic benefits. They could simply reflect the fact that distribution of NK cells in various body compartments is influenced by certain drugs, and that NK cells present in tissue and not those in the circulation are responsible for antitumor effects. The available data indicate that upregulation of endogenous NK activity and/or numbers in tumor metastases contributes to modification of the tumor microenvironment, often with therapeutically beneficial results. However, in hosts with large tumor burdens such upregulation may not be sufficient to induce tumor/metastasis regression.

5 NK Cells in Adoptive Immunotherapy of Cancer

Clinical studies (ROSENBERG et al. 1993; LOTZE et al. 1995) and those in animal models (SCHWARTZ et al. 1989; FORNI et al. 1985) have shown that AIT can induce the regression of some metastatic lesions. However, only a minority of patients achieve objective responses with this form of therapy, and it is unclear why most patients treated with AIT fail to respond. It is important to note that when responses are induced with AIT, they are often long lasting (LOTZE et al. 1995). Among factors that might influence response those likely to be particularly important include the route of delivery, the number of transferred effector cells, and their ability to localize to metastases and to sustain functional activities in vivo in the generally immunosuppressive environment. In most clinical protocols very large numbers of effector cells (e.g., 10^{10}–10^{11}) are administered systemically (ROSENBERG et al. 1992; LOTZE et al. 1995), based on an assumption that most cells with antitumor activity do not reach tumor metastases and do not survive. In vitro generation of cells for AIT has been both technically and economically demanding (ROSENBERG et al. 1993; LOTZE et al. 1995).

Our own data (SCHWARTZ et al. 1989; YASUMURA et al. 1994; BASSE et al. 1991) suggest that the number of cells used for AIT can be substantially reduced without decreasing therapeutic effects by: (a) selecting from PBMC the small subpopulation of NK cells with the ability to reach the sites of metastases and exert antitumor effects, (b) optimizing the in vivo antitumor effects of these cells, and (c) delivering them locoregionally rather than systemically to increase their chance of reaching tumor metastases in a functionally active state (VUJANOVIC et al. 1994; YASUMURA et al. 1994; RABINOWICH et al. 1992). Recent preclinical and clinical studies in our laboratories have been designed to explore these and other possibilities for improvement of

AIT, using human A-NK cells for the therapy of human tumor xenografts established in nude mice as well as of patients with advanced metastases.

6 In Vivo Localization of Adoptively Transferred A-NK Cells to Tumor Tissue

For years it has been controversial whether adoptively transferred activated lymphocytes accumulate in metastases (BASSE et al. 1991, 1992; MUKHERJI et al. 1987). Presumably, intravenously transferred effector cells cross the endothelial cell (EC) layer and the basement membrane (BM) and migrate into tissues to reach the sites of metastases (BASSE et al. 1992). The ability of effector cells to extravasate and migrate through the extracellular matrix (ECM) and to come into contact with tumor cells is thought to determine to a large extent their antitumor efficacy. The process of adhesion to EC and subsequent entry into subendothelial tissues is mediated by CAMs (WHITESIDE and HERBERMAN 1992). Adoptively transferred effector cells cultured in the presence of cytokines and expressing an abundance of β_1 and β_2 integrins, N-CAMs (WHITESIDE and HERBERMAN 1992; RABINOWICH et al. 1993a,b; MAENPAA et al. 1993), and other adhesion molecules (GISMONDI et al. 1991; RABINOWICH et al. 1995; RABINOWICH et al. 1994), are likely to interact efficiently with both EC and ECM.

It is not clear which CAMs are important for migration of A-NK cells across the EC layer and BM, but IL-2-activated effector cells seem to migrate with different kinetics than nonactivated lymphocytes (WHITESIDE and HERBERMAN 1992). Studies with LAK, TIL, or A-NK cells indicate that only a fraction, at most 5%–10% of the effector cells transferred intravenously, localize at the tumor site (BASSE et al. 1991; KUPPEN et al. 1994). Most of infused cells are eliminated when they reach the first capillary bed, and only few appear to recirculate. Thus the likelihood of these cells reaching tumors growing in downstream capillary beds is limited. However, our data indicate that a single locoregional infusion of 1×10^7 A-NK cells/liver results in rapid elimination (within 24 h) of most 3-day established metastases of human gastric carcinoma (named HR) in nude mice (YASUMURA et al. 1994; OKADA et al. 1996). For example, in the liver, few A-NK cells relative to the number of tumor cells in 3-day metastases eliminated most of the metastases and significantly improved survival. Similarly, in a syngeneic rat model of MADB106 breast carcinoma with 3-day established lung or liver metastases, systemically transferred A-NK cells did not appear to substantially infiltrate metastases, but they mediated antitumor effects (SCHWARTZ et al. 1989).

The ability of A-NK cells to localize in vivo to tumors or metastases has been studied in various animal models with divergent results (SCHWARTZ et al. 1989; BASSE et al. 1991). In our own experiments, the transfer of 1×10^7 human A-NK cells fluorescently labeled with DiO and delivered intravenously or by the intrasplenic route to nude mice bearing 3-day established liver metastases of HR resulted in elimination of metastases (OKADA et al. 1996). Most of the transferred cells were found in the liver 12 or 24 h later and were randomly distributed throughout the liver tissue. Only some A-NK cells were found by electron microscopy to have penetrated into metastases and to have come in direct contact with tumor cells (OKADA et al. 1996). In the HR gastric carcinoma model the presence of a modest number (e.g., 5×10^6) of transferred A-NK cells was associated with significantly prolonged survival of the mice with established liver metastases (OKADA et al. 1996).

Although localization of effector cells to the sites of metastasis may be essential for control of tumor spread (BASSE et al. 1991, 1992; KUPPEN et al. 1994), the mere presence of effector cells in metastases does not always indicate that these cells are therapeutically effective. In a syngeneic model of B16 melanoma in mice with established pulmonary metastases (BASSE et al. 1991), large accumulations of adoptively transferred A-NK cells were present around pulmonary metastases but did not substantially contribute to elimination of metastases (BASSE et al. 1991). Later BASSE et al. (1994) showed that delivery of polyethylene glycol–IL-2 (which has a longer half-life in vivo than IL-2) sustains antitumor activity of the transferred cells and improves their therapeutic effectiveness. In addition, localization of transferred A-NK cells or their ability to eliminate metastases in vivo appears to depend on the characteristics of the metastases. Recently NANNMARK et al. (1995) reported the presence of “dense” and “loose” metastases in the lungs of mice with B16 melanoma, which were, respectively, not infiltrated or well infiltrated with transferred syngeneic A-NK cells. At this time, it remains to be determined to what extent the number, route of delivery, state of activation, and expression of CAMs on A-NK cells, their functional status in situ, and the heterogeneity of metastases contribute to the efficacy of AIT. Among the various factors likely to influence results of AIT those which may play a major role include the differences in size, degree of vascularization or content of the matrix in metastases. Successful delivery of therapeutic cells to tumor sites represents a challenge, and more studies are needed to define optimal conditions for such transfers.

7 Antitumor Effects Mediated by A-NK Cells

Several mechanisms may be responsible for antitumor activities in vivo and therapeutic efficacy of A-NK cells. Direct lysis of tumor targets (“necrosis”) is the most frequently proposed mechanism. In vitro A-NK cells can induce death of cultured or freshly isolated tumor cell targets, as measured in 4-h ^{51}Cr release assays (VUJANOVIC et al. 1994b), causing a release of perforin and granzymes from lysosomal granules and rapid perforin-mediated cell membrane damage (YOUNG 1989). We have recently shown that adoptively transferred A-NK cells also can induce DNA damage and apoptosis in vivo (Fig. 4). In T cells, this process requires direct contact between effector and target cells, is mediated by membrane-bound cytokines of the TNF family (BEUTLER and VAN HUFFEL 1994) and might involve interactions of the death-transducing molecule Fas (APO-1) on the target with its ligand on the effector cells (SMITH et al. 1994; KAGI et al. 1994; SUDA et al. 193; SUDA and NAGATA 1993).

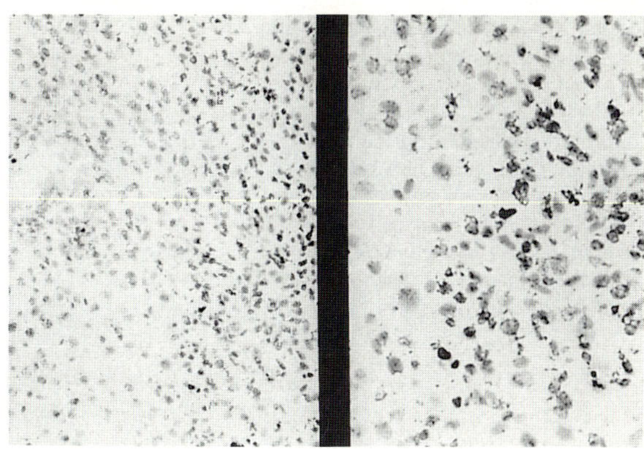

Fig. 4. A cryostat section of the murine liver stained for DNA fragmentation (TUNEL). The nude mouse with established metastases of HK, a human gastric carcinoma, was treated with human A-NK cells and IL-2 (78). A low-power (×200, *left*) and high-power (×450) views show TUNEL+(dark) tumor cells within metastases. TUNEL assay is negative on control cryostat sections of liver metastases in mice sham treated with phosphate-buffered saline

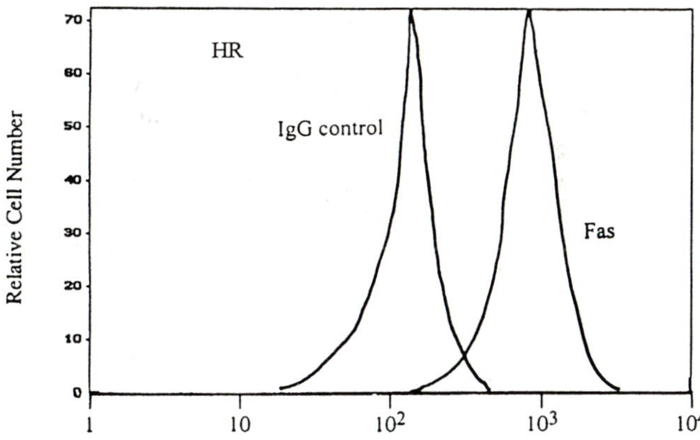

Fig. 5. Expression of Fas on the surface of HR, human gastric carcinoma determined by flow cytometry

We have demonstrated expression of Fas as well as TNF-R on human HR cells used to establish liver metastases in our model (Fig. 5). Yet another cytotoxic mechanism, which is mediated by soluble cytokines and leads to DNA fragmentation and apoptosis, has also been observed with A-NK cells (Fig. 6).

Thus these cells appear to be able to mediate various types of cytotoxicity in vitro and might utilize diverse mechanisms for elimination of metastases in vivo. Also, human A-NK cells may alter biological behavior of the tumor in situ by delivery and release of soluble factors. They have been shown to express mRNAs for and to secrete a broad spectrum of cytokines (Whiteside and Herberman 1994; N.L. Vujanovic, unpublished data) which mediate recruitment to the tumor of endogenous effector cells and upregulate their antitumor activity. A-NK-cell derived cytokines might be cytostatic to the tumor, alter its growth characteristics or induce susceptibility to lysis by effector cells as a result of changes in expression of, for example, class I or II MHC

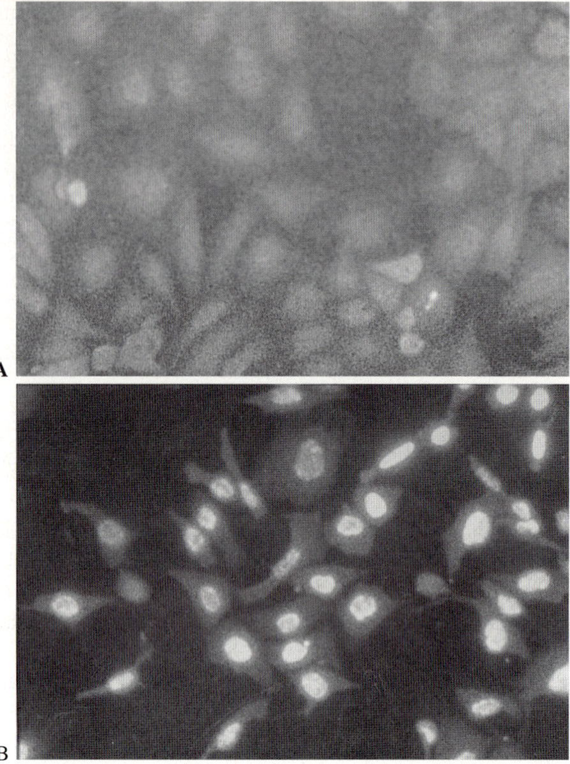

Fig. 6A,B. An in situ terminal deoxynucleotide transferase (TdT) break and extension assay with Cy3-labeled dUTP olignucleotide confirms that human A-NK cells can utilize apoptotic mechanisms to kill HR tumor cells. **A** Control. The HR monolayer incubated with medium. **B** The HR monolayer incubated for 1 h with the supernatant of human A-NK cells. ×450

antigens or CAMs on the tumor cell surface (WHITESIDE and HERBERMAN 1992). Alternatively, products of A-NK cells may have pronounced effects on the vascular elements in the tumor (SASAKI et al. 1991). Even short-term contact of A-NK cells with vascular EC in the tumor has been shown by us to result in vascular stasis and subsequent tumor necrosis (SASAKI et al. 1991). Interestingly, A-NK cells do not appear to harm EC, as shown in our HR liver metastasis model, using anti-CD31 antibody which stains murine EC (Whiteside et al. unpublished data). In our hands, some human carcinomas induce and sustain activation of A-NK cells in vivo (RABINOWICH et al. 1992), and this is correlated with elimination of established subcutaneous tumors in one of our xenograft (SCCHN) models (SACCHI et al. 1991; RABINOWICH et al. 1992). In contrast, other human tumors are known to produce immunosuppressive factors which are likely to partially or completely inhibit antitumor functions of transferred A-NK cells. Thus immunosuppressive factors present in the tumor milieu may profoundly influence the outcome of AIT.

It seems likely that the in vivo behavior of adoptively transferred effector cells, including the ability to release cytokines, perhaps selectively in response to the tumor, will be important for their therapeutic efficacy. Some of the multiple antitumor mechanisms that A-NK cells might utilize in vivo may be more important for therapeutic effects than others. In situ activities of A-NK cells might depend on the ability of the tumor to either activate or inhibit them. To optimize therapeutic benefits of A-NK cell delivery it appears to be necessary to identify and optimize those mechanisms that are most likely to lead to elimination of metastases and improved survival. Since these mechanisms may vary in different types of human tumors or at different tissue sites, the choice of strategies for achieving effective AIT is difficult but extremely important for therapeutic success.

8 IL-2 Dependency of A-NK Cells

IL-2 is necessary not only for generation of A-NK cells in vitro but also for survival in vivo and support of antitumor activities of transferred effector cells (BASSE et al. 1994). Although A-NK cells express high-affinity IL-2R, they depend on high doses of IL-2 (2.2–22 n*M*) for proliferation and other functions in vitro (VITOLO et al. 1993). Removal of IL-2 from A-NK cell cultures leads to a loss of ability to proliferate and mediate cytotoxicity (N. Vujanovic et al. unpublished data). In vivo studies in rats (VUJANOVIC et al. 1987; SCHWARTZ et al. 1989; KUPPEN et al. 1994) and mice (BASSE et al. 1994) indicate that both antitumor functions and trafficking of adoptively transferred syngeneic A-NK cells are dependent on concomitantly administered IL-2. Similar results were obtained in our nude mouse model (Fig. 7).

In humans the systemic administration of high-dose IL-2 has been associated with undesirable toxicity (ROSENBERG et al. 1989; LOTZE et al. 1986). It would therefore be desirable to restrict high IL-2 concentrations in vivo to the regions of effector cell accumulation and to minimize the systemic levels. This might be achieved by

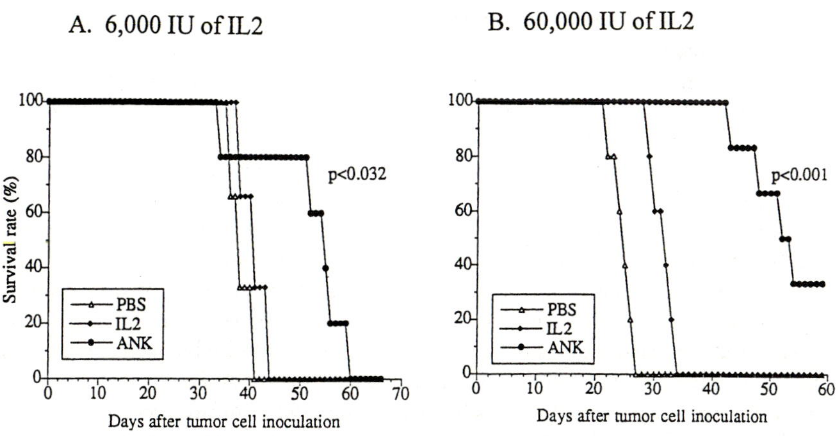

Fig. 7A,B. Survival curves for nude mice with established 7-day liver metastases of HR (groups of five to ten animals) treated intrasplenically with A-NK cells together with low (**A**) or high (**B**) doses of IL-2 delivered i.p. (66). Kniskal-Wallis test was used to calculate significance of the data

engineering local production of IL-2 by, for example, tumor cells and/or fibroblasts transduced with the IL-2 gene (BUBENIK et al. 1988; GANSBACHER et al. 1994) thus allowing for its continuous release (ANDERSON et al. 1994). Overall, data from several experimental in vivo systems indicate that both localization and antitumor functions of A-NK cells in tissues are critically dependent on IL-2 available in situ (BASSE et al. 1994; YASUMURA et al. 1994), and that substantial therapeutic benefits would be achieved if high levels of IL-2 could be maintained locally for prolonged periods of time. Alternatively, it might be possible to use cytokines other than, or in addition to, IL-2 to stimulate antitumor activities of transferred effector cells. In this respect IL-12 has been shown by us (RABINOWICH et al. 1993b) and others (NAUME et al. 1992) to be able to augment NK activities in vitro at doses five- to tenfold lower than IL-2. Also, IL-12 has been recently shown to mediate antitumor effects in vivo in animal models of tumor growth (NASTALA et al. 1994).

9 AIT of Human Cancer with A-NK Cells

Our preclinical studies in syngeneic and xenograft animal models of tumor metastasis suggest that human tumors could be successfully treated with AIT using A-NK cells. In the past 5 years four clinical trials have been performed at our institution to evaluate therapeutic potential of autologous A-NK cells in patients with advanced cancer. While the rationale of initiating these trials was established in the animal models discussed above, concerns existed about toxicity of this therapy as well as the feasibility of obtaining a sufficient number of A-NK cells. In a phase I pilot trial performed in patients with metastatic melanoma or renal cell carcinoma several years ago, we demonstrated the feasibility of generating A-NK cells from peripheral blood of patients with advanced malignancies (WHITESIDE et al. 1990). Although therapeutic benefits of systemic AIT with autologous A-NK cells and moderate doses of IL-2 in 14 evaluable patients in this trial were modest, with only one complete remission (lasting more than 7 months) and one partial remission, we demonstrated that A-NK cells can be transferred to cancer patients safely without considerable toxicity (WHITESIDE et al. 1990).

These results were confirmed in two subsequent pilot clinical trials. In one of these, A-NK cells were delivered locoregionally using, intrahepatic catheters, plus IL-2 to six patients with liver metastases form colon carcinoma (M. Lotze et al. unpublished data). In the other, A-NK cells plus IL-2 were administered within 2 days of peripheral blood stem cell transplantation (PBSCT) to patients with bone marrow metastases from breast carcinoma (MAGALHAES-SILVERMAN et al. 1997). These studies thus used different routes of administration of A-NK cells, patients with metastases at different sites, and patients previously treated with surgery, chemotherapy, and/or bone marrow transplantation. They demonstrated that toxicity associated with this therapy is tolerable, and that highly purified A-NK cells can be generated from leukapheresis products in patients with advanced metastatic disease. In the post-PBSCT pilot trial, AIT was performed in five patients using autologous A-NK cells and IL-2

(2×10^6 IU/m^2per day for 4 days) following initial high-dose chemotherapy and stem call transfer. Two other cohorts, each consisting of five patients, were treated with high-dose chemotherapy and posttransplant granulocyte colony-stimulating factor. In one of these two cohorts, IL-2 without A-NK cells was also administered. All 15 patients who engrafted; tolerated the administration of IL-2 or A-NK cells plus IL-2 after stem cell transplanation, and the administration of these cells did not adversely affect stem cell engraftment (MAGALHAES-SILVERMAN et al. 1997).

Recently we have completed a phase I/II clinical trial in patients with relapsed or primary refactory lymphoma (*n*=37), relapsed Hodgkin's disease (*n*=3), or poor-prognosis lymphoma in first remission (*n*=2), who were infused with autologous A-NK cells immediately after PBSCT (LISTER et al. 1995, 1997). This trial documented the feasibility of generating A-NK cells from the peripheral blood mononuclear cells of patients with advanced lymphoma who were previously treated with chemotherapy (LISTER et al. 1995, 1997) and of combining PBSCT and immunotherapy with A-NK cells and IL-2 in the immediate posttransplant period. Furthermore, in a subgroup of patients who were selected for eligibility according to the PARMA criteria (PHILIP et al. 1995) and thus had especially poor prognosis, overall and progression-free survival was 65% (LISTER et al. 1997). In this subgroup of lymphoma patients the combination of PBSCT and A-NK cell transfer resulted in a better clinical outcome than historical controls and thus provided evidence, that this combination is a promising alternative to PBSCT alone for patients with poor-prognosis lymphoma. In addition, evidence was obtained for more rapid recovery of platelet counts in some of the patients treated with A-NK cells than in historical controls. Plans are underway for a subsequent clinical study to evaluate more fully the contributions of A-NK cells to improved survival by following their distribution after transfer and localization to sites of disease.

The possibility has been considered that AIT with A-NK cells is more effective in hosts rendered immunoincompetent, and more specifically, depleted of T cells. Therapeutic effectiveness of A-NK cells observed in the setting of PBSCT following ablative chemotherapy or in the HR model of hepatic metastases in nude mice, as described above, suggests that the absence of mature T cells favors antitumor functions of transferred NK cells. In patients treated with A-NK cells after PBSCT preliminary data indicate prolonged circulation of the transferred effector cells. Conversely, the immune system of immunocompetent hosts with established metastases might be able to suppress and/or destroy transferred activated NK cells, leading to a reduction in therapeutic benefits. These possibilities are now being tested in an experimental syngeneic model of lung metastases in the rat established in our laboratories.

10 Summary

Evidence has been reviewed which indicates that NK cells play a role in the control of metastasis dissemination. Both activation of endogenous NK cells in a tumor-bearing host and adoptive transfer of ex vivo activated NK cells may be therapeutically beneficial. The small number of phase I/II clinical trials of AIT with A-NK cells performed in patients with cancer so far does not allow firm conclusions, except to ascertain the feasibility and a lack of toxicity of this form of therapy. Although numerous trials have been performed with BRMs, many of which are known to upregulate NK activity in vivo, a general lack of correlations between clinical responses or survival and upregulated NK activity in the peripheral blood has dampened enthusiasm for biological therapies. However, these clinical trials have been confined largely to patients with advanced metastatic disease.

It is highly likely that tumor-induced immunosuppression plays a crucial role in neutralizing the benefits of BRM therapy, and that levels of effector cell activation sufficient for metastasis elimination are seldom achieved in this clinical setting. On the other hand, administration of BRMs in the adjuvant setting could be more effective and when combined with monitoring for effector cell functions might perhaps provide a better guide for achieving the levels of endogenous NK activity necessary for elimination of remaining or occult metastases. An improved understanding of NK cell biology in cancer patients is likely to serve as a positive reinforcement for design of a new generation of clinical trials incorporating novel approaches to NK cell mediated cancer therapy.

References

Anderson PM, Katsanis E, Sencer SF, Hasz D, Ochoa AC, Bostrom B (1992) Depot characteristics and biodistribution of interleukin 2 liposomes: importance of route of administration. J Immunother 12:19–31

Barlozzari T, Reynolds CW, Herberman RB (1983) In vivo role of natural killer cells: involvement of large granular lymphocytes in the clearance of tumor cells in anti-asialo GM1-treated rats. J Immunol 131:1024–1027

Barlozzari T, Leonhardt J, Wiltrout RH, Herberman RB, Reynolds CW (1985) Direct evidence for the role of LGL in the inhibition of experimental tumor metases. J Immunol 134:2783–2789

Basse P, Herberman RB, Nannmark U, Johansson ER, Hokland M, Wasserman K, Goldfarb R (1991) Accumulation of adoptively transferred A-LAK cells in metastases. J Exp Med 174:479–488

Basse PH, Herberman RB, Hokland ME, Goldfarb RH (1992) Tissue distribution of adoptively transferred adherent LAK cells: role of route of administration. Nat Immun 11:193–202

Basse PH, Hokland M, Ren YL, Rao V, Neufeld SK, McCaslin D, Goldfarb RH (1993) Increase in number of organ-associated natural killer (NK) cells induced by poly I:C. Proc AACR 34:448

Basse PH, Goldfarb RH, Herberman RB, Hokland ME (1994) Accumulation of adoptively-transferred A-NK cells in murine metastases: kinetics and role of interleukin 2. In Vivo 8:17–24

Beutler B, Van Huffel C (1994) Unraveling function in the TNF ligand and receptor families. Science 264:667–668

Biron CA, Su HC, Orange JS (1996) Function and regulation of natural killer (NK) cells during viral infections: characterization of responses vivo. Methods (Companion to Methods in Enzymol) 9:1–15

Bubenik J, Voitenok NN, Kieler J, Prassolov VS, Chumakov PM, Bubenkova D, Simova J, Jandlova T (1988) Local administration of cells containing an inserted IL2 gene and producing IL2 inhibits growth of human tumors in nu/nu mice. Immunol Lett 19:279–282

Caligiuri MA, Zmuidzinas A, Manley T, Levine H, Smith KA, Ritz J (1990) Functional consequences of IL2 receptor expression on resting human lymphocytes: identification of a novel NK cell subset. J Exp Med 171:1509–1513

Caligiuri MA, Murray C, Robertson MJ, Wang E, Cochran K, Cameron C, Schow P, Ross ME, Klumpp TR, Soiffer RJ et al (1993) Selective modulation of human natural killer cells in vivo after prolonged infusion of low dose recombinant interleukin 2. J Clin Invest 91:123–132

Cole BF, Gelber RD, Kirkwood JM, Goldhirsch A, Barylak E, Borden E (1996) Quality-of-life-adjusted survival analysis of interferon alfa-2b adjuvant treatment of high-risk resected cutaneous melanoma: an Eastern Cooperative Oncology Group study. J Clin Oncol 14:2666–73

Edwards RP, Gooding W, Lembersky BC, Colonello KA, Hammond R, Paradise C, Kunschner AJ, Kowal CD, Baldisseri M, Kirkwood JM, Herberman RB (1997) Comparison of toxicity and survival followingintraperitoneal recombinant IL-2 for persistent ovarian cancer after plantinum: 24h versus 7-day infusion. (15:3399–3407)

Forni G, Giovarelli M, Santoni A (1985) Lymphokine-activated tumor inhibition in vivo. I. The local administration of interleukin 2 triggers nonreactive lymphocytes from tumor-bearing mice to inhibit tumor growth. J Immunol 134:1305–1311

Garcia-Barcina M, Lukomska B, Gawron W, Winnock M, Vidal-Vanaclocha F, Biolac-Sage P, Balaband C, Olszewski W (1995) Expression of cell adhesion molecules on liver-associated lymphocytes and their ligands on sinusoidal lining cells in patients with benign or malignant liver disease. Am J Pathol 146:1406–1413

Gansbacher B, Zier K, Cronin K, Hantzopoulos PA, Bouchard B, Houghton A, Gilboa E, Golde D (1994) Retroviral gene transfer induced constitutive expression of interleukin 2 or interferon-irradiated human melanoma cells. Blood 80:2817–2825

Gismondi A, Morrone S, Humphries MJ, Piccoli M, Frati L, Santoni A (1991) Human natural killer cells express VLA-4 and VLA-5, which mediate their adhesion to fibronectin. J Immunol 146:384

Gorelik E, Herberman RB (1986) Role of natural killer (NK) cells in the control of tumor growth and metastatic spread. In: Herberman RB (ed) Cancer immunology: innovative approaches to therapy. Nijhoft, Boston, pp 151–176

Hata K, Van Thiel DH, Herberman RB, Whiteside TL (1992) Phenotypic and functional characteristics of lymphocytes isolated from liver biopsy specimens from patients with active liver disease. Hepatology 15:816–823

Herberman RB, Vujanovic N, Rabinowich H, Whiteside TL.(1992) Natural killer cells and interleukin 2-activated killer cells. In: Mertelsmann R (ed) Lymphohaematopoietic growth factors in cancer therapy. II Eur Schl Oncology. Monographs. Springer, Berlin Heidelberg, New York, pp 11–27

Ho M, Jaffe R, Miller G, Breinig M-K, Dummer S, Makowka M, Atchison RW, Karrer F, Nalesnik MA, Starzl TE (1988) The frequency of Epstein-Barr virus infection and associated lymphoproliferative syndrome after transplantation and its manifestations in children. Transplantation 45:719–727

Introna M, Montavani A (1983) Natural killer cells in human solid tumors. Cancer Metastasis Rev 2:337

Kagi D, Vignaux F, Ledemann B, Burki K, Depraetere V, Nagata S, Hengartner H, Golstein P (1994) Fas and perforin pathways as major mechanisms of T cell-mediated cytotoxicity. Science 265:528–530

Kirkwood JM, Wilson J, Whiteside TL, Bryant J, Donnelly S, Herberman RB (1997a) Phase IB trial of picibanil (OK-432) as an immunomodulator in patients with resected high-risk melanoma. Cancer Immunol Immunother 44:137–149

Kirkwood JM, Bryant J, Schiller JH, Oken MM, Borden EC, Whiteside TL (1997b) Immunomodulatory function of interferon gamma in patients with metastatic melanoma: results of a phase IIB trial in subjects with metastatic melanoma: ECOG Study E 4987. J Immunother 20:146–157

Kuppen RJK, Basse PH, Goldfarb RH, Van De Velde CJH, Fleuren GJ, Eggermont AMM (1994) The infiltration of experimentally-induced lung metastases of colon carcinoma CC531 by adoptively-transferred interleukin 2-activated natural killer cells in Wag rats. Int J Cancer 56:574–579

Lai P, Rabinowich H, Crowley-Nowick PA, Bell MC, Mantovani G, Whiteside TL (1996) Alterations in expression and function of signal transduction proteins in tumor associated NK and T lymphocytes from patients with ovarian carcinoma. Clin Cancer Res 2:161–173

Levey DL, Srivastava PK (1995) T cells from late tumor-bearing mice express normal levels of p56lck, p59lyn, ZAP-70, and CD3ζ despite suppressed cytolytic activity. J Exp Med 182:1029–1036

Lister J, Rybka WB, Donnenberg AD, de Magalhaes-Silverman M, Pincus SM, Bloom EJ, Elder EM, Ball ED, Whiteside TL (1995) Autologous peripheral blood stem cell transplantation and adoptive immunotherapy with A-NK cells in the immediate post-transplant period. Clin Cancer Res 1:607–614

Lister J, Rybka WB, de Magalhaes-Silverman M, Donnenberg A et al (1997) A-NK cell infusion immediately after autologous peripheral blood item cell transplantation for relapsed lymphoma and Hodgkin's disease. Manuscript in preparation

Lotze MT, Chang AE, Seipp CA, Simpson C, Vetto JT, Rosenberg SA (1986) High-dose recombinant interleukin 2 in the treatment of patients with disseminated cancer: responses, treatment-related morbidity and histologic findings. JAMA 256:3117–3129

Lotze MT, Rubin JT, Whiteside TL, Herberman RB (1995) Cytokine and cellular mediated immunotherapy. In: Rich RR, Thomas TA, Schwartz BD, Shearer WT, Strober W (eds) Principles and practice of clinical immunology. Mosby, St. Louis, pp 1919–1930

Maenpaa A, Jaaskelainen J, Carpen O, Patarroyo M, Timonen T (1993) Expression of integrins and other adhesion molecules on NK cells: impact of IL2 on short- and long-term cultures. Int J Cancer 53:850

Magalhaes-Silverman M, Donnenberg A, Elder E, Lembersky B, Lister J, Rybka W, Whiteside T, Ball ED (1997) Post transplant immunotherapy in metastatic breast cancer (MBC). J Immunother (in press)

Matera L, Giancotti FG (1983) Natural killer activity and low affinity E rosettes in acute leukemia. Acta Haematol 70:158–162

Matsuda M, Petersson M, Lenkei R, Taupin J-L, Magnusson I, Mellstedt H, Anderson P, Kiessling R (1995) Alterations in the signal-transducing molecules of T cells and NK cells in colorectal tumor-infiltrating, gut mucosal and peripheral lymphocytes: correlation with the stage of the disease. Int J Cancer 61:765–772

Mizoguchi H, O'Shea JJ, Longo DL, Loeffler CM, McVicar DW, Ochoa AC (1992) Alterations in signal transduction molecules in T lymphocytes from tumor-bearing mice. Science 258:1795–1798

Mukherji B, Arnbjarnarson O, Spitznagle LA, Hoffman J, Ergin MT, Spencer RB (1987) Biodistribution of ^{111}In-labeled tumor sensitized autologous lymphocytes in cancer patients. Prog Clin Biol Res 244:325–334

Nagashima S, Reichert TE, Kashii Y, Suminami Y, Chikamatsu K, Whiteside TL (1997a) In vitro and in vivo characteristics of human squamous cell carcinoma of the head and neck cells engineered to secrete interleukin-2. Cancer Gene Ther (in press)

Nagashima S, Kashii Y, Reichert TE, Suminami Y, Suzuki T, Whiteside TL (1997b) Human gastric carcinoma transduced with the IL-2 gene: increased sensitivity to immune effector cells in vitro and in vivo. Int J Cancer 72:174–183

Nannmark U, Johansson BR, Bryant JL, Unger ML, Hokland ME, Goldfarb RH, Basse PH (1995) Microvessel origin and distribution in pulmonary metastases of B16 melanoma: implication for adoptive immunotherapy. Cancer Res 55:4627–4632

Naume B, Gately M, Espevik (1992) A comparative study of IL12-, IL2- and IL7-induced effects on immunomagnetically purified $CD56^+$ NK cells. J Immunol 148:2429

Nastala CL, Edington HD, McKinney TG, Tahara H, Nalesnik MA, Brunda MJ, Gately MK, Wolf SF, Schreiber RD, Storkus WJ, Lotze MT (1994) Recombinant IL12 administration induces tumor regression in association with IFN-γ production. J Immunol 153:1697–1706

Okada K, Nannmark V, Vujanovic NL, Watkins S, Basse P, Herberman RB, Whiteside TL (1996) Elimination of established liver metastases by human IL-2 activated natural killer cells after locoregional or systemic adoptive transfer. Cancer Res 56:1599–1608

Philip T, Guglielmi C, Hagenbeek A et al (1995) Autologous bone marrow transplantation as compared with salvage chemotherapy in relapse of chemotherapy-sensitive non-Hodgkin's lymphoma. N Engl J Med 333:1540–1544

Pilaro AM, Taub DD, McCormick, Williams HM, Sayers TJ, Fogler WH, Wiltrout RH (1994) TNF-α is a principal cytokine involved in the recruitment of NK cells to liver parenchyma. J Immunol 143:372–377

Pross HF, Lotzova E (1993) Role of natural killer cells in cancer. Nat Immun 12:279–292

Rabinowich H, Vitolo D, Altarac S, Herberman RB, Whiteside TL (1992) The role of cytokines in the adoptive immunotherapy of an experimental model of human head and neck cancer by human IL2-activated NK cells. J Immunol 149:340–349

Rabinowich H, Herberman RB, Whiteside TL (1993a) Response of human NK cells to IL6: alteration of the cell surface phenotype, adhesion to fibronectin and laminin and TNFα-/β secretion. J Immunol 150:4844

Rabinowich H, Herberman RB, Whiteside TL (1993b) Differential effects of IL12 and IL2 on expression and function of cellular adhesion molecules on purified human natural killer cells. Cell Immunol 152:481–498

Rabinowich H, Lin W-C, Herberman RB, Whiteside TL (1994) The role of β_1 and β_3 integrins expressed on human NK cells in protein phosphorylation, cytokine production and cell proliferation. Nat Immun 13:218

Rabinowich H, Lin W-C, Manciulea M, Herberman RB, Whiteside TL (1995) Induction of protein tyrosine phosphorylation in human NK cells by triggering via $\alpha_4\beta_1$ or $\alpha_5\,\beta_1$ integrins. Blood 85:1858–1864

Rabinowich H, Suminami Y, Reichert TE, Crowley-Nowick P, Bell M, Edwards R, Whiteside TL (1996a) Expression of cytokine genes or proteins and signaling molecules in lymphocytes associated with human ovarian carcinoma. Int J Cancer 68:276–284

Rabinowich H, Banks M, Reichert TE, Logan TF, Kirkwood JM, Whiteside TL (1996b) Expression and activity of signaling molecules in T lymphocytes obtained from patients with metastatic melanoma before and after IL-2 therapy. Clin Cancer Res 2:126361274

Riccardi C, Santoni A, Barlozzari T, Pucetti P, Herberman RB (1980) In vivo natural reactivity of mice against tumor cells. Int J Cancer 25: 475–486

Rosen FS, Cooper MD, Wedgwood RJP (1995) The primary immunodeficiencies. N Engl J Med 333:431–440

Rosenberg SA, Lotze MT, Yang JC, Aebersold PM, Linehan WM, Seipp CA, White DE (1989) Experience with the use of high-dose interleukin 2 in the treatment of 652 cancer patients. Ann Surg 210:474–485

Rosenberg SA, Lotze MT, Yang JC, Topalian SL, Chang AE, Schwartzentruber DJ, Aebersold P, Leitman S, Linehan WM, Seipp CA, White DE, Steinberg SM (1993) Prospective randomized trial of high-dose interleukin 2 alone or in conjunction with lymphokine-activated killer cells for the treatment of patients with advanced cancer. J Natl Cancer Inst 85:622–627

Sacchi M, Vitolo D, Sedlmayr P, Rabinowich H, Johnson JT, Herberman RB, Whiteside TL (1991) Induction of tumor regression in experimental model of human head and neck cancer by human A-LAK cells and IL2. Int J Cancer 47:784–791

Sasaki A, Melder RJ, Whiteside TL, Herberman RB, Jain RK (1991) Preferential localization of human adherent lymphokine-activated killer (A-LAK) cells in tumor microcirculation: a novel mechanism for adoptive immunotherapy. J Natl Cancer Inst 83:433–437

Schwartz R, Vujanovic NL, Hiserodt JC (1989) Enhanced antimetastatic activity of lymphokine-activated killer cells purified and expanded by their adherence to plastic. Cancer Res 49:1441–1446

Soiffer RJ, Murray C, Cochran K, Cameron C, Wang E, Schow PW, Daley JF, Ritz J (1992) Clinical and immunologic effects of prolonged infusion of low-dose recombinant interleukin 2 after autologous and T-cell-depleted allogeneic bone marrow transplantation. Blood 79:517–526

Sondel PM (1989) Cellular immunotherapy of cancer: preclinical and clinical testing utilizing interleukin 2. In: Lotzova E, Herberman RB (eds) IL2 activated killer cells in cancer treatment. CRC, Boca Raton, pp 1–24

Smith CA, Farrah T, Goodwin RG (1994) The TNF receptor superfamily of cellular and viral proteins: activation, co-stimulation and death. Cell 76:959–962

Strayer DR, Carter WA, Mayberry SD, Pequignot E, Brodsky J (1984) Loco natural cytotoxicity of peripheral blood mononuclear cells in individuals with high familial incidence of cancer. Cancer Res 44:370–374

Strayer DR, Carter WA, Brodsky I (1986) Familial occurrence of breast cancer is associated with reduced natural killer cytotoxicity. Breast Cancer Res Treat 7:187–192

Suda T, Nagata S (1993) Purification and characterization of the Fas ligand that induces apoptosis. J Exp Med 179:873–879

Suda T, Takahashi T, Golstein P, Nagata S (1993) Molecular cloning and expression of the Fas ligand, a novel member of tumor necrosis factor family. Cell 75:1169–1178

Ullum H, Gotzsche PC, Victor J, Dickmeiss E, Skinhoj P, Pedersen BK (1995) Defective natural immunity: an early manifestation of human immunodeficiency virus infection. J Exp Med 182:789–799

Vitolo D, Vujanovic N, Rabinowich H, Schlesinger M, Herberman RB, Whiteside TL (1993) Rapid interleukin-2 induced adherence of human natural killer (NK) cells accompanied by expression of mRNA for cytokines and IL2 receptors. J Immunol 151:1926–1937

Vujanovic NL, Herberman RB, Maghazachi AA, Hiserodt JC (1987) Lymphokine-activated killer cells in rats. III. A simple method for the purification of large granular lymphocytes and their rapid expansion and conversion into lymphokine-activated killer cells. J Exp Med 167:15–29

Vujanovic NL, Rabinowich H, Lee YJ, Jost L, Herberman RB, Whiteside TL (1993a) Characteristic of human natural killer cells obtained by rapid interleukin 2-induced adherence to plastic. Cellular Immunol 151:133–157

Vujanovic NL, Herberman RB, Lagenaur C, Chambers WH, Whiteside TL (1993b) Precursors of the ANK cell subset in human peripheral blood. J Immunol 155:299A

Vujanovic NL, Begovic M, Herberman RB, Whiteside TL (1994a) The mechanisms of breast cancer cell killing by human natural killer cells. FASEB J 8:A209

Vujanovic NL, Yasumura S, Hirabayashi H, Lin W-C, Watkins S, Herberman RB, Whiteside TL (1994b) Antitumor activities of subsets of human IL2-activated natural killer cells in solid tissues. J Immunol 154:281–289

Vujanovic NL, Chambers WH, Lagenaur C, Shen L, Ernst L, Nagashima S, Herberman RB, Whiteside TL (1995a) Shared expression of the NC-1 (ANK-1) epitope on N-CAM and precursors of A-NK cells. Proc AACR 36: 2815

Vujanovic NL, Polimeno L, Francavilla A, Chambers WH, Starzl TE, Herberman RB, Whiteside TL (1995b) Changes of liver-resident natural killer cells during liver regeneration in rats. J Immunol 154:6324–6338

Vujanovic NL, Basse P, Herberman RB, Whiteside TL (1996) Antitumor function of natural killer cells and control of metastases. Methods (Companion Methods Enzymol) 9:394–408

Whiteside, TL (1993) Tumor-infiltrating lymphocytes in human malignancies. Medical intelligence unit, R.G. Landes Co., Austin, Texas

Whiteside TL, Herberman RB (1990) Characteristics of natural killer cells and lymphokine-activated killer cells. Their role in the biology and treatment of human cancer. Human Cancer Immunol 10:663–704

Whiteside TL, Herberman RB (1992) Extravasation of antitumor effector cells. Invasion Metastasis 12:128–146

Whiteside TL, Herberman (1994) Role of human natural killer cells in health and disease. Clin Diag. Lab Immunol 1:125–133

Whiteside TL, Herberman RB (1995) The role of natural killer cells in immune surveillance of cancer. Curr Opin Immunol 7:704–710

Whiteside TL, Bryant J, Day R, Herberman RB (1990) Natural killer cytotoxicity in the diagnosis of immune dysfunction: criteria for a reproducible assay. J Clin Analysis 4:102–144

Whiteside TL, Ernstoff MS, Nair S, Kirkwood JM, Herberman RB (1990) In vitro generation and in vivo effects of adherent-lymphokine activated killer (A-LAK) cells and IL2 in patients with solid tumors. In: Schmidt RE (ed) Natural killer cells: biology and clinical application. Karger, Basel, pp, 293–302

Whiteside TL, Letessier E, Hirabayashi H, Vitolo D, Bryant J, Barnes L, Snyderman C, Johnson JT, Myers E, Herberman RB, Rubin J, Kirkwood JM, Vlock DR (1993) Evidence for local and systemic activation of immune cells by peritumoral injections of interleukin 2 in patients with advanced squamous cell carcinoma of the head and neck. Cancer Res 53:5654–5662

Wiltrout RH, Mathieson BJ, Talmadge JE, Reynolds CW, Zhang S, Herberman RB, Ortaldo JR (1984) Augmentation of organ-associated natural killer activity by biologic response modifiers: isolation and characterizations of large granular lymphocytes from the liver. J Exp Med 160:1431–1449

Wiltrout RH, Herberman RB, Zhang S-R, Chirigos MA, Ortaldo JR, Green KM Jr, Talmadge JE (1985) Role of organ-associated NK cells in decreased formation of experimental metastases in lung and liver. J Immunol 134:4267–4275

Wiltrout RH, Pilaro A, Gruys ME, Talmadge JE, Longo DL, Ortaldo JR, Reynolds CW (1989) Augmentation of mouse liver-associated natural killer activity by biologic response modifiers occurs largely via rapid recruitment of large granular lymphocytes from the bone marrow. J Immunol 143:372–378

Yasumura S, Lin W-C, Hirabayashi H, Vujanovic NL, Herberman RB, Whiteside TL (1994) Immunotherapy of liver metastases of human gastric carcinoma with IL2-activated natural killer cells. Cancer Res 54:3808–3816

Young JD-E (1989) Killing of target cells by lymphocytes: a mechanistic view. Physiol Rev 69:250–314

Ziegler H, Kay NE, Zarling JM (1981) Deficiency of natural killer cell activity in patients with chronic lymphocytic leukemia. Int J Cancer 27:321–327

Zier KS, Salvadori S, Cronin KC, Gansbacher B (1994) Vaccination with IL2-secreting tumor cells stimulates the generation of IL2-responsive T cells and prevents the development of unresponsiveness. Cancer Gene Ther 1:43–50

Subject Index

Printing: Saladruck, Berlin
Binding: Buchbinderei Lüderitz & Bauer, Berlin

Current Topics in Microbiology and Immunology

Volumes published since 1989 (and still available)

Vol. 191: **ter Meulen, Volker; Billeter, Martin A. (Eds.):** Measles Virus. 1995. 23 figs. IX, 196 pp. ISBN 3-540-57389-5

Vol. 192: **Dangl, Jeffrey L. (Ed.):** Bacterial Pathogenesis of Plants and Animals. 1994. 41 figs. IX, 343 pp. ISBN 3-540-57391-7

Vol. 193: **Chen, Irvin S. Y.; Koprowski, Hilary; Srinivasan, Alagarsamy; Vogt, Peter K. (Eds.):** Transacting Functions of Human Retroviruses. 1995. 49 figs. IX, 240 pp. ISBN 3-540-57901-X

Vol. 194: **Potter, Michael; Melchers, Fritz (Eds.):** Mechanisms in B-cell Neoplasia. 1995. 152 figs. XXV, 458 pp. ISBN 3-540-58447-1

Vol. 195: **Montecucco, Cesare (Ed.):** Clostridial Neurotoxins. 1995. 28 figs. XI., 278 pp. ISBN 3-540-58452-8

Vol. 196: **Koprowski, Hilary; Maeda, Hiroshi (Eds.):** The Role of Nitric Oxide in Physiology and Pathophysiology. 1995. 21 figs. IX, 90 pp. ISBN 3-540-58214-2

Vol. 197: **Meyer, Peter (Ed.):** Gene Silencing in Higher Plants and Related Phenomena in Other Eukaryotes. 1995. 17 figs. IX, 232 pp. ISBN 3-540-58236-3

Vol. 198: **Griffiths, Gillian M.; Tschopp, Jürg (Eds.):** Pathways for Cytolysis. 1995. 45 figs. IX, 224 pp. ISBN 3-540-58725-X

Vol. 199/I: **Doerfler, Walter; Böhm, Petra (Eds.):** The Molecular Repertoire of Adenoviruses I. 1995. 51 figs. XIII, 280 pp. ISBN 3-540-58828-0

Vol. 199/II: **Doerfler, Walter; Böhm, Petra (Eds.):** The Molecular Repertoire of Adenoviruses II. 1995. 36 figs. XIII, 278 pp. ISBN 3-540-58829-9

Vol. 199/III: **Doerfler, Walter; Böhm, Petra (Eds.):** The Molecular Repertoire of Adenoviruses III. 1995. 51 figs. XIII, 310 pp. ISBN 3-540-58987-2

Vol. 200: **Kroemer, Guido; Martinez-A., Carlos (Eds.):** Apoptosis in Immunology. 1995. 14 figs. XI, 242 pp. ISBN 3-540-58756-X

Vol. 201: **Kosco-Vilbois, Marie H. (Ed.):** An Antigen Depository of the Immune System: Follicular Dendritic Cells. 1995. 39 figs. IX, 209 pp. ISBN 3-540-59013-7

Vol. 202: **Oldstone, Michael B. A.; Vitković, Ljubiša (Eds.):** HIV and Dementia. 1995. 40 figs. XIII, 279 pp. ISBN 3-540-59117-6

Vol. 203: **Sarnow, Peter (Ed.):** Cap-Independent Translation. 1995. 31 figs. XI, 183 pp. ISBN 3-540-59121-4

Vol. 204: **Saedler, Heinz; Gierl, Alfons (Eds.):** Transposable Elements. 1995. 42 figs. IX, 234 pp. ISBN 3-540-59342-X

Vol. 205: **Littman, Dan R. (Ed.):** The CD4 Molecule. 1995. 29 figs. XIII, 182 pp. ISBN 3-540-59344-6

Vol. 206: **Chisari, Francis V.; Oldstone, Michael B. A. (Eds.):** Transgenic Models of Human Viral and Immunological Disease. 1995. 53 figs. XI, 345 pp. ISBN 3-540-59341-1

Vol. 207: **Prusiner, Stanley B. (Ed.):** Prions Prions Prions. 1995. 42 figs. VII, 163 pp. ISBN 3-540-59343-8

Vol. 208: **Farnham, Peggy J. (Ed.):** Transcriptional Control of Cell Growth. 1995. 17 figs. IX, 141 pp. ISBN 3-540-60113-9

Vol. 209: **Miller, Virginia L. (Ed.):** Bacterial Invasiveness. 1996. 16 figs. IX, 115 pp. ISBN 3-540-60065-5

Vol. 210: **Potter, Michael; Rose, Noel R. (Eds.):** Immunology of Silicones. 1996. 136 figs. XX, 430 pp. ISBN 3-540-60272-0

Vol. 211: **Wolff, Linda; Perkins, Archibald S. (Eds.):** Molecular Aspects of Myeloid Stem Cell Development. 1996. 98 figs. XIV, 298 pp. ISBN 3-540-60414-6

Vol. 212: **Vainio, Olli; Imhof, Beat A. (Eds.):** Immunology and Developmental Biology of the Chicken. 1996. 43 figs. IX, 281 pp. ISBN 3-540-60585-1

Vol. 213/I: **Günthert, Ursula; Birchmeier, Walter (Eds.):** Attempts to Understand Metastasis Formation I. 1996. 35 figs. XV, 293 pp. ISBN 3-540-60680-7

Vol. 213/II: **Günthert, Ursula; Birchmeier, Walter (Eds.):** Attempts to Understand Metastasis Formation II. 1996. 33 figs. XV, 288 pp. ISBN 3-540-60681-5

Vol. 213/III: **Günthert, Ursula; Schlag, Peter M.; Birchmeier, Walter (Eds.):** Attempts to Understand Metastasis Formation III. 1996. 14 figs. XV, 262 pp. ISBN 3-540-60682-3

Vol. 214: **Kräusslich, Hans-Georg (Ed.):** Morphogenesis and Maturation of Retroviruses. 1996. 34 figs. XI, 344 pp. ISBN 3-540-60928-8

Vol. 215: **Shinnick, Thomas M. (Ed.):** Tuberculosis. 1996. 46 figs. XI, 307 pp. ISBN 3-540-60985-7

Vol. 216: **Rietschel, Ernst Th.; Wagner, Hermann (Eds.):** Pathology of Septic Shock. 1996. 34 figs. X, 321 pp. ISBN 3-540-61026-X

Vol. 217: **Jessberger, Rolf; Lieber, Michael R. (Eds.):** Molecular Analysis of DNA Rearrangements in the Immune System. 1996. 43 figs. IX, 224 pp. ISBN 3-540-61037-5

Vol. 218: **Berns, Kenneth I.; Giraud, Catherine (Eds.):** Adeno-Associated Virus (AAV) Vectors in Gene Therapy. 1996. 38 figs. IX,173 pp. ISBN 3-540-61076-6

Vol. 219: **Gross, Uwe (Ed.):** Toxoplasma gondii. 1996. 31 figs. XI, 274 pp. ISBN 3-540-61300-5

Vol. 220: **Rauscher, Frank J. III; Vogt, Peter K. (Eds.):** Chromosomal Translocations and Oncogenic Transcription Factors. 1997. 28 figs. XI, 166 pp. ISBN 3-540-61402-8

Vol. 221: **Kastan, Michael B. (Ed.):** Genetic Instability and Tumorigenesis. 1997. 12 figs.VII, 180 pp. ISBN 3-540-61518-0

Vol. 222: **Olding, Lars B. (Ed.):** Reproductive Immunology. 1997. 17 figs. XII, 219 pp. ISBN 3-540-61888-0

Vol. 223: **Tracy, S.; Chapman, N. M.; Mahy, B. W. J. (Eds.):** The Coxsackie B Viruses. 1997. 37 figs. VIII, 336 pp. ISBN 3-540-62390-6

Vol. 224: **Potter, Michael; Melchers, Fritz (Eds.):** C-Myc in B-Cell Neoplasia. 1997. 94 figs. XII, 291 pp. ISBN 3-540-62892-4

Vol. 225: **Vogt, Peter K.; Mahan, Michael J. (Eds.):** Bacterial Infection: Close Encounters at the Host Pathogen Interface. 1998. 15 figs. IX, 169 pp. ISBN 3-540-63260-3

Vol. 226: **Koprowski, Hilary; Weiner, David B. (Eds.):** DNA Vaccination/Genetic Vaccination. 1998. 31 figs. XVIII, 198 pp. ISBN 3-540-63392-8

Vol. 227: **Vogt, Peter K.; Reed, Steven I. (Eds.):** Cyclin Dependent Kinase (CDK) Inhibitors. 1998. 15 figs. XII, 169 pp. ISBN 3-540-63429-0

Vol. 228: **Pawson, Anthony I. (Ed.):** Protein Modules in Signal Transduction. 1998. 42 figs. IX, 368 pp. ISBN 3-540-63396-0

Vol. 229: **Kelsoe, Garnett; Flajnik, Martin (Eds.):** Somatic Diversification of Immune Responses. 1998. 38 figs. IX, 221 pp. ISBN 3-540-63608-0

Vol. 230: **Kärre, Klas; Colonna, Marco (Eds.):** Specificity, Function, and Development of NK Cells. 1998. 22 figs. IX, 248 pp. ISBN 3-540-63941-1

Vol. 231: **Holzmann, Bernhard; Wagner, Hermann (Eds.):** Leukocyte Integrins in the Immune System and Malignant Disease. 1998. 40 figs. XIII, 189 pp. ISBN 3-540-63609-9